FROM CRAFT
TO SPECIALTY

FROM CRAFT TO SPECIALTY

A Medical and Social History of Anesthesia and Its Changing Role in Health Care

David Shephard

In association with

Alan Sessler, Francis Whalen, and Tuhin Roy

York Point Publishing
Thunder Bay, Ontario

To order additional copies of this book, contact:
Xlibris Corporation
1-888-795-4274
www.Xlibris.com
Orders@Xlibris.com
56457

CONTENTS

For Rosemary

Foreword

It is an honor to write a foreword to *From Craft to Specialty: A Medical and Social History of Anesthesia and Its Changing Role in Health Care* by Dr. David Shephard in association with Drs. Alan Sessler, Francis Whalen, and Tuhin Roy. This unparalleled volume offers an insightful narrative of the development and evolution of anesthesiology from a craft to a discipline and, finally, to a medical specialty. Unlike many earlier historical works that concentrated on a rather truncated time frame, Dr. Shephard's chronicles the history of anesthesia from its inchoate stages to its contemporary status as a distinguished medical specialty in its own right. He relates the expansion of its scope beyond the operating room into intensive care units, pain clinics, and resuscitation venues. Indeed, the practice of anesthesiology is now so diverse that it has an eminent role in the broader health care delivery system.

A distinguished medical historian and writer, Dr Shephard was twice the recipient of fellowships from the Wood Library-Museum of Anesthesiology (WLM). The WLM has long believed that its *raison d'être* is to build a sense of professionalism and community by preserving and publicizing the rich heritage of our past. We can be inspired by exemplary examples of ingenuity and integrity and be cautioned by illustrations of scientific folly and human foibles. The WLM fervently strives to fulfill the vision so powerfully articulated by Goethe who exhorted us to "Make the future better by making the most out of the past."

As the author of this comprehensive and illuminating volume, Dr. Shephard has uniquely contributed to the historiography of our specialty. He deftly traces the progress of anesthesiology from its humble beginnings to its current status as an intellectual and clinical specialty devoted to continuously improving patient safety and to advancing knowledge at both the molecular and the societal level. Instructive themes emerge, such as the ability of anesthesiologists to adapt to evolving needs in surgery, medicine, and society. As a result of these exigencies, subspecialty care has developed, for example, and anesthesiologists often have led the way in navigating the mine fields of thorny ethical issues. Notably, Dr.

Henry Knowles Beecher shaped not only anesthesia but the milieu in which every specialty in medicine is practiced. He more than any other individual deserves credit for initiating peer review of experimental protocols and ensuring that informed consent is obtained in clinical research. Moreover, Beecher was largely responsible for transforming our thinking about death by redefining the endpoint from cardiovascular to neurologic, eventually enabling organ transplantation to thrive. By educating us about the past, David Shephard has provided us with the context and perspective to empower us to make informed and wise decisions about the future.

Kathryn E. McGoldrick, M.D.
Past President (2001-2004), WLM
Professor and Chair of Anesthesiology
New York Medical College
Director of Anesthesiology
Westchester Medical Center

Donald Caton, MD
2004 Laureate of the History of Anesthesia
Past President (1998-2001), WLM
Professor Emeritus of Anesthesiology
University of Florida, Gainesville

Mary Ellen Warner, MD
President (2008-present), WLM
Associate Professor of Anesthesiology
College of Medicine, Mayo Clinic
Medical Director, Outpatient Centers
Mayo Clinic, Rochester MN

Prefatory Note

A word is in order to clarify the authorship of this book. Initially, I considered the desirability of revising Tom Keys' classic work, *The History of Surgical Anesthesia* (New York: Henry Schuman, 1945), but it soon became clear that the enormous advances in anesthesia in the second half of the twentieth century made a revision impractical. I therefore planned a new history, one that was as comprehensive as Keys but brought up-to-date and emphasizing the fact that anesthesia had become a medical specialty in its own right.

The research and parts of the first draft were accomplished in Prince Edward Island, Canada, and Greenville, North Carolina. In 2006, I had the opportunity of completing the project at the Mayo Clinic in Rochester, Minnesota. There, I was able to discuss the manuscript, as a work in progress, with three anesthesiologists who are closer to current practice than I am in retirement: Alan Sessler, Francis Whalen, and Tuhin Roy. Because their invaluable suggestions exceeded those that warranted just acknowledgments, I came to regard my three colleagues as associates, though they did none of the research or writing. The final responsibility for what is written in this book, of course, rests with me, and any faults of omission or commission are mine alone.

David Shephard
Thunder Bay, Ontario, Canada

Acknowledgments

In researching and writing this book, I have had the assistance and advice of many individuals and institutions, though I cannot recognize all here. But I do thank the staff of the Health Sciences Library, Brody School of Medicine, East Carolina University, for access to microfilm holdings and various texts. I thank Dr. Alan Sessler, of the Mayo Clinic, for making it possible for me to use office space in the History of Medicine Library in the Plummer Building of the Mayo Clinic, which I appreciated as a Mayo Clinic alumnus and former denizen of that building. I thank the staff of the Health Sciences Library there for always graciously helping me access essential documents and making available necessary facilities. I am especially grateful to Pat Erwin, MLS, head reference librarian, and Larry Prokop, MLS, for helping me verify certain sources. I also acknowledge the ability to access texts and bound issues of past anesthesia journals owned by Dr. Alan Sessler, which, like microfilms, have become rare as space limitations rule and so prevent invaluable browsing. I thank Patrick Sim, MLS, librarian at the Wood Library-Museum of Anesthesiology, for responding to various requests and permitting me to visit the museum and the library. I am greatly indebted too to Judith Robins, collections supervisor there, for acceding to my requests for illustrative material and for discussing points of detail she has made herself uniquely familiar with.

It is a particular pleasure to thank Hilary Lane, coordinator of the History of Medicine Collection of the Mayo Clinic Library. Hilary was never fazed by my requests for research material and never failed to obtain them. The proximity in the library to volumes written by such luminaries as Andreas Vesalius, William Harvey, John Hunter, and Humphry Davy was, of course, an additional stimulus to my research, which gave me a sense of continuity with individuals who loom large in the history of anesthesia.

Finally, I acknowledge the osmotic value of my association over the years with members of the Canadian Society of the History of Medicine. As a physician, I learned much that, though indefinable and unwritten, imbued in me an interest in, and awareness of, the methodological aspects of the history of medicine. I hope that this history repays, in small measure, the intellectual debt of that association.

David Shephard
Thunder Bay, Ontario, Canada

Introduction

The history of anesthesia is principally the history of an idea. The idea is a simple one: that pain in patients having surgical operations might be relieved. It's also a very old idea. The ancient Incas, for example, are said to have chewed coca leaves and then dribbled the saliva on the skull before making a hole in it in the operation of trephining.[1] Long before William Thomas Green Morton introduced ether for "modern" clinical anesthesia in 1846,[2] surgeons were always concerned about pain in their patients, but their methods of pain relief were not very efficacious. Only from 1846 onward, when practitioners took up the new field of "etherization"—later termed *anesthesia**—could the pain associated with a surgical operation be relieved effectively and consistently. Therefore, the term *anesthesia* traditionally denotes the abolition of the pain associated with a surgical operation, and one aspect of the history of anesthesia concerns the way pain relief in the operating room has been managed over the years.

However, two other aspects of anesthesia, and therefore of its history, must be considered. One concerns the different types of care that, beginning in the second half of the twentieth century, anesthesiologists provided for many types of patients besides those in operating rooms. Women in labor, people with chronic pain, patients in intensive care units, and even those who are victims of sudden collapse and have to be resuscitated outside the hospital—all these types of patients may be cared for by anesthesiologists. How these different activities developed is also part of the history of anesthesia.

A third aspect of anesthesia is that of anesthesia as a medical specialty—the focus of this history. For the first fifty years, anesthesia was a *craft*, with an empirical base of practice, but lacking in both a rigorous scientific foundation and an organizational and professional structure. That changed in the twentieth century. First, beginning in about 1900, the practice and the study of anesthesia

---

*For definitions and usage of the large linguistic family of terms such as *anesthesia*, *anaesthesia*, and *anesthesiology*, see the glossary in appendix B.

became more objective and scientific, so that it may be thought of as a *discipline*. Then, late in the 1930s, both in the United States and the United Kingdom, after professional societies were created and educational programs devised, anesthesia was recognized as a *specialty*. That evolutionary process was a lengthy and complex one and, as the emergence of *subspecialties* in the second half of the twentieth century shows, a continuing one. How anesthesia passed through these three stages is emphasized, not only for its relevance to the history of anesthesia but also because it helps to explain the process of medical specialization. Therefore, the evolutionary process in shaping the development of anesthesia from craft to specialty runs like a thread throughout this history.

Although those three aspects of the development of anesthesia are the primary topics in this history, still others must be considered. Because they form the background to this history of anesthesia, they will be discussed here. Three sets of factors are particularly significant. They are advances in science and technology, the growth of professionalism, and the engagement of anesthesia with society. In addition, the terms *craft*, *discipline*, and *specialty* will be further defined, and the need for a comprehensive history of anesthesia and its relevance will be discussed.

Anesthesia and Science, Professionalism, and Society

One factor that shaped the development of anesthesia was the *growth of scientific knowledge and of technology*. New drugs and techniques certainly altered the practice and understanding of anesthesia, but many of the changes that modified anesthesia were due to progress in many fields outside surgery and medicine besides anesthesia itself. Thus physiology, pharmacology, chemistry, physics, biochemistry, electronics, engineering, and even the plastics industry all had an impact. At the same time, the new knowledge yielded by work in those fields did not obscure a core of older knowledge. Drugs like morphine and hyoscine, for example, were first used centuries ago; and some of the basic knowledge of physiology was established in the seventeenth century, and that of chemistry, in the eighteenth century. There is thus a "prehistory" of anesthesia, as well as a more recent history. Moreover, that prehistory is a significant one, and it needs to be recounted for a simple reason that relates to that older knowledge.

Much of that prehistory, as is discussed in chapter 1, was created by scientists like William Harvey, Robert Boyle, and Joseph Priestley. All of them laid a foundation of knowledge that would benefit not only future anesthesia practitioners but also medical scientists. Furthermore, after anesthesia was introduced in 1846, that early scientific knowledge was all that the first anesthesia practitioners could fall back on, *because until October 1846, there was no body of knowledge that was unique to anesthesia*. At first, that older knowledge—together with empirical knowledge, based on experience—did help the first practitioners understand anesthesia: for example, how a volatile chemical like ether could be taken into the lungs and circulated to the brain to induce anesthesia. But as anesthesia developed, knowledge specific to anesthesia was required, which was one of the first tasks of the earliest anesthetists. It is in that context that the contributions of Londoner John Snow,[3] an epidemiologist as well as an anaesthetist, must be understood.

Though what was established in the prehistory of anesthesia, and its links to the present, may not be obvious, they do demonstrate interesting historical tendencies. We see, for example, how a specific body of knowledge of a new field is sometimes grafted on the old. We see how valuable the continuity of growth of knowledge was to certain areas of anesthesia, and how important a role a specific matrix of knowledge and technology played in the evolving process that led to specialty recognition of anesthesia. Yet the continuity of the linkage between past and present may be tenuous, indeed; from 1800 to 1840, for example, as chapter 2 makes clear, "nonevents" rather than actual events are what is evident.

Once anesthesia had been introduced, it was necessary to build a foundation specifically for the art and science of the new field of anesthesia. How that was created in the first half century of anesthesia we examine in chapter 3. That foundation was built on the study and use of ether, chloroform, and nitrous oxide, and on the design and use of apparatus that was simple, small, and portable, for in the nineteenth century, anesthesia was given in people's homes, as well as in hospitals. In the next century, many other anesthetic agents were introduced (all of which are discussed in chapters 4, 5, and 9), while the technical aspects of anesthesia became steadily more complex (many being discussed in chapters 6, 7, and 10).

All these innovations, which reflect changes in medicine, and to some extent in society, changed the practice of anesthesia, particularly in the second half of the twentieth century. Not only did surgery become increasingly complex, but anesthesiologists extended their work to areas beyond the operating room, as in labor suites, intensive care units (as discussed in chapter 11), and even outside the hospital itself, as in pain clinics (chapter 12) and resuscitation medicine (chapter 13). Anesthesia became more closely integrated with medicine, and society benefited.

One outcome of some of these developments was the *growth of professionalism in anesthesia*. As practitioners became involved in education and research, as well as clinical practice, the approach to anesthesia became more professional. An *ethos* grew among anesthesia practitioners: they were identified with anesthesia as a special field, and their need was recognized by other physicians. They became de facto specialists long before anesthesia was formally recognized a specialty.

Early on, the practice of anesthesia as a separate professional activity was identified with physicians. In England, they included with Joseph Clover,

Frederic Hewitt, and Dudley Buxton besides Snow, and in the United States, T. S. Buchanan, Thomas L. Bennett, and Adolph Erdmann among others. This development was enhanced by the founding of two early professional societies: the Society of Anaesthetists in London in 1893[4] and the Long Island Society of Anesthetists in 1905.[5] The appointment of physicians as anesthetists to some hospitals also illustrates the development of professionalism.[6] In the more sparsely populated United States, pioneer nurse-anesthetists like Florence Henderson, Edith Graham, and Alice Magaw at the Mayo Clinic[7] also played a part, and their work wove a separate organizational thread in the practice of anesthesia.

The development of a professional *ethos* was also enhanced as anesthesia expanded in nature and scope. As anesthesia emerged from its traditional locus of the operating room, it became increasingly an important part of surgical and medical care. The image that surgeons, obstetricians, and internists, as well as practitioners of anesthesia themselves, had of anesthesia then changed significantly.

Professionalism, while shaping the practice of anesthesia, was, however, just one of many forces that led to anesthesia being recognized as a medical specialty. Specialty recognition, besides being a lengthy and complex process, was circular and often stagnant. Obstacles had to be overcome and challenges met, many of which are discussed in chapter 8. Even so, the process was an evolutionary one, for anesthesia passed successfully through the stages of craft and discipline first, before becoming a recognized specialty, and much later, as discussed in chapter 14, spawning subspecialties.

A third general factor that influenced the evolution of anesthesia was *the relationship between anesthesia and society*. Though the impact on anesthesia has been less than the two foregoing influences, this relationship has existed since the early days of anesthesia. Thus, very soon after ether and chloroform were used to relieve childbirth pain, the public was vociferous in airing its views on anesthesia. Some physicians and many clerics objected to the artificial abolition of pain in laboring women, but their sisters, including Queen Victoria in England, forcefully countered those objections, and anesthesia for delivery was eventually accepted.[8] Society also articulated its feelings in the 1960s, and the stress that it laid on accountability induced anesthesiologists to take a closer look at the problem of human error.[9] (See also chapter 10.)

In turn, anesthesia has benefited society. The growth of diversity of anesthesia has meant that it has come to play a greater role in health care. Anesthesiologists are no longer confined to the operating room; they care for many different types of patients. The spectrum of anesthetic care today is far broader than it was when anesthesia was a craft. As it evolved toward being a specialty, it increasingly benefited society.

Often this resulted from individual initiatives. Three examples of dedication to society illustrate this. First, English anaesthetist Edgar Pask was anesthetized.

A breathing tube was inserted in his trachea, and he was ventilated, all this being part of a research project that was directed to developing a life jacket that would help downed air force pilots in World War II float faceup in the water.[10] Second, after the war, American anesthesiologist Scott Smith received curare, while conscious, to determine whether it affected the central nervous system.[11] A third example is of Danish anesthesiologist Bjorn Ibsen; his initiative in 1952 changed the way poliomyelitis was treated[12] and led to the new field of critical care.

Craft, Discipline, and Specialty: The Terms Defined

As already noted, the central theme of this history is the transition of anesthesia from a craft to a specialty. Because the terms *craft*, *discipline*, and *specialty* are used in a particular sense, they are defined at some length here. (Other terms that may be unfamiliar in this book are defined in the glossary in appendix B.) Other aspects of this evolutionary process are also discussed here.

Anesthesia as a craft. For the first fifty years, anesthesia was a craft. Ether or chloroform was poured onto a rag or a mask to make the patient pain free and to adhere to the surgeon's wish to operate on an immobile patient. The practice of anesthesia was wholly service oriented; there was art but little science. Since anesthesia was brand-new, a critical question was this one: *what* was anesthesia? While that question was addressed both clinically and in the laboratory by Snow,[13] most early practitioners were content to take an empirical approach to anesthesia, without being especially interested in the physiological and pharmacological responses to anesthesia. That approach served well most of the time, particularly as surgical operations were relatively simple and very brief in the first half century, though the high mortality associated with anesthesia was of concern. Minimalism and simplicity, clinical competence and dexterity, vigilance and inventiveness characterized the practice of anesthesia, and these features characterize anesthesia as a craft.

Anesthesia as a discipline. From 1900 to the mid-1930s, anesthesia was shaped more by objective knowledge and by a critical attitude. However, the knowledge was still mainly applied to clinical practice; it was not *created* for its own *academic* value. In this book, the term *discipline* indicates an approach to anesthesia that was midway between art and science, between practice and theory. The basic question that anesthetists asked was this: *how* was anesthesia to be achieved?

The work of two individuals shows how this question shaped their work and how they answered it. One was Hewitt in London. He was interested in nitrous oxide, especially in the way nitrous oxide anesthesia could be achieved and made safer by adding certain proportions of oxygen. This he did systematically in a series of investigations beginning in 1885.[14] The other individual was the American Walter Boothby, who determined inhaled ether concentrations[15] while he was asking himself how to design an anesthesia machine.[16] Hewitt's and Boothby's investigations are considered in chapter 7. They reflect anesthesia as a discipline.

The stage of a discipline also illustrates the concept of the evolution of anesthesia as being part of a *process*. Many factors shaped this, and as a result, no single device or drug, and no single person or event is in itself evidence for the stage of anesthesia as a discipline. Rather, the evidence is collective. Anesthesia as a discipline was characterized by the development of an *attitude* to anesthesia that derived from the need to formally solve clinical problems. Technical, investigative, and professional factors contributed to this; and all laid the basis, and provided the justification, for anesthesia as a specialty.

Anesthesia as a specialty. Although the stage of anesthesia as a specialty was not attained until the latter 1930s, the quest was of long standing. Though the concept of specialist anesthesia was espoused first by Snow in 1852,[17] the actual process took nearly a century. The process was a complex one, factors including research and education, as well as clinical practice and the need for an organizational structure for anesthesia. Much had to be accomplished, many obstacles had to be overcome, and the vectors of many factors had to be directed in the right direction. The twentieth-century pioneers had to show that anesthesia had matured sufficiently to justify specialty recognition. Thus it is simplistic to equate specialization just with full-time practice, which Hewitt had called for in 1896,[18] which S. Ormond Goldan stressed in 1901,[19] and which some historians do even today.[20] Specialization comprised many facets of an organizational structure that were designed to support anesthesia as an autonomous, peer-governed branch of medicine that embraced the three components of education, research, and clinical practice—all, ideally, directed toward providing excellence of health care. All that took many years to achieve. Much later, the process of specialization was taken farther still as the subspecialties developed.

If the two previous stages of anesthesia were concerned with the *what* and *how* of anesthesia, the question now was *why*. This question may be considered further by looking at the contributions of two other individuals who practiced around the time when anesthesia was moving toward specialty status.

One of those individuals was Ralph Waters. He joined the University of Wisconsin in 1927, and over the next ten years, he did a great deal in the struggle to have anesthesia recognized as a specialty. Waters was self-educated in anesthesia, for when he first showed an interest in anesthesia, there were no training programs that he could turn to. Therefore, this self-made anesthetist answered the question as to *why anesthetics worked* by relying on his own experience, together with a modicum of experimental study. So he looked at chloroform and cyclopropane, for example, from a clinical point of view. He also had a well-developed vision for anesthesia that embraced research and teaching for what they could give to clinical practice.[21] Both his innovative residency program and his cooperative research program did much to shape the movement for specialty recognition. Waters himself personified anesthesia for those of his medical colleagues, especially his surgical peers, who had important roles in accepting or rejecting anesthesia as a potential candidate for specialty recognition. By showing what anesthesia could achieve in terms of clinical practice, teaching, and research, Waters was a potent force in the quest to have anesthesia recognized as a specialty.

The other individual of note was Waters' younger contemporary Henry Beecher, of Harvard University.[22] Since he entered anesthesia in the 1940s, his impact on anesthesia was different from Waters'. It was different in part because he entered anesthesia after the battles for specialty recognition had been won and because he came from an academic background. Beecher therefore answered the question as to *why* in a different way from the way Waters had.

Originally trained in surgery and then physiology, Beecher brought to anesthesia the perspective and the benefits of an academic background, and his answer was formulated in terms of physiology and pharmacology. Beecher also extended the vision of what anesthesiologists could contribute. For example, he took an active role in the ethics of the diagnostic criteria of death, his physiological background guiding him there; he was also interested in morphine and curare, and his pharmacological understanding, similarly, was helpful to him.

In those respects, Waters and Beecher are contrasting figures: Waters brought to the university environment the practical background; Beecher did the opposite. They reflect the fact that, as anesthesia evolved, it did so along two lines: that of clinical practice and that of the academic milieu, that of town and gown.

Since much of this history is concerned with anesthetic agents, it is appropriate here to provide just one example of the way an answer to the question *why* is found. Although the mechanism by which drugs cause anesthesia has not yet been elucidated, it is probable that the chemical and geometric aspects of the structure of anesthetic agents are significant. Each drug exerts specific pharmacological effects on the body, and these effects are derived from the chemical structure of each drug. This relationship is analogous to the relationship between a key and the lock it opens by virtue of having been cut to a specific pattern. While this aspect of anesthesia lies behind the discussion of each of the drugs that are discussed in this history, it is appropriate to stress the contributions that chemists and also pharmacologists have made to anesthesia. In particular, much of the developmental work in anesthesia, particularly in research, has been made by chemists and pharmacologists, and though the goal of finding the perfect drug, the holy grail in anesthesia, has not yet been reached, the research that is governed by that search has been essential.

The Need for a Comprehensive History of Anesthesia

The history of anesthesia is therefore complex, and all of the foregoing considerations buttress the need for a history that is comprehensive. An additional consideration is the fact that a history that reviews the full spectrum of the development of anesthesia up to the twenty-first century is lacking. Many valuable texts on the history of anesthesia have been written, but none presently is both current and comprehensive. However, six books that have value as significant resources must be noted.

The first is Thomas Keys' classic, a comprehensive survey of anesthesia up to 1940, but published as long ago as 1945.[23] It is still a valuable resource. Barbara Duncum's study of 1947 is also invaluable, even though it deals only with inhalational anesthesia from 1846 to 1900.[24] A third text is Bryn Thomas' survey of anesthesia apparatus, though it is mainly concerned with anesthesia machines in the United Kingdom up to 1970.[25] The detailed study of anesthesia history by Norman Bergman, published in 1996, is another important source, but it does not deal with events after 1846.[26] Two other histories cover a good deal of ground, and they are excellent introductions to the history of anesthesia; however, they are not comprehensive in that some topics are dealt with quite briefly and some others not at all. One book is *A Short History of Anaesthesia: The First 150 Years*, by G. Rushman, N. Davies, and R. Atkinson, which was published in 1996[27]; the other is *Anaesthesia and the Practice of Medicine: Historical Perspectives* by Keith Sykes and John Bunker, published in 2007,[28] which provides a transatlantic perspective.

Besides the foregoing, a number of other histories of anesthesia have been written over the years. They are listed in the bibliography. However, they are not as authoritative.

The Relevance of the History of Anesthesia

Several themes, then, run through this history. How may their significance be judged? History is to some extent subjective, and a historian's perspective differs from that of readers. Although both may share an interest in the work of our predecessors, readers may argue that knowing the history of anesthesia makes no difference to the way they practice anesthesia. That is true, and a historian must answer the objection. Here, it may be said that while, similarly, one could argue that knowing the history of the Model T Ford is equally irrelevant to one's ability to drive a car, that objection misses the point. History is not utilitarian; its context, while partly technical, is cultural or professional. In the history of anesthesia, the context is mainly professional. Knowing the history of anesthesia will give anesthesiologists a broader perspective of the specialty. Some will be interested in drugs and techniques; others, in anesthesiologists and their ideas and how they shaped anesthesia and smoothed the way to the present for us; and still others, in the development of the practice of anesthesia and of the *ethos* in being an anesthesiologist.

Like readers, historians vary in their preferences and in their prejudices, their interests, and their objectives. The approach that one historian will take in writing a history will differ in some respects from that of other historians; the perspective varies, as does the selection and interpretation of material. Nor is there any one way to write history, for it is dependent on the subject, as well as on the historian. John Burnham, for example, saw the history of medicine as the intertwining of the dramas of the healer, the sick, diseases, knowledge, and society,[29] and some elements of that may be seen in the history of anesthesia. Anesthesia historian Rene Fulop-Miller's perspective too was individual: with his own experience of pain, he found that it was the nature of the content of the history of anesthesia that influenced the way he chose to present the subject,[30] though he also saw himself as a creative artist who breathed life into "dry facts" and the "dead past."

Each historian attempts to make dry facts come alive, but the history of anesthesia is much more than a catalog of facts, as interesting as they are. The history of anesthesia shows us much drama and a great deal of human interest. There are so many whom we remember for what they achieved and for the links history provides us with: the personal sufferings of the pioneers Horace Wells, Charles Jackson, and William Morton; the too-short lives of original thinkers like Hickman and Snow; the vision of Ralph Waters and John Lundy; the initiatives of Ivan Magill, Bjorn Ibsen, and Virginia Apgar; and the dedication in the more recent past in the self-experimentation of Edgar Pask and Scott Smith. All these anesthesiologists and their varied contributions, and those of so many others, are part of the cultural history of anesthesia. They have all had roles on the stage that is anesthesia. Their task was frequently to solve the problems of the day, and in doing so, they paved the way to the present and thus made the work of today's anesthesiologists—and patients—much easier than in days of yore.

The purpose of this history is not only to provide a narrative of how anesthesia developed but also to depict the past so that we can benefit by learning from it and from those who shaped it. The history of anesthesia is a panorama that shows how our forbears went about their daily work, faced challenges and overcame them, adding new drugs and techniques to their armamentarium, and so smoothing the path to the less-taxing present so that today's practitioners can overcome yet other challenges. It is a panorama that helps us understand our links to the past and to the men and women whose efforts paved the way to the present. Reading about them alters our perspective, sometimes minimally, but frequently to a considerable extent. History is for each of us, its value to be appreciated individually.

Chapter 1

The Beginnings to 1800

Long before ether was first used as an anesthetic in the 1840s, various means were tried to relieve the pain of a surgical operation. Someone with a gaping wound or a fracture, for example, might receive an anodyne (or analgesic) derived from a plant, or supportive words from a shaman or a priest, or, later, a physician. Plants were always available, and though the medicaments obtained from them varied in potency, their use maintained the idea of surgical pain relief down the ages. Indeed, some of the pain-relieving substances of plant origin, such as morphine-containing opium and scopolamine-containing henbane, were efficacious enough to remain in use long after ether anesthesia was introduced in 1846.

Ether is not of plant origin but a chemical substance. It was discovered in the Middle Ages, perhaps by the Arabian Jabir in the eighteenth century or by the Spaniard Raymond Lully in the thirteenth, though the evidence in either case is slim.[1] More definite evidence of the effects of ether came in the sixteenth century with the work of two others: Valerius Cordus,[2] in his text of 1561, and Paracelsus, whose text of 1605 stated that it made chickens sleep.[3] However, in these years, no one conceived the idea of sleep, or hypnosis, *as a means of inducing anesthesia*. It was used as a remedy for headache, toothache, and earache,[4] and for chest ailments,[5] but never as a surgical aid.

Ether was used as an anesthetic only after the ground work in physiology and chemistry was laid in the seventeenth and eighteenth centuries. Key events then included William Harvey's proof in 1628 that the blood circulates round the body[6] and the studies of Robert Boyle and a group of natural scientists on respiration and the blood later in the seventeenth century.[7] Other significant advances, a century later, included Joseph Priestley's discovery in the 1770s of nitrous oxide[8] and oxygen.[9]

These discoveries were key because they provided the basis for anesthetic procedures such as the injection of hypnotic or analgesic substances into veins and the inhalation of hypnotic or anesthetic gases. They have historical value in two ways. First, they introduced the important element of the experimental method into medicine; and second, they invalidated and outdated the ancient ideas of the humors and qualities that had buttressed medical thought since Greek and Roman times.

Though this new knowledge bears only indirectly on the introduction of anesthesia, it is a significant part of the prehistory of anesthesia. For that reason, it is discussed in this chapter.

Ancient Anodynes

Because the earliest records of pain relief are those of myth and legend, we cannot be sure of the validity of the earliest accounts of what might have been anesthesia. To treat pain, always a common human complaint, physicians and others likely sought analgesia (absence of pain) and sedation rather than deep anesthesia (absence of feeling). Over time, the term *anesthesia* denoted deep sleep as well, though it had other connotations. In the fourth century before the Common Era (CE), Plato used it to connote a moral quality rather than a physical one.[10] In the first century CE, Dioscorides noted that after mandragora was given, "the knife or the actual cautery . . . may not be felt,"[11] thus using the term in the modern sense. Today we think of anesthesia as a reversible state of mental and physical "insensibility." Oliver Wendell Holmes defined it thus for William Thomas Green Morton on November 21, 1846,[12] which is how the term is used in this book.

The earliest accounts of medication before surgery were oral. Some of those accounts have been favored by some historians and some by others.[13] Fact was sometimes distorted or embellished, or usurped by myth or legend. Single vegetable agents, such as mandragora or poppy, were used; but usually several were given together, which suggests that no one drug was wholly efficacious. Some accounts certainly indicate that a measure of efficacy was attained. The fourth-century account of Saint Hilary, of France, for example, suggests that, with drugs, "limbs can be cut off without pain: the flesh is dead to all feeling and does not heed the deep thrust of the knife,"[14] even though we do not know which drugs were given. That account is certainly suggestive of positive efforts to relieve surgical pain, but since many of these early accounts were oral while the few written ones cannot be cross-checked against other accounts, two questions must be asked when assessing early accounts of pain relief. The first: how sound does the evidence seem? The second: how reliable does the account seem?

Initially, pain was thought to be the work of the devil or evil spirits, and numerous techniques were used to repel them, such as skin tattooing, rings in the ears and noses, and talismans and amulets.[15] In time, early peoples found that remedies derived from plants such as the poppy, mandragora, henbane, Indian hemp, corn, and potato were efficacious; the first four had hypnotic and analgesic properties, while the latter two, when fermented, induced alcoholic stupefaction. But because such remedies likely did not consistently prevent or abolish the acute pain of a surgical operation, other techniques were used. The Chinese used acupuncture; the Incas chewed coca and dribbled coca-laden saliva over the site of trephining (though the evidence for this is not firm[16]); and some surgeons compressed the carotid vessels to induce loss of consciousness.[17]

The Poppy and Opium

The most reliable of the plant anodynes was raw opium, which was produced by the poppy. It is mentioned in the earliest literature. In the *Odyssey*, Helen, daughter of Zeus, may well have prepared opium as an anodyne. She dissolved it in wine to assuage her grief and anger and to forget her pain: "Straightway she cast into the wine of which they drank a drug which quenches pain and strife and brings forgetfulness of every ill."[18] This, however, is likely to be the stuff of myth. More realistic is Celsius, in the first century CE:

> Those pills which alleviate pain by causing sleep are called anodynes in Greek. It is bad practice to employ them except in cases of urgent necessity, for they are compounded of powerful drugs and are bad for the stomach. However, one may be used, which contains a denarius [i.e., equivalent to the weight of the Roman coin of that name], each of tears of poppy and galbanum, and two denarii each of myrrh, castoreum, and pepper. It is enough to swallow a piece the size of a bean.[19]

Opium would have certainly been of value in surgical cases. Nepenthe, a form of opium, is said to have been favored by Aesculapius, the god of medicine, to make his patients insensible before they were operated on.[20] Moreover, opium was readily available in and around the Middle East and Asia.

Mandragora

Mandragora is frequently mentioned in the literature, though it is uncertain how potent it was—or indeed, whether it is entirely mythical. English anaesthetist Armstrong Davison, for example, stated that "no such plant exists, or ever did exist."[21] Myth does, indeed, flavor references to mandragora. With its forked limblike roots, it seemed to have human form, which fitted in with primitive peoples' anthropomorphic ideas about nature and the world. The naming of a plant of the Solanaceae family as *Atropa mandragora* increases the uncertainty, for mandrake plants are members of the nightshade family. However, Theophrastus, in the third century BCE, described a mandragora plant that was identified with belladonna,[22] which would be consistent with stories of the soporific effect of mandragora. Thus Shakespeare's Cleopatra:

> Give me to drink Mandragora . . . .
> That I might sleep out this great gap of time
> My Antony is away.[23]

The preparation and use of mandragora was described by Dioscorides. "Some persons," he wrote, "boil down the roots in wine to a third, strain it, and put it away, using one cyathus in the case of persons suffering from insomnia or severe pain, or those to be cut or cauterized, when they wish to produce anesthesia."[24] (One cyathus was somewhat more than 1½ ounces.)

Henbane

Henbane (*Hyoscyamus niger*) also is a source of belladonna alkaloids, and its seeds and leaves are used in preparing the medicinal compound. As it contains scopolamine, it may have induced preoperative sleep; and scopolamine was used in the twentieth century as part of the preparation given to induce 'twilight sleep' in the management of childbirth.[25] Henbane seems to have been used as a constituent along with other anodynes, as, for example in *Spongia somnifera*, or soporific sponge.

Cannabis indica and Indian Hemp

Hemp has been used for recreational purposes and in medical and surgical administration for centuries. According to Herodotus, the Scythians, for example, used hemp.[26] The dried leaves that are burned and smoked are familiar as marijuana, and the resin derived from the flowering tops of hemp produces hashish, which can be chewed or drunk as well as smoked. As *ma*, hemp was used by the Chinese when acupuncture did not seem suitable.[27] Hemp is another constituent of the soporific sponge.

Spongia somnifera

In the ninth-century Bamberg *Antidotarium*, a preparation known as *Spongia somnifera* was described in detail. It was prepared as follows:

> Take . . . of opium thebaicum, juice of hyoscyamine, unripened berry
> of the blackberry, lettuce seed, juice of hemlock, poppy, mandragora,
> ivy . . . . Put all these together in a vessel and plunge therein a new
> sea-sponge just as it comes from the sea, taking care that fresh water

does not touch it. And put this in the sun during the dog-days until all the liquid is consumed. And when there is need, dip it a little in water not too warm, and apply it to the nostrils of the patient, and he will quickly go to sleep. When, moreover, you want to awaken him, apply juice from the root of the fennel and he will soon bestir himself.[28]

There's another interesting account of a soporific draught in Boccaccio's *Decameron*:

> There came to the attention of the physician a patient with a gangrenous leg, and when the master had made an examination he told the relatives that unless a decayed bone in the leg were removed either the entire leg would have to be amputated or the patient would die; moreover, if the bone were removed, the patient might recover, but he refused to undertake the case except as if the man were already dead. To this the relatives agreed and surrendered the patient to him. The doctor was of the opinion that without an opiate the man could not endure the pain and would not permit the operation, and since the affair was set for the evening, he distilled that morning a type of water of his own composition which had the faculty of bringing to the person who drank it sleep for as long as was deemed necessary to complete the operation.[29]

Three points are relevant to a discussion of ancient soporific preparations and anodynes. First, the medical attendants doubtless did what they could to relieve pain in surgical patients, though we do not know how effectively. Pain may have been perceived as being God's judgment, but shamans and physicians did give such medicated preparations that were available. Second, the multiplicity of substances in the soporific sponge, for example, indicates polypharmacy, which suggests reliance on a shotgun effect and implies that no one drug was very potent. And third, there are good reasons why many of the ancient anodynes lacked efficacy and might even have been dangerous. None was standardized or prepared in pure form, dosage was not regulated, and no controlled experiments were carried out to determine the greater efficacy of one remedy over another. Hence some doubt abounds. Anesthesiologist Norman Bergman believed that "anesthetics of the Ancients . . . simply did not work!"[30] Howard Raper, citing the testing of a soporific sponge as reported by Theodoric in the thirteenth century, stated that it wouldn't even make a guinea pig nod.[31]

Ether as a Hypnotic Anodyne

Because ancient anodynes either were inefficacious or acted inconsistently, the search for anodynes continued. Ether was part of that search, even though it was used for purposes other than pain relief. Cordus, for example, in describing the synthesis of "sweet oil of vitriol" from a sulfurous compound in 1540, said that it "consumes phlegm and assuages the thirst and dryness in fevers."[32] But with respect to ether as a hypnotic, it is instructive to cite Paracelsus' observations on chickens:

> The following should be noted here with regard to this sulphur, that of all things extracted from vitriol it is most remarkable because it is stable. And besides, it has associated with it such a sweetness that it is taken even by chickens, and they fall asleep from it for a while but awaken later without harm. On this sulphur no other judgment should be passed than that in disease which needs to be treated with anodynes it quiets all suffering without any harm, and relieves all pain, and quenches all fevers, and prevents complications in all illnesses.[33]

Whether Cordus or Paracelsus has priority in discovering the analgesic effect of ether is, however, not clear. The two worked together. The text in which Cordus described ether was not published until 1561, long after his death; and Paracelsus' book, in which he had referred to sleeping chickens, was also published posthumously, in 1605. Either, or both, of these two individuals may, therefore, be credited with discovering ether (so named in 1730 by Johannes Frobenius[34]).

In terms of priority of description of anesthesia with ether, Paracelsus' observations are significant, even though the subjects were chickens and not humans. The statement that ether "relieves all pain" is the first description of such an effect, though Paracelsus did not suggest that ether might be of use in surgical operations. (In 1800, in a similar wink at history, Humphry Davy noted that nitrous oxide could relieve pain, and so he went farther than Paracelsus in suggesting—but just en passant—that the gas might be of surgical use[35] [see also chapter 2].)

Despite such a near-miss, the older remedies remained in use. In 1562, William Bullein referred to Dioscorides and mandragora when he had a fictional character say, "This bringeth slepe, it casteth men into a trauns on a depe tirrible dreame, untill he be cutte of the stone."[36] Even so, despite the many references to the concept of pain relief down the ages, in the sixteenth century, pain was still regarded as punishment to be stoically borne. Otherwise, poor pregnant Eufaemia MacCalyan would not have been burned at the stake in 1591 for conspiring, with the "witch" Agnes Sampson, to attempt to relieve the pain of childbirth.[37] Thus, the time was not yet ripe for anesthesia; nor would it be for another two centuries and a half.

The Sixteenth and Seventeenth Centuries: Early Modern Science

Great progress was made with the scientific revolution of the sixteenth century, for a sea change occurred in the thinking about science. This affected ideas about the relationship of human beings to the world; they had to adapt to the heliocentric ideas of Nicolaus Copernicus, Galilei Galileo, and Johannes Keppler, for example. In medicine, the best-known figure of change is Andreas Vesalius (fig. 1.1). His anatomical dissections set him apart from the outmoded and bookish teachings in medicine of Galen, whose ideas were based on studies of animals. In contrast, Vesalius emphasized the importance of *human* anatomy. This was the age too of experimentation and measurement—qualities that would be essential when it became necessary to unlock the mysteries of anesthesia.

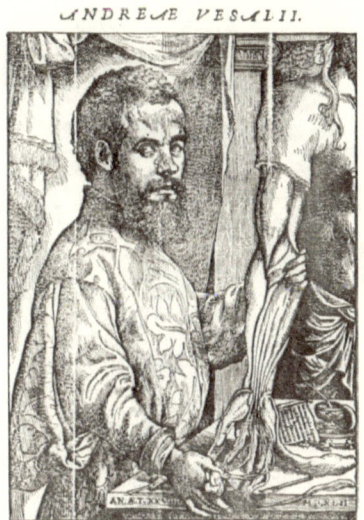

Fig. 1.1. Andreas Vesalius (1514-1564)
Andreas Vesalius, born in Brussels, studied medicine in Louvain and Paris and was appointed professor of anatomy at the University of Padua when only twenty-three. His dissections of the human body, rather than of animals, taught him (and others) human anatomy in a way that the Galenic tradition of dissecting animals did not. Though he did not break with Galen's teaching and was not in that sense a revolutionary, Vesalius showed that blood certainly did not pass from the right ventricle to the left through pores in the interventricular septum. In 1543, Vesalius published *De humani corporis fabrica*, a classic of the Renaissance in looking forward rather than back. It represented the belief that accuracy in anatomical knowledge was essential to progress in medicine in the sixteenth century, as was accuracy in physiology to progress in the sixteenth century and accuracy in chemistry to progress in the eighteenth century. Vesalius rejuvenated the study of anatomy. However, in his own day, Vesalius was regarded as dangerously unorthodox, and because of that, he left the dissecting table and Padua and joined the court of the Spanish king Charles V. He died while returning from a pilgrimage to Jerusalem.

In medicine, the new attitude can be discerned in three books of this era. One was Jean Fernel's *De naturali parte medicinae*[38] (1542), which contained the first original observations on physiology since the days of Galen. The second was Vesalius's *De humani corporis fabrica*[39] (1543; fig. 1.2), which was the first modern and objective study of anatomy. The third revolutionary text was by another Padua student: William Harvey (fig. 1.3), the author of *De motu cordis*[40] (1628; fig. 1.4). Harvey's proof that the blood circulated around the body is characteristic of the new attitude. With Vesalius, Harvey did much to help overthrow ancient doctrines in medicine, such as those of the four humors and the pneuma.

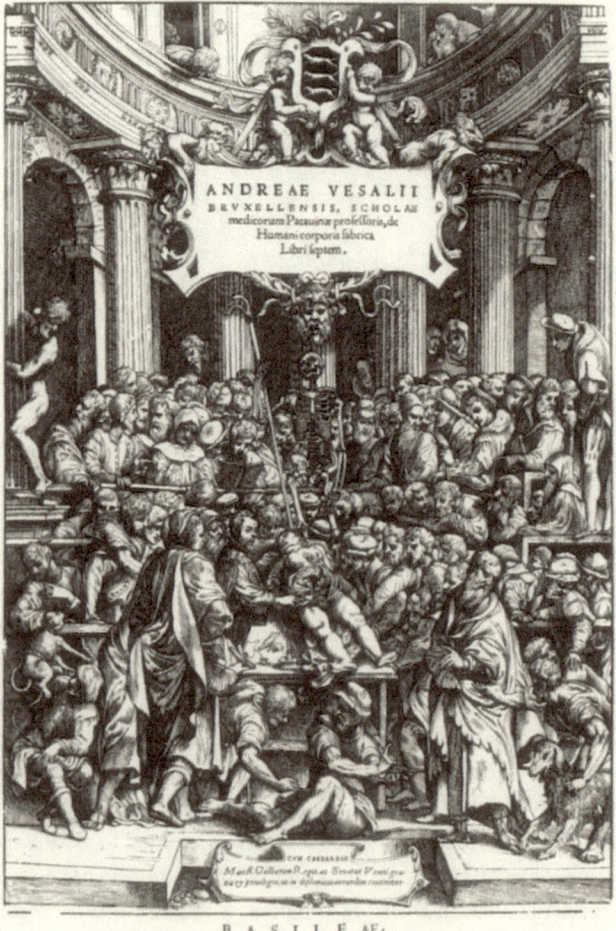

Fig. 1.2. Title page of Vesalius's *De humani corporis fabrica libri septem* (1543). (Mayo History of Medicine Library Collection.)

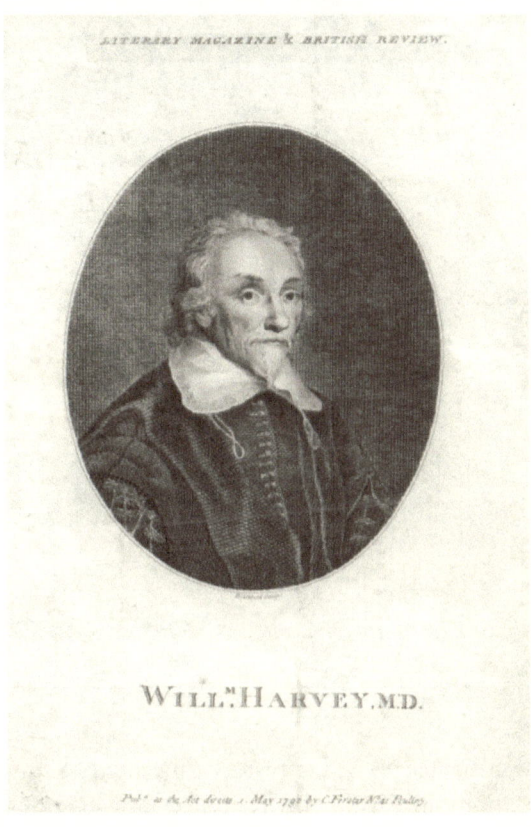

LITERARY MAGAZINE & BRITISH REVIEW.

WILL.ᵐHARVEY.MD.

Fig. 1.3. William Harvey (1578-1657)

William Harvey was born in Folkestone, England. He studied at Cambridge and Padua. He obtained his MD degree in 1602, and then returned to England. He became prominent in the Royal College of Physicians of London, and was appointed Lumleian Lecturer in 1615 and president in 1654. He believed that the blood constantly passed through the lungs into the aorta and proved that the blood perpetually moves in a circle as the heart pulsates. He amplified these innovative ideas, which were first expressed in his Lumleian Lecture of 1616, in *de motu cordis*, which was published in 1628. He explained that blood circulates to the limbs in arteries and that it returns through veins, the valves of which are consistent with unidirectional flow. Like many great innovators, Harvey was regarded as "crack-brained" by some, though he was highly regarded by others. Harvey was not alone in believing that the blood circulated around the body—Ibn al-Nafis, Realdo Colombo, and Michael Servetus also did so—but he did provide the proof, and so argued that Galen was incorrect in his ideas about the circulation. As well as being interested in the circulation, Harvey was deeply interested in embryology and published *Excercitationes de genaratione animalium* in 1651.

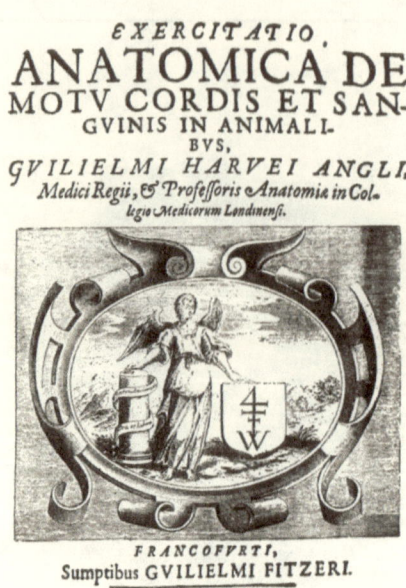

EXERCITATIO,
ANATOMICA DE
MOTV CORDIS ET SAN-
GVINIS IN ANIMALI-
BVS,
GVILIELMI HARVEI ANGLI,
Medici Regii, & Profeſſoris Anatomiæ in Col-
legio Medicorum Londinenſi.

FRANCOFVRTI,
Sumptibus GVILIELMI FITZERI.
ANNO M. DC. XXVIII.

Fig. 1.4. Title page of *Exercitatio anatomica de motu cordis* (1628). (Mayo History of Medicine Library Collection.)

Harvey is a pivotal figure in the history of anesthesia. In laying the basis for intravenous injection, his work determined how anesthesia practitioners would think about the circulation two centuries later. All previous writings on the movement of the heart and arteries, Harvey wrote, had been "penned with an eye upon the lungs"; it was believed that "in diastole the arteries take air into their cavities and in systole expel sooty vapours through the same pored of flesh and skin."[41] Harvey corrected such ideas by proving that the heart simply drove the blood around the body. However, he did not formulate any new ideas on respiration, and his thinking was still influenced by the ideas of the ancients. But Harvey was a good-enough scientist to acknowledge that he had left some questions unanswered, which others would have to answer. Harvey's indecision was valuable precisely because it left the unsolved problem of respiration to be solved by other scientists.[42]

Representative of those scientists was Robert Boyle (fig. 1.5). He and other Oxford University virtuosi conducted fundamental studies on respiration[43] that, together with Harvey's, were the first bricks in the edifice that is part of the intellectual foundation of anesthesiology. Those studies marked a paradigmatic shift in scientific thought. One result of that was the emergence of pneumatic medicine (the medicinal use of gases) at the end of the eighteenth century, and this in turn was a factor in the later development of anesthesia.[44]

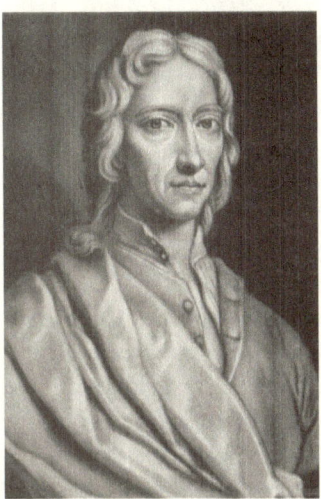

Fig. 1.5. Robert Boyle (1627-1691)
Robert Boyle, son of the Earl of Cork, was born in Linsmore, Munster in Ireland. Educated at Eton College and by a private tutor, Boyle traveled widely in Europe. He became interested in the experimental method of science, as enunciated by Francis Bacon, in 1649. In London in the early 1660s, he was one of a group of men for whom the study of "natural philosophy" engaged their attention and who founded the Royal Society. Boyle began writing on science—*The Spring and Weight of the Air* (1660) and *The Sceptical Chymist* (1661) were early books among the forty-two that he wrote—and set an example of what independent scientists and scholars could do. In 1665 or 1666, Boyle moved to Oxford, though not as a member of any college. He led a group of individuals, known as the Oxford virtuosi, who clarified the physiology of the respiration and the blood, and who fostered the scientific revolution of the seventeenth century. Boyle was fortunate in being assisted by Robert Hooke, particularly in performing those experiments that led to what became Boyle's law concerning the inverse relationship between the volume of a gas and the pressure acting on it. He also held to the view that matter has an atomic structure. In 1668, Boyle returned to London, where he continued to advocate the new science that the Royal Society would foster.

The virtuosi formed a large group. Besides Boyle, they included Richard Lower, Robert Hooke, and John Mayow. As a group, they generated enormous intellectual ferment.[45] Profoundly interested in many problems of science and medicine, they had an iconoclastic attitude to centuries-old dogma, they sought knowledge by conducting methodical experiments, and they each had the intelligence and the position in society to devote their time and energy to grappling with the problems they recognized.

Boyle, author of the *The Sceptical Chymist*,[46] (1661) was very much in tune with the scientific revolution of the seventeenth century[47] and its innovative experimental approach to problem solving.[48] He traveled in Europe, knew several languages, and became familiar with scientific progress that was being made on the Continent. Though best known for the law that relates gas volume and external pressure, Boyle is also known for his belief that chemical actions occur between particles that are in motion. His forty-two books covered science, philosophy, and theology. He helped incorporate the Royal Society in London in 1662 and supported its activities.

Boyle moved to Oxford in 1665 or 1666. Some of his work, and his encouraging his fellow virtuosi, led to new knowledge in medicine, particularly in connection with the respiration and the blood. Thus, Boyle stated that "there is in the air a little vital Quintessence . . . which serves to the refreshment and restauration of our vital Spirits,"[49] a statement whose value can only be appreciated in the context of the times, when old ideas such as the pneuma and "vital spirits" were entrenched in physiological thought. Boyle's ideas on respiration were shared by the other virtuosi, thus contributing to their own ideas on respiration. Later, Boyle returned to London, but he remained interested in natural science.

Hooke, a student at Christ Church, was skilled in making scientific instruments, and as a talented microscopist, he was the first to use the term *cell* in connection with body tissues. He helped construct the air pump that Boyle used in studying the relationship between the volume and the pressure of a gas, or Boyle's law. Boyle concluded that a gas is not just an invisible expanse but a collection of particulate matter, which became relevant in the study of respiration. Hooke shared Boyle's interest in respiration. Both believed that respiration had some things in common with combustion: the flame of a lighted combustible substance in the receiver of the pump was extinguished when the source of the air was removed.[50] Hooke went on to make his own discoveries in both natural science and respiration, and it may be difficult to distinguish Boyle's from Hooke's contributions. However, in an experiment he reported in 1667 to the Royal Society, Hooke certainly showed his own initiative in advancing the understanding of respiration. After opening the chest of a dog, he made openings in the lung surfaces and secured a pair of bellows in the trachea. The lungs became still, yet as long as air was supplied via the bellows, the heart continued to beat, and the animal remained alive.[51] Thus Hooke demonstrated the value of artificial ventilation (which Vesalius and Leonardo da Vinci had done earlier[52]) and proved that it was not just the motion of the lungs but a supply of fresh air that was essential to life.

Hooke's experiment came after Marcello Malpighi, a Bologna anatomist and a corresponding member of the Royal Society, had carried out his own significant work. Malpighi followed up Harvey's proof that the blood circulates round the body by demonstrating two other phenomena: first, the lungs are made up of membranes surrounding minute air spaces, and second, the blood circulates through capillaries in these membranes.[53] This sharpened the understanding of respiration.

Despite these various studies, the interaction in the lungs between the air and the blood was not clear. Clarification, however, came with the work of Lower and Mayow. Physicians by vocation but physiologists by nature, they consolidated the foundations of the knowledge of respiration. Lower noticed that the blood was bright red when an animal was ventilated but blue when ventilation was discontinued.[54] That is, the color of blood changed when it circulated through the lungs and so was in contact with air. Mayow then capped the work of the Oxford group by showing that a part of the air breathed is taken up during respiration.[55] The purpose of respiration was to ensure that that vital "quintessence" of air was taken up by the blood during breathing—just as some of the air is consumed in combustion.

The Oxford scientists, with Malpighi in Bologna, provided a new understanding of respiration. As Leonard Wilson noted, the Galenic concept of physiology "had been dismantled and its debris removed."[56] This was a prerequisite for the introduction, and later the understanding, of anesthesia. The new experimental knowledge stood in marked contrast to the empirical knowledge that had guided those who had, much earlier, relied on remedies without ever understanding the basis for their action.

Though in some respects the results of this work lay fallow until taken up toward the end of the eighteenth century by Joseph Priestley and Thomas Beddoes, they do link knowledge in the middle of the seventeenth century, through that in the eighteenth century, to the advent of anesthesia in the nineteenth. As Bergman observed, "It was during the course of investigating gases that the first steps were taken which would ultimately lead to the introduction of anesthesia into clinical practice."[57]

The Eighteenth Century: Pneumatic Medicine and Chemistry

Understanding of respiration was further enhanced by the discovery of a number of gases in the eighteenth century. That work too was central to ideas that were eventually basic to anesthesia,[58] for gases like carbon dioxide, nitrogen, nitrous oxide, and oxygen—all of which are basic to anesthesia—became part of the matrix from which anesthesia would later develop. Prominent among the scientists who made these discoveries were Hermann Boerhaave in the Netherlands; Stephen Hales, Henry Cavendish, Joseph Priestley, Daniel Rutherford, Thomas Beddoes, and Humphry Davy in England; Joseph Black in Scotland; Carl Wilhelm Scheele in Sweden; and Antoine Lavoisier in France. Their researches led to the discovery of oxygen, carbon dioxide, and nitrous oxide, among other gases, and to the clarification of the composition of air. The interest and excitement resulting from the discovery of these gases led some physicians later to believe that gases might be useful in medicine, and it was Beddoes who opened up the new field of pneumatic medicine. Though the value of pneumatic medicine was never validated in Beddoes' day, it was based on the inhalation of gases and vapors—a principle it shares with anesthesia.

As far as anesthesia is concerned, the work of the eighteenth century concluded with the work of Humphry Davy, Beddoes' assistant at the Pneumatic Medical Institution near Bristol. Davy is another pivotal figure in the history of anesthesia, for two reasons: he pioneered research into the physiological effects of nitrous oxide, including its effects on respiration and nitrous oxide; and in his *Researches . . . Concerning Nitrous Oxide . . .* , which was published in 1800, he suggested that nitrous oxide "may probably be used with advantage during surgical operations."[59] However, his suggestion was not acted on, by Davy himself or by anyone else. Yet it does extend the bridge from the link between the research on the physiology of respiration in the mid-seventeenth century through investigations into the chemistry of gases to Wells' use of the gas *as an anesthetic* two centuries later. Davy's suggestion on nitrous oxide is considered further in chapter 2, but here, other work on gases is first considered.

Carbon Dioxide: Hales, Boerhaave, and Black

Hales' work on blood pressure and on air indirectly connects it with the history of anesthesia. While at Cambridge, Hales was influenced by lectures on chemistry and by demonstrations of experiments based on the work of Boyle and Hooke. Natural science intrigued him, and he described his investigations in *Statical Essays* in 1733.[60] His experiments influenced later scientists. Hales estimated the blood pressure of animals from the height of a liquid in a tube in the carotid artery, though in the context of the history of anesthesia, his work on the analysis of air is more significant. He also liberated air from various substances by heat and fermentation, and he confirmed the belief that air was absorbed during respiration and combustion. Air that was contained within certain substances was "fixed," but when it was released, it regained the property of elasticity that characterized airs in general. His conclusions on air as a binding principle[61] and on the alveolar-capillary membrane as the site of absorption of air during breathing[62] were significant aspects of eighteenth-century physiology. And his apparatus, including the pneumatic trough,[63] is representative of the technology of that era and its importance to scientific investigation at the time.

Boerhaave also forged a link between the seventeenth and eighteenth centuries. A graduate in medicine and then professor at Leiden University in 1693, he pointed out the difference between "fixed air" and air that was only dissolved.[64]

The nature of fixed air, or carbon dioxide, was better understood after Black carried out his studies of chemistry in Edinburgh. Carbon dioxide may have been known in the seventeenth century to Jean Baptiste van Helmont, who wrote of a gas formed by the fermentation of wine, though to him, this *gas sylvestre* was identical to that formed by the burning of charcoal.[65] Black, in contrast, actually identified carbon dioxide by chemical investigation. A physician, Black wrote a thesis on calcium and magnesium, which was extended in his formal text of 1756.[66] Heating limestone (calcium carbonate) and also magnesia alba (magnesium carbonate) liberated fixed air; effervescence was apparent. When Black placed limewater (a solution of slaked lime [Ca $(OH)_2$]) in a vacuum, it also effervesced and generated additional air when treated with acid. Black created the first successful model of quantitative chemical investigation, which was as important in chemistry as Newton's work was in physics.[67]

Hydrogen and Nitrogen: Cavendish and Rutherford

The next gas to be discovered was hydrogen, which was described in 1766 by Cavendish.[68] An aristocrat who, like Boyle, preferred a life in science rather than in society, Cavendish initiated the systematic study of gases.[69] He discovered nitrogen in 1772. Rutherford reported this in the MD thesis that he presented in Edinburgh.[70] Son of one of Boerhaave's students and uncle of Sir Walter Scott, Rutherford studied under William Cullen and Joseph Black. After Black suggested that fixed air be studied further, Rutherford analyzed the air in which animals were confined. As the animals breathed this air, the volume of the air in the chamber diminished; and eventually, the remaining air could not support their life. Furthermore, after the carbon dioxide had been absorbed from this "residual air" with caustic alkali, the air still remaining was still incapable of supporting life. The air was thus additional to plain air and fixed air. This was the first account of nitrogen. Priestley called it "phlogisticated air"; Scheele, "vitiated air"; and French chemists, "azote."

Nitrous Oxide and Oxygen: Priestley's Discoveries

Two gases of the closest relevance to anesthesia—nitrous oxide and oxygen—were discovered toward the end of the eighteenth century by Joseph Priestley (fig. 1.6). A polymath, a clergyman with dissenting views, a teacher, and a natural scientist, Priestley was another key figure in the history of anesthesia. He discovered at least eight gases besides nitrous oxide and oxygen. He also suggested that "in time, very great medicinal use will be made of the application of these different kinds of air to the animal system."[71]

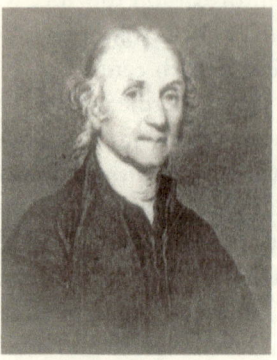

Fig. 1.6. Joseph Priestley (1733-1804)
Joseph Priestley, who was born in Fieldhead near Leeds in Yorkshire, was educated in theology and classical languages. A minister in a dissenting sect, he became interested in education and was initially a teacher. One of the subjects he taught was natural science. Encouraged by Benjamin Franklin, Priestley did experiments on electricity and wrote a standard book on the subject. In Leeds, where he continued to minister to dissenters, Priestley attended lectures on chemistry by Matthew Turner and experimented on various types of airs. Among the many gases Priestley investigated were hydrogen, nitrous oxide (which he discovered), and carbon dioxide (which was readily available in a neighboring brewery). He was also interested in hydrochloric acid. With Carl Scheele, Priestley is regarded as the co-discoverer of oxygen. Though he was an inspired chemist, Priestley was also politically active, and his activist tendencies led to his immigrating to the United States in 1794. The problem that Priestley had for some people was that he sympathized with the French revolutionaries. His chapel was burned down, and his house was ransacked. Priestley spent the last ten years of his life in Northumberland, Pennsylvania.

A fellow teacher of Priestley's was Matthew Turner, who, in 1743, suggested that sniffing "a little of the aether up the nostrils" was good for headache.[72] He also prepared ether commercially. Priestley's interest in chemistry grew as he read the principal books on chemistry, especially those of Hales and Black. He began working on gases in 1767, when the only "airs" that were known to chemists were atmospheric air, fixed air (carbon dioxide), and inflammable air (hydrogen).

Priestley described nitrous oxide in 1772,[73] when he exposed nitrous air to iron. This new gas supported combustion, but not life. He evidently conducted no experiments to determine its effects on animals other than observing that "they die the moment they are put into it."[74]

It is uncertain when Priestley discovered oxygen, and priority for the discovery of oxygen is debated. Priestley may have discovered it in 1771, when he heated potassium nitrate.[75] He noted then that a candle burned readily in the gas he obtained.[76] In August 1774, using a burning lens, he liberated a gas of uncertain nature by heating mercuric oxide.[77] He suspected that the mercuric oxide might have been impure, and in Paris, where he met the great French chemist Antoine Lavoisier, he obtained some mercuric oxide that was certainly pure. After further experiments, he read a paper on his work before the Royal Society on March 15, 1775, which is when Priestley publicly announced his discovery of oxygen,[78] though he did not name it as such.

Scheele too is credited with the discovery of oxygen, in 1771, but he did not publish his account, in German, until 1777.[79] Lavoisier's work on *le principe oxygene* must also be considered because his careful research and interpretive powers led him to name the gas that Priestley had termed "dephlogisticated air" as the "oxygen principle," or oxygen.[80] Lavoisier's ideas on respiration were correct,[81] and his *Traité' élémentaire de chemie*,[82] published in 1789, put the study of chemistry on a sound footing. Since Lavoisier's ideas inspired Beddoes and Davy, among many others, he is one more link in that chain of figures who contributed to the early history of anesthesia.

The Use of Gases in Medicine: Beddoes

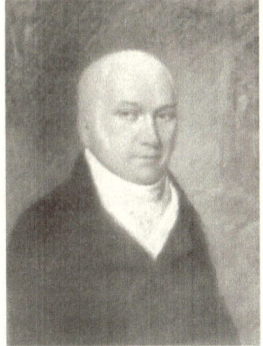

Fig. 1.7. Thomas Beddoes (1754-1808)
Thomas Beddoes, who was born in Shifnal in Shropshire in England, obtained his MD degree at Oxford in 1786. Besides being a noted lecturer in chemistry, Beddoes was a medical author, a poet, a translator, and editor—and an excellent cardplayer. His natural superiority made him intolerant of lesser mortals but friendly with men of diverse talents such as the poet Samuel Taylor Coleridge, the engineer and inventor James Watt, and the physician Erasmus Darwin; he also knew Antoine Lavoisier well. Like Joseph Priestley, Beddoes sympathized with the aims of the French Revolution and was listed as one of a number of 'disaffected and seditious persons, and was forced to leave Oxford University in 1792. He set up practice in Bristol, a city that was known for its "salubrious" health effects. At that time, partly because of Lavoisier's work on oxygen, there was a good deal of interest in "pneumatic medicine, " and Beddoes decided to open a Pneumatic Institution near the Hotwells spa in Clifton near Bristol. He opened it in 1798 and recruited Humphry Davy to be its medical superintendent. The institution enjoyed some success in the early years, but pneumatic cures did not become evident to any significant extent, and Beddoes gave up control in 1807, the year before his death.

Thomas Beddoes (fig. 1.7) also has a unique place in the history of anesthesia. In Bergman's opinion, Beddoes is in "the first rank of those individuals who set the stage for the introduction of clinical anesthesia."[83] Beddoes was convinced that gases might have a therapeutic use, and William Brownrigg, David MacBride, Thomas Henry, Thomas Percival, William Withering, Edmund Goodwyn, and Richard Pearson agreed with him. Brownrigg believed that the value of mineral waters in spas was derived from the volatile part, including carbon dioxide.[84] MacBride held that this "fixed air" prevented putrefaction.[85] And Pearson recommended ether vapor for patients with phthisis,[86] the "hectic heat" being relieved and the dyspnea often diminished.

Beddoes was the most enthusiastic and most optimistic of the pneumatic physicians. In 1798, he opened the Pneumatic Medical Institution near Bristol in England. He influenced medicine directly and, indirectly, anesthesia. He has been described as a man of science and a medical pioneer who worked at the critical time when chemistry was building its truths on unshakable experimental and mathematical foundations.[87] Thought to be "one of the most remarkable of medical men," he was the leader of the school of pneumatic physicians, the father of preventive medicine, and the discoverer of Humphry Davy and responsible for Davy's first publications.[88] Beddoes' "discovery" of Davy is certainly notable, as are his emphasis on the respiratory tract for the administration of medications and his assessment of the effects of oxygen and nitrogen.

Two years of Beddoes' work, however, failed to provide any evidence of definite and indisputable cures of diseases like consumption. Yet in the long term, even its failure served a purpose. Thus Joseph Cottle: "By its failure, it established the useful negative fact (however mortifying) that medical science was not to be improved through the medium of factitious airs."[89]

Cottle's statement suggests that the time was still not ripe for the advent of anesthesia. Yet two developments at Beddoes' establishment illustrate how people's minds were being prepared for the concept of anesthesia. One was Beddoes' investigations into the application of medication via the respiratory tract. Though, for example, the treatment of a patient with inflammation of the chest with one-eighth of an atmosphere of hydrogen may not seem today to be impressive, Beddoes did open up a new field to scientific inquiry. His simple statement about this form of therapy was impressive too: "The acute pain entirely subsided while the patient was breathing this mixture, and the febrile symptoms disappeared."[90] Beddoes also exposed his own blistered finger to carbon dioxide, whereupon he found that "the pain in two minutes quite subsided, and returned when . . . exposed . . . to the atmosphere."[91] Beddoes' work contributed to "the first foreshadowing of the idea that it might be possible to obliterate pain by means of a gas."[92] It represents one more way in which the concept of anesthesia was being developed.

The other important development at the Pneumatic Medical Institution was Beddoes' hiring Davy as medical superintendent. It is Davy's work on nitrous oxide that closes the chapter on the beginnings of anesthesia and opens the new one in which a number of factors, including new ideas on pain, combined to introduce anesthesia as a means of relieving surgical pain.

Chapter 2

THE INTRODUCTION OF ANESTHESIA
THE GERMINAL PERIOD, 1800-1846

In 1800, Humphry Davy suggested that nitrous oxide might be "be used with advantage during surgical operations in which no great effusion of blood takes place."[1] This suggestion is intriguing, but what precisely did he mean? Having found that the gas relieved toothache[2] and headache,[3] did he think it might be useful in minor surgery? If he did, why did he not follow up his own suggestion? Why did no one else, particularly a surgeon? And why was it not until 1844 that Horace Wells, a Hartford dentist, should be the first to use nitrous oxide as an anesthetic?[4]

Those questions, and others to be discussed, suggest that the early nineteenth century is of interest partly because of what did *not* happen. As anesthetics, both ether and nitrous oxide were not used until the 1840s. Yet as noted in chapter 1, the hypnotic property of ether had long been known.[5] So were its medical indications. Just before Davy made his suggestion, Richard Pearson recommended ether for the treatment of various respiratory ailments.[6] And similarly, Thomas Beddoes, with whom Davy worked in 1800, built his Pneumatic Medical Institution specifically to treat chest diseases with gases and vapors.[7] Like nitrous oxide, ether was known to affect the nervous system, producing euphoric effects in recreational inhalation,[8, 9] yet no one went so far as to recommend ether or nitrous oxide to relieve the pain of surgery.

That recommendation was not made even in 1842, when two events would have warranted it. In January of that year, student William Clarke, in Rochester, New York, gave ether to a young woman for a tooth extraction.[10] On March

30, physician Crawford Long, in Jefferson, Georgia, used ether for anesthesia in a young man with a neck tumor.[11] However, Clarke never wrote about ether, and Long didn't do so until 1849. With the exception of the abortive attempt of Henry Hickman, an English physician, to use carbon dioxide in 1824,[12] a historical vacuum persisted.

Even after 1842, anesthesia was not formally introduced in surgery for another four years. Then on October 16, 1846, William Thomas Green Morton, a dentist, showed *convincingly and publicly* that ether was a potent anesthetic.[13] That raises more questions. One: why was ether introduced only in steps in the 1840s? Two: why is it that the introduction of anesthesia is associated primarily with the use of ether (and Morton rather than Long) as opposed to nitrous oxide (Davy and then Wells), or even carbon dioxide (Hickman)? And three: why were the two most prominent individuals in the story of the introduction of anesthesia, in terms of publicity, two *American dentists*—Wells and Morton—rather than either *British chemists*, who had done so much of the original work on gases, or *surgeons*, who daily had to accept the fact that their patients were hurting?

The last point gives Hickman's experiments with carbon dioxide great significance. It was precisely because Hickman was concerned about the suffering endured by his fellow human beings, and because he explicitly said so,[14] that he tried the effects of carbon dioxide in small animals. He wished to know if this would enable him to perform minor operations, *painlessly*. In fact, *Hickman was able to do exactly that*. In this pre-anesthesia period, Hickman was unique in both *conceiving* the idea of what was later termed "anesthesia" and *carrying* it out. He went farther than Davy: he stated that he was concerned about relieving the "excruciating" pain that surgical patients suffered. Whether Hickman had other motives is unknown, and the actual impact of his experiments on the eventual advent of clinical anesthesia is not apparent. Like the initiative of Long, they did not, in fact, bring it about.

Three more questions must be asked. One is why was anesthesia introduced in the *1840s* but not before? A second relates to the actual *first use of inhalational substances*: can we say that Hickman or Clarke or Wells, besides Morton, was the very first? And third, perhaps of lesser interest, how was the news of ether spread beyond Boston?

All these questions and the context of their setting, together with accounts of the work of the *dramatis personae*, are discussed in this chapter.

1800: Davy's Suggestion of Nitrous Oxide for Surgery

Assessing the value of various gases for medical therapy was one of the tasks Humphry Davy (fig. 2.1) carried out when he worked at the Pneumatic Medical

Institution. One of those gases was nitrous oxide, which he wrote about in his classic monograph of 1800[15] (fig. 2.2). Of all the gases he and others in the eighteenth century studied, nitrous oxide is the one that is most obviously a part of the history of anesthesia, and Davy's ideas in relation to anesthesia demand elucidation.

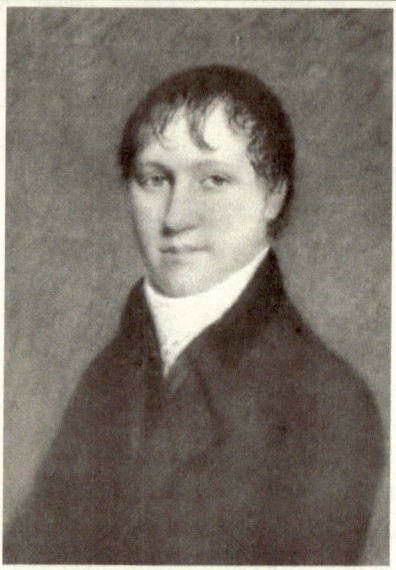

Fig. 2.1. Humphry Davy (1778-1829)
Humphry Davy was born in Penzance, England. Although he was interested in poetry, literature, philosophy, and religion, he became appreciated to a local surgeon-apothecary. His early interest in science intrigued Thomas Beddoes, who was looking for a medical superintendent who would assist him in the study of "factitious airs" at his new Pneumatic Medical Institution near Bristol. Davy accepted Beddoes's offer of a job and, thinking it might help him in medicine, accepted. He joined Beddoes in October 1898. Nitrous oxide was one of the "airs" that he and Beddoes studied with a view to its therapeutic use, and his study led to his publishing his *Researches* . . . in 1800. Davy suggested that because it was analgesic, nitrous oxide might be used during surgical operations "in which no great effusion of blood takes place." In 1801, Davy joined the staff of the Royal Institution and did not study the gas further. He is more widely known for the miners' safety lamp, electrolysis, and the isolation of some of the earth elements. His researches were of value in several different fields, including mining, agriculture, and tanning. Davy was a brilliant lecturer, and he was one of the first to join brilliant scientific work with education of the public. Davy was knighted in 1812 and became president of the Royal Society in 1820.

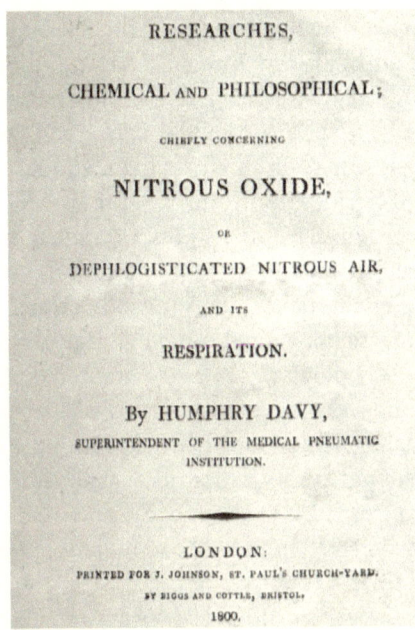

RESEARCHES,

CHEMICAL AND PHILOSOPHICAL;

CHIEFLY CONCERNING

NITROUS OXIDE,

OR

DEPHLOGISTICATED NITROUS AIR,

AND ITS

RESPIRATION.

By HUMPHRY DAVY,
SUPERINTENDENT OF THE MEDICAL PNEUMATIC
INSTITUTION.

LONDON:
PRINTED FOR J. JOHNSON, ST. PAUL'S CHURCH-YARD.
BY BIGGS AND COTTLE, BRISTOL.
1800.

Fig. 2.2. Title page of Davy's *Researches; Chemical and Philosophical, Chiefly Concerning Nitrous Oxide* . . . (1800). (Mayo History of Medicine Library Collection.)

It is essential to understand Davy's thinking on pain relief and surgery. Despite his being aware of the analgesic property of nitrous oxide vis-à-vis toothache and headache, there is, however, no evidence that he thought about pain relief in surgery beyond suggesting the possible use of nitrous oxide, "with advantage," in surgical operations. That intriguing statement is the only one in his writings that indicates any such an interest. Nor is there any evidence that Davy ever expressed the revulsion for the pain of an operation that Hickman did—the feeling that led Hickman actually to try using a gas to abolish that pain. As Norman Bergman said of Davy, "The thought of patient comfort probably never crossed his mind at any stage of his life."[16]

Nor did anyone else at this time formulate the concept that nitrous oxide might relieve the pain of an operation.[17] Rather, people thought in terms of standard anodynes such as opium and alcohol. They did not think of *substances that might induce anesthesia*, because that was an alien concept. Davy, then, thought of nitrous oxide as an anodyne; and his suggestion was just that: a *suggestion*. It was *not*, as Hickman's was, a *concept of anesthesia* that led to action, albeit in animals.

This lack of vision might be surprising. Davy lived when the Enlightenment bred the hope that suffering might be lessened; and society does seem to have been more sensitive to human ills than earlier. By 1840, society manifested a greater sensitivity to pain.[18] Historian Derek Beales, for example, wrote of the greater concern for "helpless living things: animals, children, prisoners, emigrants and slaves." In 1802, an English statute protected children working in cotton factories. In 1803, one safeguarded emigrants; and in 1807, one abolished the slave trade where the United Kingdom was concerned.[19] Davy himself was a sensitive person, as were others of his circle, like Beddoes and the essayists and poets Samuel Taylor Coleridge and Robert Southey. The philosophical Davy might have been a poet himself if he had not become a chemist.[20] He and his friends were men of sensitivity and did not ignore suffering.

As far as abolishing the pain of surgical operations is concerned, Davy believed that medicine was not yet concerned with finding a definite means of pain relief in surgery. Physiology was not yet "interested in teaching the means of procuring pleasure and relieving pain."[21] Moreover, like others, Davy held that pain was valuable, signaling a return of vitality to previously "exhausted" organs.[22] Excessive action of the gas could be harmful. As historian Stephanie Snow suggests, Davy was concerned also about the suspension of sensibility, which he saw as a potentially lethal form of suffocation, and therefore physiologically unsupportable.[23] The time was not yet ripe.

What, then, explains Davy's intriguing suggestion about nitrous oxide?

Davy was influenced by the ideas of Scottish physician John Brown. Health was a balance between *sthenia* (a state of overstimulation) and *asthenia* (a state in which the body was unable to respond to stimulation).[24] Bergman summarized Davy's belief in this way: the stimulus of pain led to a sthenic state; hemorrhage would counteract this and tend to cause asthenia. If nitrous oxide was breathed, excitability might be produced, but asthenia might be aggravated as the excitability wore off; and if hemorrhage occurred during surgery, then oxygen would be lost; and then the insensibility caused by nitrous oxide might threaten a patient's life.[25] Or, knowing that nitrous oxide could relieve the pain of toothache, Davy may have thought that nitrous oxide might be useful just in minor surgery. Davy did not go any farther.

Though Davy did no further work on the therapeutic aspects of nitrous oxide after he left the Pneumatic Medical Institution in 1801, by 1828, he had consolidated his view about nitrous oxide somewhat: he concluded that nitrous oxide couldn't support human life. Thus it has been inferred that he thought that the gas should not be used to induce sensibility.[26]

1800-1842: The Non-use of Nitrous Oxide and Ether

Though ether and nitrous oxide (the latter known as "laughing gas") were used by the public for recreational purposes, physicians and chemists advised against their use in more serious settings. They thought them toxic and possibly dangerous. Samuel Latham Mitchill, an American, thought that the toxic nitrous oxide caused plague and contagion.[27] Englishman Michael Faraday in 1818 reported that ether had induced a "very lethargic state" for thirty hours in one man, who was feared might die; he advised "caution" in any experiments.[28]

Surgeons also had negative views. Benjamin Brodie, the London surgeon who was interested in toxicology, found that some of the guinea pigs who were placed in jars together with ether did not survive, and he attributed death to the ether[29] rather than to suffocation. That is, ether seemed to be a narcotic poison.[30] Others found the coma-like state of ether insensibility distasteful since it might compromise one's being. Scottish surgeon John Bell asked, "Who would lose, for fear of pain, this intellectual being?"[31] This implies the acceptance of the inevitability of the pain of operations and the fear of the loss of consciousness.[32] To deliberately endanger a patient's life by inducing "coma" could be thought reckless. There were other ways to abolish pain: by giving opium or laudanum or alcohol; by bleeding a patient to the point of syncope; by compressing a main nerve, or even the carotid artery; by refrigerating a limb; by hypnotizing a patient; and by performing acupuncture. The trouble was that none was invariably efficacious or reliable. In total contrast, some surgeons believed that pain was actually essential to healing.[33] Others, such as Louis Velpeau, argued that "to obviate pain in operations is a chimera which it is to-day no longer permissible to seek after."[34] Many people held that pain was part of God's plan.

In short, early in the nineteenth century, the moral climate was not compatible with the idea of inducing unconsciousness for surgical purposes. Patients needing surgery just had to withstand the pain, perhaps with the aid of established anodynes. Some were able to do so, often in an astonishing manner; others just collapsed; and others simply succumbed. Three representative accounts follow:

- A woman had surgery for a tumor of the jaw. The surgeon used a chisel and a mallet. It was said that the courage she displayed was "almost incredible." After the operation, she "fell into a slight swoon," but speedily recovered and left the hospital, apparently in "perfect health."
- A second woman had cancer of the uterus. After half an hour, by which time the surgeon had made little progress, the patient lost her "fortitude." Enfeebled by loss of blood and "irritated" by the dissection and by the agony, she made an expulsive movement that caused the intestines to protrude from the vagina. After this operation, she took "small doses of wine, ether, and tincture of opium." Three hours later, she was "better."
- A man required a lithotomy, but this was "unduly prolonged" because the stone kept slipping from the forceps. Several surgeons "tired themselves" in attempting to extract the stone. A physician watching the procedure "urged that the prayer of the patient for release should be listened to . . . but the operator . . . would neither abandon the altar nor the victim . . . . The patient, at length, could only utter feeble groans, and his life was ebbing fast when, after two hours of horrible torments, he was unbound and put to bed, where he expired in an hour.'[35]

1824: Henry Hill Hickman's Research on Carbon Dioxide

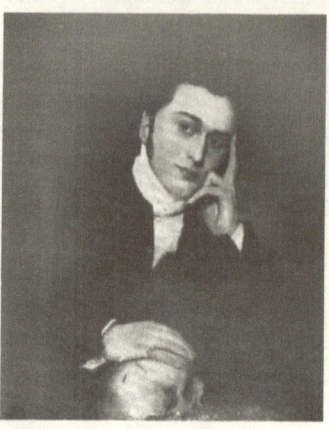

Fig. 2.3. Henry Hill Hickman (1800-1830)

Henry Hickman was born in Bromfield, near Ludlow in England. He studied in Edinburgh, became a member of the Royal College of Surgeons of England in 1820, and began his medical practice in 1821 in Ludlow. Recent knowledge of gases—their potential as therapeutic agents, and their absorption from the lungs into the blood—formed the background for Hickman's idea that inhaled gases might induce a pain-free state for surgery. He tested his idea beginning in 1823, when he gave some small animals carbon dioxide to breathe and denied others access to atmospheric air. He performed minor operations on them without inflicting pain. He termed this state of anesthesia "suspended animation, " which perhaps had negative connotations. His work failed to generate any interest among members of the Royal Society (in 1824) and the French Royal Academy of Medicine (in 1828). Yet Hickman advanced well beyond Humphry Davy on the track of a method whereby patients' "fears may be tranquillised and suffering relieved, " believing that the human body might be "rendered insensible by means insensible by means of the introduction of certain gases into the lungs." Surely, Hickman stood on the cusp of the concepts and the method on induction of anesthesia, but he was ahead of his time. Only much later was the basis of Hickman's idea proved sound.

While Hickman (fig. 2.3) was not alone in being distressed by the thought of operations in the preanesthetic era, he was unique in acting on his feelings. He studied medicine in Edinburgh in 1819 and 1820, so he was probably familiar with the recreational aspects of nitrous oxide and ether, the opinions of Davy and Faraday, and probably the earlier work of Beddoes and Priestley. Hickman also worked in Shifnal in Shropshire, England, where Beddoes was born, which may have stimulated Hickman to think about the medicinal uses of gases. Beddoes knew that nitrous oxide could cause "perfect intoxication without subsequent debility"[36] and that hydrocarbonate had been used for "throwing the patient into syncope" so that a strangulated hernia could be reduced.[37] Beddoes also knew that carbon dioxide had analgesic properties[38]—and it was carbon dioxide that Hickman used in his animal experiments beginning on March 20, 1823.[39] And Hickman conducted his study in the same year that J. J. Berzelius, a Swedish contemporary, wrote about the use of gases. In 1824, when Hickman wrote to T. A. Knight about his own experiments on what he termed "suspended animation"[40] (fig. 2.4), Berzelius reported that hydrogen, administered to men or animals, "throws them into a profound sleep."[41] Thus, it is reasonable to argue that Hickman's vision was formed by positive ideas, in contrast to the negative ideas of Davy and Faraday, and of surgeons Bell, Brodie, and Velpeau. Hickman even discounted the proviso in Davy's suggestion concerning cases when hemorrhage was likely, for, he suggested, in contrast, his method was "particularly advisable in Cases where haemorrhage would be dangerous."[42]

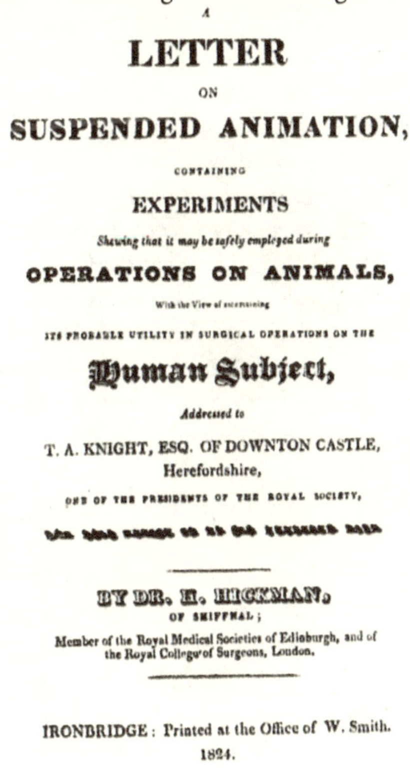

A

LETTER

ON

SUSPENDED ANIMATION,

CONTAINING

EXPERIMENTS

Shewing that it may be safely employed during

OPERATIONS ON ANIMALS,

With the View of ascertaining

ITS PROBABLE UTILITY IN SURGICAL OPERATIONS ON THE

𝕳𝖚𝖒𝖆𝖓 𝕾𝖚𝖇𝖏𝖊𝖈𝖙,

Addressed to

T. A. KNIGHT, ESQ. OF DOWNTON CASTLE,
Herefordshire,

ONE OF THE PRESIDENTS OF THE ROYAL SOCIETY,

███ ████ █████ ██ ██ ██ ████████ ████

BY DR. H. HICKMAN,
OF SHIFFNAL;

Member of the Royal Medical Societies of Edinburgh, and of
the Royal College of Surgeons, London.

IRONBRIDGE : Printed at the Office of W. Smith.
1824.

Fig. 2.4. Cover page of Hickman's letter to T. A. Knight, 1824. (Source: Souvenir Henry Hill Hickman Centenary Exhibition 1830-1930 [London: Wellcome Foundation, 1930].)

Hickman was a true pioneer. His vision took him beyond the belief that pain was essential to healing and that deliberately inducing unconsciousness was reckless. He did not think that pain and suffering were positive qualities but took the opposite view. As he told Knight in 1824, he would "shudder at the idea of an operation . . . knowing the great pain that must be endured."[43]

Hickman was a pioneer in acting on his vision. He thought that it was "rather singular that no experiments have hitherto been made with the object of ascertaining whether operations could successfully performed upon animals whilst in a torpid state." So he anesthetized small animals with carbon dioxide to see whether he could perform minor operations on them without inflicting observable pain. This affirmed his vision; he suggested that "animation in the human subject could be safely suspended by proper means, carefully employed." A patient's mind, Hickman believed, should be relieved of "the anticipation of suffering" and the body from "the actual suffering" imposed by the surgeon's knife. Stephanie Snow concluded that Hickman, in contrast to Davy, could support a separation between the functions of the mind and the body.[44]

In the history of anesthesia—in that period when no one else had conceived the idea of anesthesia—Hickman stands alone. Unlike anyone else, he believed in the validity of the *principle* of inducing unconsciousness so that painless surgery could be performed. However, his work was ignored: partly because he was ahead of his time, partly because his term *suspended animation* had negative connotations,[45] and partly because negative views about vivisection were becoming more evident.[46] His work was even scorned.[47] Even Hickman's appeal to Charles X of France had no effect.[48] Though Hickman's initiative was, in a sense, an anomaly, he was unable to carry out further work because he died in 1830. Like John Snow later, Hickman died prematurely; and as with Snow, the work of an original thinker was unfinished. After Hickman, no research was done on substances that might induce anesthesia until the fact of clinical anesthesia was demonstrated.

The 1840s: Why Was Anesthesia Introduced Then?

Hickman also provides a link between Davy and Wells and the years 1800 and 1844. In that interval, human thinking and feeling in society, with Hickman in the van, seems to have reached the point when the idea of anesthesia could be accepted. The greater sense of humanity in this era was one factor in this process of evolution, while the development of new social and cultural attitudes was another. Other factors include advances in science and technology and nuances in the personal and psychological beliefs of some individuals—of which Hickman's beliefs are an example. Still, why so many years elapsed in the nineteenth century before anesthesia was finally introduced, and why it was introduced in the 1840s and not earlier, has some of the elements of what anesthesiologist Emanuel Papper called a "historical puzzle."[49]

There are several facets of this puzzle in addition to Papper's own conclusion that sensitivity to pain and the romantic movement in the arts were linked.

One facet comprises new beliefs about pain and the relief of pain. Jeremy Bentham thought that pain was "inherently evil"[50] and not God-given, the

Devil's work; and John Stuart Mill, that pain resulted from the cruelty of Nature, and that the Word of God had no part in this.[51] The concept that each of us is responsible for the welfare of others was, in Nicholas Greene's view, the first prerequisite for the discovery of anesthesia,[52] though it did not come overnight. The development was that of a new social conscience, not just an attitude.

Donald Caton had another perspective.[53] He pointed out that until comparatively recently, pain had a religious connotation: as the will of God or, alternatively, as a form of punishment. It just had to be accepted. This view began to change once the ideas of the Enlightenment led society, as philosopher René Descartes put it, to "improve health, lengthen life, and banish the terrors of old age."[54] Pain had a biological rather than a religious or philosophical quality; that which could be managed with drugs. Pain was secularized. The utilitarian philosophy of Bentham and Mill furthered the idea that it could be treated.

Ray Fink suggested another line of reasoning.[55] In the 1820s and 1830s, there were spectacular advances in science and technology, chemistry, geology, engineering, physics, and astronomy, as well as medicine. Combined with the social reforms of the 1830s, they instilled confidence in a brighter and progressive future. They broadened people's mental horizons and generated new concepts. That explains the wider use of ether, nitrous oxide, and carbon dioxide in medicine, especially in the treatment of conditions like asthma and consumption.[56] Hickman had used carbon dioxide, a known analgesic, to obtund sensibility in his animal experiments in 1824[57] and Wright, in 1825, used it to treat middle-ear pain.[58] Nitrous oxide was used for asthma in 1829,[59] for cholera in 1832,[60] and for hydrophobia in 1834.[61] But still, no one in the 1830s seems to have conceived the idea of using either nitrous oxide or ether for anesthesia. No one followed up on the ideas of Davy and Hickman; no one applied the idea of the medicinal use of ether and nitrous oxide to pain relief during surgical operations.

As anesthesiologist Ralph Waters observed, there is always a delay between conception of an idea and its application, and then between that application and its incorporation into clinical practice.[62] The delay in using nitrous oxide as an anesthetic is a good example of this. Even if a medical scientist had taken up Davy's suggestion about nitrous oxide soon after 1800, physicians might have been slow to respond to such a medical advance, despite its possibility of surgically useful insensibility. Hickman was ignored in England and in France, but he alone envisioned the possibility of anesthesia. All this suggests that before the 1840s, the time was not ripe for anesthesia.

Even surgeons themselves were devoid of vision concerning insensibility as the solution to the problem of pain; they were unable to think beyond the concept of standard anodynes. To deliberately induce coma in order to abolish the pain associated with surgery was too far-fetched, even foolhardy. Only Hickman had thought of that. There was no concept of anesthesia, which was not named as such until it was actually witnessed and people were convinced of the phenomenon in 1846. A similar state of affairs existed with respect to the phenomenon of energy, which was formulated in the third great law of nature presented in the 1840s.[63]

The word *force* had to be used instead to connote the concept of the variety, interconvertibility, and equivalence of the energies of Nature. All this took time. So it was with anesthesia. Until 1846, various terms were used. Davy spoke of "the destruction of pain"; Hickman, of "suspended animation"; Long, in failing to report the phenomenon in 1842, seems not to have been aware of its significance; Wells referred to the "influence of gas"; and Morton, to "ether sleep."

The time, then, had to be right for the introduction of anesthesia. Hickman, Clarke, Long, Wells, and Morton found themselves on the cusp of the movement that sanctioned the use of ether and nitrous oxide to induce anesthesia. Wells and Morton, in particular, forged the path that led from that cusp. The contributions of those two individuals, in particular, need to be looked at more closely.

The Key Roles of Wells and Morton

Why was it that, at last, it should have been two American dentists (Wells in 1844 and Morton in 1846)—rather than surgeons, or even chemists in England—who introduced *clinical* anesthesia in the 1840s? The answer lies in the difference between the practices of surgeons and dentists.

Surgeons operated primarily because emergencies endangered life; they, and their patients (if they plucked up enough courage to consult a surgeon), knew that an operation (if successful—and if a patient did not die!) would relieve their pain. Patients went to surgeons precisely because the pain of an acquired life-threatening condition called for surgery. Legs continued to be broken and had to be cleansed and straightened, and cancer of the breast or a strangulated hernia continued to mandate surgical treatment. Surgeons knew that pain would not keep their patients away for long; and that, as a result, they would not lose income. But surgeons were by no means indifferent to pain. Robert Liston, for example, the first London surgeon to operate on a patient under ether, argued that "The infliction of unnecessary pain through want of adroitness . . . and consequent protraction of the operative procedure—cannot be defended."[64] So most welcomed the advent of anesthesia on the grounds that pain now could, and indeed should, be abolished.

Dentistry was practiced in the context of a different set of patient responses. Patients saw dentists in order to have teeth removed or dental plates fitted, and while that was painful, it was not lifesaving. So patients often stayed away from dentists, preferring to suffer in their own homes rather than endure the pain of dental work. So dentists lost income when fear of pain trumped reason's call for treatment. They had a special need to find a potent analgesic.

For dentists Horace Wells (fig. 2.5), of Hartford, Connecticut, and William Morton (fig. 2.6), of Boston, who did a good deal of bread-and-butter prosthetic work, those factors were important. Fear of dental pain, especially, limited their practice. But they also knew that America was a good place for dentists. The population was growing, and the nation valued knowledge and inventions that were practical and useful. In the 1820s and 1830s, many useful inventions made life easier. While advances in science and technology continued to flow from Europe, devices such as the electromagnet, the electric telegraph, the transformer, the reaping machine, and the sewing machine demonstrated American inventiveness. Other "Yankee dodges" included the vulcanization of rubber and the manufacture of the collapsible metal tube. As historian Samuel Morison remarked, "The tide of invention had risen higher in the United States than in the Old World."[65] He observed that the Americans' "pleasure came from doing."[66] Fink concluded that "the discovery itself came in the new world and not in the old because that is where the incentives and the "can do" spirit of the age most insistently beckoned on the horizon."[67]

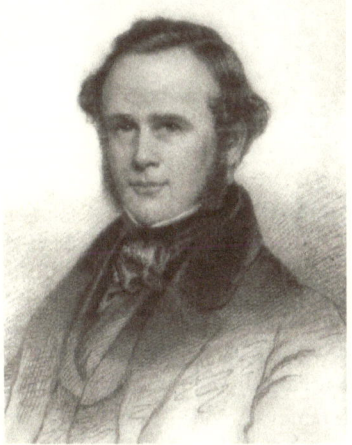

Fig. 2.5. Horace Wells (1815-1848)

Horace Wells was born in Hartford, Connecticut. In 1834, he was apprenticed to some Boston dentists so he could learn dentistry, and set up practice in 1836 in Hartford. His inventive genius and mechanical talent gave him a reputation beyond the extraction of teeth. Wells taught dentistry to William Morton, and in 1842 and 1843, they shared a practice and endeavored to construct gold plates. The partnership was dissolved in 1844. On December 10 that year, Wells watched itinerant lecturer Gardner Quincy Colton demonstrate nitrous oxide, which changed Wells' life; it also brought the concept of anesthesia closer to realization. The next day, Colton administered nitrous oxide to Wells, who had a wisdom tooth removed by fellow dentist John Riggs. Wells thereupon exclaimed, "A new era in tooth-pulling!" Wells then gave the gas to some fifteen patients in his own practice. By mid-January 1845, Wells was ready to demonstrate the method, and in Boston, before Morton and a medical audience, he anesthetized a medical student for the extraction of a tooth. However, the demonstration was not wholly successful, probably because Wells gave too little nitrous oxide, even though the student said that he had suffered less pain than was to be expected. Wells admitted that for some of the audience, it was "a humbug affair." He became depressed, was jailed after he threw acid at a prostitute, and committed suicide in jail.

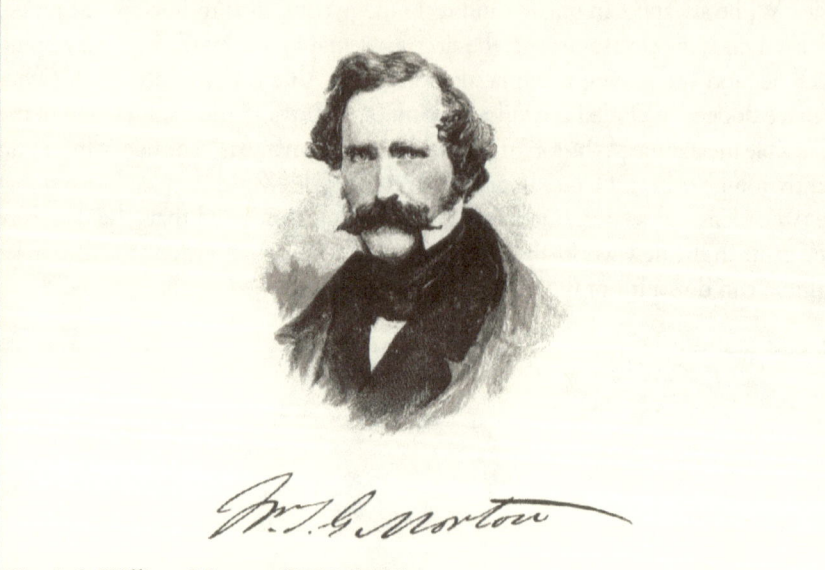

Fig. 2.6. William Morton (1819-1868)

William Thomas Green Morton was born in Charlton, Massachusetts. After failing to succeed in business, he studied dentistry in Baltimore and practiced in Farmington, Connecticut. In 1842 and 1843, Morton worked as a partner with Horace Wells, and then on his own in Boston. He also enrolled as a medical student at Harvard, though he never graduated. He believed that dental plates should not be fitted until all carious teeth had been removed, which made him search for a way to abolish or relieve pain. Nitrous oxide in Wells's hands seemed a poor choice, and ether, which he learned, from Charles Jackson and others, had analgesic properties, seemed more promising. Morton first used ether topically in liquid form, and the stupefying effect of the vapor form led him to investigate it further. After testing ether on himself, his assistants, and a dog, and endeavoring to learn more from Jackson, Morton etherized a patient on September 30, 1846, and thirty-seven others operated on by surgeon Henry Jacob Bigelow. On October 16, 1846, Morton proved to the world that ether was an anesthetic, and the new medical field of anesthesia was born. Morton tried to patent and license ether (as Letheon) and to gain recognition, and remuneration, for his perceived status as the sole discoverer of ether anesthesia. He ended his life, however, as a broken man living in poverty.

It was in this environment that Wells and Morton in New England went beyond Hickman in Old England in seeking the real-life goal of a wholly effective anodyne. Their objective was the practical one of finding a means of pain relief to enable them to carry on their daily work; it was not part of any academic research into analgesics and hypnotic substances. This is what enabled them to succeed where others had failed.

Who Discovered Anesthesia? Some Guides to a Discussion

Discoveries are seldom made by single individuals working alone, and anesthesia was "discovered" as the result of numerous steps taken by many individuals from the seventeenth century onward. As Cartwright points out, "In the last analysis, any and all of the experiments that were done with the gases and with ether were dependent upon some work that had gone before."[68] It is, therefore, fruitless to debate the question of who discovered anesthesia. It is better to ask how key events unfolded and to establish links between the events and the individuals. The nub of the discussion is this: what concepts of anesthesia did each individual have of anesthesia, and how were they applied?

Yet the human interest of the claims of the principals in the drama continues to fascinate, even though Davy, Hickman, Clarke, Long, Wells, and Morton, as well as Boston physician and chemist Charles Jackson are long gone from us. So complex is the maze of competing arguments that it is difficult to assign merit to the priority claims fairly and justifiably. The United States Congress certainly found that when they tried to evaluate the claims on several occasions; "confused Congressmen threw up their hands in despair of ever getting at the truth."[69]

Part of the problem is that the discovery of anesthesia can be interpreted in different ways. The topic of priority is full of semantic pricks and thorns. If we consider just the *idea* of what was discovered, Davy has priority, for he first stated the *idea* of nitrous oxide as a surgical anesthetic. If we discuss the *principle* of anesthesia, credit must go to Hickman, who envisioned surgery being made pain-free. But Davy did not follow up his suggestion and carried out no experimental research; and Hickman's research was on animals rather than on humans, and he did not write it up in a scientific journal. Should, then, priority be related to the *demonstration* of the principle of anesthesia in human beings? If so, does not Wells' use of nitrous oxide, initially on himself in December 1844 and then on others in January 1845, merit the crown of laurel leaves? Yet a fourth way of assessing priority is related to the ability to *convince others of the phenomenon* of anesthesia, which is what Morton certainly did.

Confusion has arisen also because the debate often concerns the first use of *ether*, rather than the use of nitrous oxide or carbon dioxide. Morton's demonstration of ether, witnessed by a sophisticated medical audience, was so dramatic that Wells' earlier use of nitrous oxide was pushed into the background, as was Hickman's of carbon dioxide. Both historically and psychologically, Morton trumped Wells and Hickman. Morton also trumped Clarke and Long; Clarke never reported his use, and Long only did so after seven years. Or Long, who used it in Jefferson, Georgia, two months later, and had witnesses but didn't report it until 1849. Clarke, a medical student, never wrote about his experience, and Long may have been concerned about other physicians' opinions of his use of ether.

The topic is almost as complex as that of angels dancing on the head of a pin. Let us, therefore, look at the dramatis personae and events more closely.

Carbon Dioxide: Hickman and Wright

In the context of Hickman's original experiments with carbon dioxide, three points may be made. First, he alone was traveling on the right road. Only he actually devised an experimental method to prevent pain during minor operations. Though he did this on animals, he ultimately was concerned about suffering in human beings. He thought of the need to "tranquilize" the fears and to relieve the suffering of surgical patients; the purpose of his experimental approach was to "to ascertain the practicability of such treatment on the human subject."[70] Hickman's vision was of nothing less than *the state that would later become known as anesthesia.*

Second, in thinking about extrapolating his animal research to clinical practice, Hickman inferred that his "salutary" results might allow him to render humans *"insensible by the introduction of certain gases into the lungs"*[71] [italics added]. It is not clear what gases Hickman was thinking of, but he worked in a period in which the studies of Beddoes and Davy were quite recent, and he may indeed have been thinking about nitrous oxide, as well as carbon dioxide. This makes Cartwright's opinion that Hickman's experiments link the parent pneumatic medicine to its descendant anesthesia[72] a logical one.

Third, the lack of any response to Hickman's research, in both England and France, confirms that the time was not ripe for the introduction of anesthesia. Physicians did not share Hickman's conception of a surgically applicable state of suspended animation.'

Aurist William Wright also used carbon dioxide in the 1820s, as well as ether, though he used neither to induce anesthesia. Working in Bristol, Wright might have known about the inhalation of gases in pneumatic medicine, though he was reluctant to take it up.[73] Wright found that blowing carbonic acid gas into the ear in chronic otitis relieved the pain, which he reported in 1829.[74] He thought carbonic acid gas relieved a number of conditions by acting as an antiseptic. He recommended ether to suppress the cough induced by instrumentation of the ear canal, which reemphasizes the fact that ether was well known as a remedy for a miscellany of conditions before it was used as an anesthetic.

Nitrous Oxide: Colton and Wells

Although no one appeared to have a medical use for nitrous oxide for years after Davy's researches, its effects on the nervous system were taught to students of medicine and chemistry.[75] Its euphoric effects made laughing gas a recreational drug and the subject of public lectures and demonstrations by self-styled chemical lecturers. One of those was Gardner Quincy Colton.[76] Once a medical student at the Columbia University College of Physicians and Surgeons in New York, he was well read on nitrous oxide. He gave up the bedside for the stage, and his familiarity with the gas gave him an air of authority when he lectured. His role, though a minor one, was, historically, a key one.

One of Colton's demonstrations was given in Hartford, Connecticut, on December 10, 1844, and it was then and there that he and the bright young local dentist Horace Wells met.[77] Wells had studied dentistry in Boston, and he too would have learned about nitrous oxide as a student, though there is no evidence that he knew about Davy's researches. A conscientious and competent dentist, he was knowledgeable enough to publish *An Essay on Teeth* . . . in 1838.[78] Wells was concerned about the pain of dentistry, and as early as 1840, according to dental student Linus P. Brockett, Wells was "deeply impressed with the idea that some discovery would yet be made by which dental and other operations might be performed without pain."[79] The idea, doubtless, remained in his mind, to be activated by Colton's demonstration.

On that December day in 1844, the practical lesson of Colton's demonstration and Wells' idea came together. Colton's advertised "entertainment" for that evening was to include "a few of the most surprising Chemical Experiments,"[80] but what occurred that evening would surprise Colton himself and amaze Wells. Wells noticed that when pharmacist's assistant Samuel Cooley danced around under the influence of the laughing gas and bumped his legs against the wooden furniture on the stage badly enough to draw blood, he *appeared to feel no pain*.[81] He felt pain only after the effects of the gas vanished.

A eureka moment followed from the recognition that pain relief was reversible. Wells asked Colton, "Why cannot a man have a tooth pulled while under the gas and not feel it?" Colton said he did not know. Wells started thinking about the possibility. He described his thinking this way:

> Reasoning by analogy, I was led to believe that surgical operations might be performed, without pain, by the fact, that an individual, when much excited from ordinary causes, may receive severe wounds without manifesting the least pain; as, for instance, the man who is engaged in combat may have a limb severed from his body . . . after which he testifies that it was attended by no pain at the time; and so the man who is intoxicated with spirituous liquor may be treated severely without his manifesting pain, and his frame, in this state, seems to be more tenacious of life than under ordinary circumstances. By these facts I was led to inquire if the same result would not follow, by the inhalation of some exhilarating gas, the effects of which would pass off immediately, leaving the system none the worse for its use.[82]

Wells later that evening asked Colton to come to his office next morning, along with a gasbag and some nitrous oxide, so that he could find out more about the gas. Wells would breathe the gas while fellow dentist John Riggs would extract a troublesome wisdom tooth from Wells himself. Thus, Wells would test his own hypothesis. Colton duly gave the nitrous oxide while Riggs extracted the molar tooth. The autoexperiment was a success. Wells dramatically said that "it is the greatest discovery ever made. I didn't feel it so much as the prick of a pin."[83] He reportedly added, "A new era in tooth-pulling."[84] Wells thus linked himself with Davy and his 44-year-old suggestion, though he went farther than Davy and also Hickman.

Convinced by autoexperimentation of the analgesia of nitrous oxide, Wells used the gas on patients over the next few weeks. By mid-January 1845, he had extracted teeth from fifteen patients under its influence,[85] and he was ready to make his discovery known by demonstrating his method of painless dental extractions in the premier medical city of Boston. However, Wells may have been too anxious then to make known the humanitarian benefits of nitrous oxide and too confident of his experience, and he failed to convince his medical audience.

Wells was in Boston by the end of January 1845, with permission to put on a demonstration. One can see the problem that loomed: on the one hand, his audience included ever-critical medical students; on the other, the sensitive and retiring Wells had to introduce a new therapy not simply as dentist but combining the roles of lecturer, anesthetist, and operator. A medical student volunteered to take the gas and have his tooth extracted. Though the demonstration was not a complete failure, it was not satisfactory either. The medical student said later that he had felt virtually no pain, but he groaned as the tooth was loosened, and the audience concluded that the gas had not made the dental nerve insensible. The unfortunate Wells was laughed out of the room, noting later that his unsuccessful demonstration was derided as a "humbug affair."[86] He criticized himself too for having removed the gasbag prematurely, though it might have contained insufficient gas, or the gas might have been impure. The anesthesiologist of today knows that anesthesia with nitrous oxide often *appears* to be incomplete, even though pain is not perceived by the patient under those circumstances. The failure of the demonstration was personally unfortunate for Wells, and he never recovered from it. Historically, it meant that priority in the discovery of anesthesia would not be his.

One of those who observed Wells was Morton, then a medical student. He had studied under Wells and partnered him in practice for a while in 1844. He even loaned Wells the dental instruments he needed in Boston.[87] Afterward, Wells talked to Morton and Jackson, who was well known not only as a physician but also as a chemist. He told them about nitrous oxide, and both admitted that nitrous oxide anesthesia was new to them.[88] This is why Wells has been credited priority in the discovery of anesthesia by some individuals. The meaning of his work was summarized by Charles F. Heywood on January 14, 1853, who had seen Morton give ether on October 16, and he thought about Wells and the discovery of anesthesia. He noted,

> We observe in the first period, an indefinite search after *some* method of producing insensibility to pain, and animal magnetism was tried and failed; opium and other anodynes were then made use of, but the result was unsatisfactory. The came a *second period*, when a great advance was made, *which is beyond all dispute*, due to Dr. Horace Wells. In this period was made known the great fact that substances applied to the pulmonary surfaces by inhalation produced a sudden and concentrated effect quite different form that of the same agent when taken into the stomach. The method of administration required that the same substances should be in the state of vapor or gas, and *Dr. Wells soon discovered by experimentation that certain intoxicating agents* would produce, when inhaled, insensibility to pain, and this was the first important step in the history of anesthesia.[89]

Wells must have convinced his fellow dentists in Hartford of the efficacy of nitrous oxide, because they soon started using it, as did surgeons as well.[90, 91]

Wells also used ether during 1844 and 1845,[92] though he preferred nitrous oxide. Though it was less potent than ether, it seemed more suitable for short procedures such as teeth extraction. However, he backed the wrong drug.[93] Several other factors conspired against Wells. Hartford, where he worked, was much smaller than Boston; it had fewer physicians, and none with the authority of those in Morton's medical world; he was handicapped by his unconvincing demonstration of nitrous oxide in Boston in January 1845; and he was quieter and more modest than Morton, his brash nemesis. Wells and nitrous oxide lost out to Morton and ether. Wells lost out in another way, being jailed for throwing acid at a prostitute and then died after consuming a large dose of chloroform.

Ether—I: Jackson, Clarke, Long, and "Jump-up-behinders"

According to historical convention, modern anesthesia really begins with Morton on October 16, 1846. However, if the first use of ether as an anesthetic is what is being considered, there is a case for Clarke in January 1842,[94, 95, 96] and an even stronger one for Long in March 1842.[97] Apart from their contributions, Jackson's must be considered, because it was so closely tied to Morton's[98] and extends back farther in time. The dubious claims to priority of Walter Channing,[99] R. H. Collyer,[100] E. R. Smilie,[101] and William Wheeler[102] also have to be assessed. All these claims will be discussed before Morton's successful demonstration, and his unethical adventures in the ether trade are recounted.

Charles Jackson. The Boston physician and chemist Charles Jackson claimed to have known about ether long before Morton, and his knowledge of chemistry, as well as medicine—together with a forceful personality—made his claim credible. Jackson was Morton's main rival during the lengthy period when Morton was trying to convince his fellow Americans that it was he, and no one else, who discovered anesthesia. What points fired the relationship between the two men?

Jackson, according to his brother-in-law Edward Waldo Emerson, had known, since 1837 and before Morton ever met him, that ether could be inhaled as an antidote to chlorine.[103] Thus, he knew what to do when, in 1842, he accidentally inhaled chlorine in his laboratory: he found that ether relieved the distress caused by the chlorine. He even found that breathing ether resulted in insensibility.[104] In 1843, Jackson told apothecary H. D. Fowle and D. J. Browne that ether was suitable for surgical operations.[105] In 1841, Jackson had given Fowle a vial of ether to relieve toothache,[106] and in 1842, he told John Blake that ether would relieve headache.[107] Jackson also said that he told several people about this pain-relieving property of ether. Jackson then gave up medicine for geology and chemistry, so he did not test ether further but wished others to test what he'd told them.

When Jackson tried to convince others that he had discovered anesthesia, his personality quirks worked against him. Previously, he had believed that he had conceived an idea and that others went on to use it in inventing devices that became widely used, such as Samuel Morse's electric telegraph. He tended to regard observations as facts without attempting to test them. As T. T. Bouve, a student of Jackson's, said about him, "From some peculiarities hard to comprehend," he often expressed "what he recognized as fact, without striving to substantiate it."[108] It does appear, though, that Jackson passed on to Morton knowledge about ether; as Richard Wolfe noted, Jackson did give Morton the essential clue to the discovery. He pointed Morton in the right direction.[109] As far as the actual *use* of ether as an anesthetic is concerned, however, Jackson never tested his suggestion clinically. This weakens his claim to priority.

Jackson met Morton first in 1844, when he acted as an informal preceptor. As a medical student for two courses, Morton boarded with Jackson. Morton benefited from his relationship with Jackson, for he learned about the use of chloric ether in deadening the sensitivity of dental nerves and about the intoxicating effects of sulfuric ether, which Jackson gave him.[110] Jackson appears to have served as a responsible preceptor, and in Wolfe's opinion, Jackson served as the stabilizing force for Morton. He gave Morton the essential clue, and by doing so, he pointed Morton in the right direction and steadied his path.[111] Thus Morton was in Jackson's debt. He left the Jackson household sometime before the end of September 1946, and the story of the claims of Jackson on the one hand and Morton on the other becomes less clear.

On "about" September 30, 1846, Morton went to see Jackson.[112] He borrowed a bag made of India rubber; dissimulating, he said that he wished to inflate it with air and tell a nervous patient that it would help her. When he returned the bag, Jackson told Morton about something that really would work, by inducing insensibility in patients. He told him where Morton could obtain some sulfuric ether and how it could be used. Morton confirmed this meeting, but he didn't tell Jackson that, as we shall see, he had already observed some satisfactory results with sulfuric ether and had visited him to obtain information about the chemistry of ethers; and he pretended to be ignorant about sulfuric ether in order to keep quiet about his own schemes for its use.[113] While Jackson likely did influence Morton's thinking to some extent, there is no clear evidence that Jackson should have priority for the first use of ether.

William E. Clarke. At about the time that Jackson was making his early observations on ether, two other individuals actually used ether to make patients insensible prior to surgery. Clarke was one. He was familiar with "ether frolics" as a medical student, and late in January 1842, Clarke administered ether, on a towel, so that Elijah Pope could painlessly extract a tooth from a Ms. Hobbie.[114] The problem with this incident is that Clarke never reported it himself. It did not become known until Henry Lyman noted it in his textbook of 1881.[115] Clarke may have neglected to report it because his preceptor, E. M. Moore, told him that Ms. Hobbie was a hysterical "freak" and not to make any more experiments with ether.[116] As one commentator put it, "One must have an alert mind and the will to champion one's own observations" for a claim to priority to be supported.[117] Clarke never went that far.

Crawford Williamson Long (fig. 2.7). More credible is Long, who is reasonably claimed to have used ether in 1842, and thus to be the first physician to administer ether as an anesthetic for surgical purposes.[118] Long—a Philadelphia-trained physician who practiced at that time in Jefferson, Georgia—was familiar with the recreational use of ether. Like Wells later, he realized that while under its effects, he had bruised himself without feeling any pain, and he made the same observations of others. His friend James Venable also had taken ether, so when he asked Long to remove two tumors from the back of his neck, Long agreed to do so, and to use ether. Long excised the first tumor on March 30, 1842, which is the basis of the argument that Long discovered anesthesia. *Long was the first person to use ether deliberately to induce anesthesia for surgical purposes.*

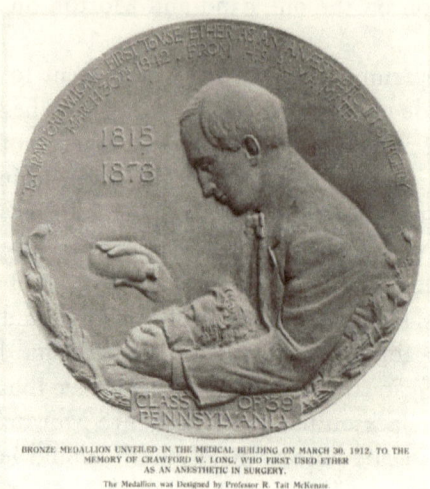

BRONZE MEDALLION UNVEILED IN THE MEDICAL BUILDING ON MARCH 30, 1912, TO THE
MEMORY OF CRAWFORD W. LONG, WHO FIRST USED ETHER
AS AN ANESTHETIC IN SURGERY.

The Medallion was Designed by Professor R. Tait McKenzie

Fig. 2.7. Crawford Long (1815-1878)

Crawford Williamson Long was born in Danielsville, Georgia. He learned medicine as an apprentice to Dr. George Grant, in Jefferson, Georgia, and studied in Transylvania University in Lexington, Kentucky, and the University of Pennsylvania. After graduating in 1839, Long took further training in surgery in New York. Thus, as a practitioner in Jefferson, Long was unusually well trained and familiar with the academic life. He was also familiar with the recreational use of both ether and nitrous oxide and their effects. When Long was asked by some of his friends to make some nitrous oxide, he declined, not having the apparatus, but he suggested that they try ether. Long observed the analgesic effect when partying people painlessly hurt themselves. On March 30, 1842, Long suggested to James Venable, one of his friends and who had cysts in his neck, that ether could prevent the pain of surgery and could make surgery painless. One cyst was removed that day, and a second one on June 6. Long used ether in several other patients, sometimes also withholding its use to confirm that ether did make surgery painless. Long anesthetized his wife in her labor on December 17, 1845. With good reason, many people believed that Long was the first to use ether; and certainly, Long was the only one of the pioneers of anesthesia who enjoyed a long and happy life.

The case for Long is strong for two other reasons: he provided statements from several other individuals, including Venable, testifying to what had happened in March 1842; and he used ether on other occasions. One who was convinced by Long was Jackson.[119] Long's case is weak, however, because he did not report his use of ether until 1849,[120] nearly three years after Morton's demonstration in Boston. This might suggest that Long did not understand the significance of what he had done. Or this failure of Long's can be attributed to the lack of medical colleagues with whom he could discuss his use of ether, to his having a busy single-handed practice, and perhaps to his thinking that other physicians might accuse him of being reckless in using ether when many physicians advocated mesmerism for the management of persons undergoing surgery.

Long's case for priority was, however, supported by some physicians. In 1853, Long read an abstract of his 1849 paper, and the Georgia Medical Society endorsed his claims and urged him to present his case to the American Medical Association (AMA).[121] Next year, Georgia senator William Dawson presented letters from Long and Jackson, hoping to convince his fellow U.S. senators when the appropriations bill, in which Morton's claim was then considered, was up for the final reading. The bill did not pass, the Civil War came about a few years later, and the opportunity for Long's case to be followed up was missed. Long's legacy is like Hickman's: his early work on anesthesia may have served to accustom people to the idea of anesthesia in this early period.

Channing, Collyer, Smilie, and Wheeler. The advent of ether anesthesia led a number of individuals in the 1840s to claim priority in using it. However, these minor actors in the drama of the ether controversy had no effect on the evolution of anesthesia. Stanley Sykes labeled them as "jump-up-behinders."[122] Obstetrician Walter Channing, for example, reported that a patient of his had been given ether by her husband during childbirth in 1833, though he did not write about it for nineteen years. Collyer may have used ether in 1843, though his report did not impress anyone, Sykes dismissing him as eccentric and unconventional.[123] Smilie, in 1846, claimed to have used a mixture of ether and opium in 1844. As for Wheeler, who stated that he administered ether in 1845, his experience was reported by surgeon John Collins Warren in a memorandum among his family papers, but not until 1919.[124] Wheeler's story was that as a chemistry student, he had obtained ether from his physician father's supply and gave it to a young man, who promptly became unconscious and only recovered after some time. Wheeler reportedly believed that this was "probably one of the first cases of complete anesthesia ever accomplished."

Ether—II: Wells and Morton

Horace Wells. Though Wells is linked to the first anesthetic use of nitrous oxide, in 1847, he stated that when he "first made the discovery, rectified ether was used, as well as nitrous oxide gas."[125] Whether Wells used ether is not clear from the letter that he wrote in 1847 to the *Boston Medical and Surgical Journal*, but other evidence suggests that he did. Hartford surgeon P. W. Ellsworth said that Wells "debated for some time which to use, the gas or ether, but preferred the former as he thought it less liable to injure the system."[126] E. E. Marcy, also of Hartford, stated that in the latter part of 1844, he suggested the use of ether to Wells, and that Wells used it to anesthetize a man who was to have a tumor removed from his head.[127] Further evidence of Wells's familiarity with ether and of his use of it *before its introduction in Boston by Morton* was provided by New York surgery professor Valentine Mott in a deposition dated December 23, 1852. Mott stated that Wells had discussed both nitrous oxide and ether as anesthetic agents at a time before any publication was made on the subject.[128] Wells never formally presented any priority claim himself. His suicide on January 22, 1848, prevented that.

William Thomas Green Morton. Morton's claim is much stronger than that of his perceived rivals, for his use of ether was witnessed and documented. He was the first to publicly and successfully show that inhalation of a chemical substance would induce insensibility that was practical for use in surgery. It was he who, on October 16, 1846, performed the *experimentum crucis* that proved, to the satisfaction of critical onlookers, that ether would abolish the pain of surgery, and that it was complete and safe. *Morton was the first to demonstrate the fact of anesthesia convincingly and publicly*. What sort of man was one who has been dubbed as a "tarnished idol"[129]?

It is uncertain when and where Morton was born. It may have been on August 9, 1819, in Charlton, Massachusetts,[130] or on August 19.[131] Or he may have been born in Burrillville, Rhode Island, the site of Morton's Quaker ancestors.[132] What is certain is that at 10:25 a.m. on Friday, October 16, 1846, Morton did administer ether in Boston's Massachusetts General Hospital so that John Collins Warren could excise a vascular tumor from the neck of Gilbert Abbott—and without inflicting significant pain.[133]

Understandably, Morton valued his contribution to surgery highly. His self-assurance convinced an early biographer that he was a "public benefactor."[134] Since Morton was inducted into New York University's Hall of Fame of Great Americans in 1920,[135] many people shared his own opinion regarding priority. Yet Morton is not universally regarded as a hero; Wolfe gave his biography of Morton the title *Tarnished Idol*.[136] The pendulum of opinion has swung back to the days when his unseemly rush to patent his discovery and his persistence in staking his claim for priority (and for consequent compensation) before the United States Congress and Senate antagonized many people. He seemed to be interested more in making money than in making pain relief as freely available, to paraphrase Horace Wells, as the air.[137]

This is not the place to detail the reasons why Wolfe, for example, has labeled Morton—admittedly in his wayward youth—as unscrupulous, scurrilous, a liar, a thief, a plagiarist, and even a scoundrel.[138] But these character defects must be borne in mind when Morton's own accounts of the ether story are examined. They are not infrequently self-serving, and on a particular topic, they vary from one account to another. In addition, the cases made by Morton's rivals to the claim for priority must be considered. This is laborious. Wolfe, after examining the Morton extensive archive, concluded that the evidence is so "muddled and confusing"[139] that the truth is hard to discern. It is, therefore, necessary to cross-check with other contemporary accounts in discerning which is accurate.

When Morton studied dentistry from 1841 to 1843, he knew that it was possible, with a minimum of training, to call oneself a dentist. He also knew that, with a minimum of money, he could set up an office. His practice in 1841 and 1842 with Wells,[140] who by then was a successful dentist who fitted many patients with dental plates, showed Morton that "mechanical dentistry" was potentially lucrative. Morton learned two other things as he worked under and then with Wells. One was the magnitude of the problem of pain. To fit dental plates, you first had to extract teeth, which was painful. The second thing, then, was to find a way of making dental procedures less painful. For the sensitive and humane Wells, that was why finding a way to lessen or abolish pain was urgent; for the ambitious and entrepreneurial Morton, finding a painless approach to dentistry was more of a business matter.

Wells' unsuccessful demonstration of nitrous oxide showed Morton that he would need a substance that was preferable to nitrous oxide if he was to find a way of abolishing pain. Ether seemed to be one answer. Although the admission by Jackson and Morton that the subject of painless surgery was "entirely" new to them[141] was probably spurious, Jackson had claimed that he had been thinking along these lines since the early part of the 1840s, and according to William Leavitt, Morton appeared secretive when he was requested to obtain some ether without letting anyone know it was for Morton.[142] Morton wanted the holy grail—and the money—for himself.

Morton had used ether in liquid form as early as July 1844, and so he was probably thinking even then about the problem of pain. That was when a Ms. Parrot had asked Morton to attend to a tooth that was giving her a lot of pain.[143] The tooth needed to be filled, and to allay the pain of the procedure, Morton applied liquid ether to the adjacent gum—a trick he had learned from Jackson. Morton would also have recalled that when he had used liberal amounts of ether, surrounding parts of the face went numb. If the effect of the ether spread thus, might it not spread to all of the body if enough ether was used?

The idea of generalized insensibility was mentioned in Rice's *Trials of a Public Benefactor*, which, though written under Rice's name, contains much material supplied by Morton. *Trials* stands as part of Morton's own testament, but it did not appear until a decade after the ether controversy had been inaugurated. It is therefore reasonable to be cautious in accepting Morton's own explanation for the origin of his ideas about anesthesia. Moreover, in the first half of the nineteenth century, people knew about ether and the insensibility it could induce. Furthermore, there is no evidence that Morton was an original thinker, and from 1844 to 1846, he would probably have gleaned ideas from

current books on *materia medica*. And so by June 1846, when Morton asked
Dr. Grenville Hayden to superintend his office, "he had an idea in his head,
connected with dentistry," which he thought would be "one of the greatest
things ever known," and which he wished to perfect by giving all his time and
attention to developing it.[144] Morton, who had tried to test the effects of ether
on his spaniel, said that he told Hayden, Francis Whitman, his brother-in-law,
and Richard Henry Dana, his lawyer, that he believed he could find a means of
extracting teeth painlessly.[145]

By now, Morton had concluded that ether was not as dangerous as he'd
been led to believe. Consequently, about the beginning of August 1846, he
was able to persuade his two dental assistants, William Leavitt and Thomas
Spear, to inhale ether.[146] Spear said that Morton often conducted experiments
in the little room adjoining the office, and it was in that room that he had the
following experience:

> I felt a numbness in my limbs [Morton related], with a sensation
> like nightmare, and would have given the world for someone to
> come and arouse me. I thought for a moment I should die in that
> state, and the world would only pity or ridicule my folly. At length,
> I felt a slight tingling of the blood in the end of my third finger, and
> made an effort to touch it with my thumb, but without success. At
> a second effort, I touched it, but there seemed to be no sensation.
> I gradually raised my arm, and pinched my thigh, but I could see
> that sensation was imperfect. I attempted to rise from my chair,
> but fell back. Gradually, I regained power over my limbs, and full
> consciousness. I immediately looked at my watch, and found that I
> had been insensible between seven and eight minutes.[147]

According to Hayden, by August 1846, Morton was "continually talking
about his discovery," though toward the end of September, he had to admit
that "his discovery did not work exactly right."[148] Consulting books had not
provided all the answers, but according to Hayden, Morton did believe he was on
the track of finding something that no one else had ever used. Hayden advised
Morton to see a chemist, and "about the last of September 1846" Morton saw
Jackson. Evidently blinded by his conviction that he was the sole discoverer of
anesthesia, he did not at first acknowledge having obtained significant clues
from both Jackson and Wells. Morton did later admit his debt to Jackson, from
whom he had "derived from him a hint by which . . . [he] thought he could
remove the only remaining difficulty."[149]

In view of the fact that both Morton and Jackson had the reputation for
bending the truth if it should serve them, the versions of the two men about the
evening's events should be compared, even though they were made sometime

after the initial demonstration at the Massachusetts General Hospital. First, Morton's account, which is indicative of his studied nonchalance in an attempt to keep from Jackson what he had on his mind:

> I asked Dr. Jackson for his gas-bag. He told me it was in his house. I went for it, and returned through the laboratory. He said, in a laughing manner, "Well, Doctor, you seem to be all equipped, minus the gas. I replied, in the same manner, that perhaps there would be no need of having any gas, if the person who took it could only be made to believe there was gas in it . . . . He . . . said . . . that I had better not attempt such an experiment, lest I should be set down as a greater humbug than Wells was with his nitrous oxide gas. Seeing that there was an opportunity to open the subject, I said, in as careless a manner as I could assume, why cannot I give the ether gas? He said that I could do so, and spoke again of the students taking it at Cambridge. He said the patient would be dull and stupefied, that I could do what I pleased with him, that he would not be able to help himself. Finding the subject open, I made the inquiries I wished as to the different kinds and preparations of ether. He told me something about the preparations, and thinking that if he had any it would be of the purest kind, I asked him to let me see his. He did so, but remarked that it had been standing for some time, and told me that I could get some highly rectified at Burnett's. As I was passing out, Dr. Jackson followed me to the door, and told me that he could recommend something better than the gas-bag, to administer the ether with, and gave me a flask with a glass tube inserted in it.[150]

Jackson's account, written by his lawyers soon after October 23, 1846, implied that Morton was virtually acting under his instructions and his agent. He wrote as follows:

> Dr. W. T. G. Morton called on him near the latter part of last month to obtain the loan of a gas-bag, which he said it was his intention to use for the purpose of administering atmospheric air, or something else, to a patient quiet her fears in order that he might extract one of her teeth . . . . Dr. Morton stated that he was desirous of operating on the imagination of the person . . . . Dr. Jackson . . . told Dr. Morton that such an experiment would prove a failure . . . that he had better let her breathe some ether . . . which would put her to sleep, and then he could pull her tooth . . . that Dr. Morton inquired of him as to the danger and mode of using it. He replied to him, that he might saturate a sponge or cloth with it, and apply it to her mouth or nose.[151]

Morton was now ready for clinical experimentation. A test came on September 30, 1846. Eben Frost had asked Morton to extract a very sore tooth, but dreading the operation, he said he wished to be mesmerized. Morton told him that he had something better, and induced him to take ether. The operation was a success. The *Boston Daily Journal* for October 1, 1846, related an account that had supposedly come from an eyewitness to the operation. It was said that "an ulcerated tooth was extracted from the mouth of an individual, without giving him the slightest pain. He was put into a kind of sleep, by inhaling a preparation . . . which lasted for about three quarters of a minute . . . just long enough to extract the tooth."[152] This account also points up the manner in which the report was obtained. Slyly and somewhat unethically, Morton had arranged for a reporter to be present, so that, in Wolfe's words, "he could utilize the story for advertising and profit."[153]

Morton followed up the Frost operation with several others. According to William James Morton, Morton's son, thirty-seven of these operations were performed privately by Dr. Henry J. Bigelow, before ether was first used at the Massachusetts General Hospital.[154] Morton's son, a professor of diseases of the mind and nervous system and electrotherapeutics, stated that his father used to administer laudanum (40 minims) before beginning etherization. However, because Morton fils did not document his statement and because Dr. Bigelow never referred to these operations, this intriguing story cannot be confirmed. As to whether Morton administered ether to some patients before October 16, though, we do have Dr. Hayden's testimony[155] and a statement by Morton's son.[156] Hayden stated that the glass tube that Jackson loaned Morton was of no help, and it was replaced by a conical glass tube obtained from Mr. Wightman, an instrument maker. Even then, his success was not uniform. Morton wondered if part of the problem was rebreathing, and he asked Nathan Chamberlain, another instrument maker, for assistance. Chamberlain's inhaler, Hayden said, gave "almost uniform success . . . the results of which are known to the world."[157]

Now Morton was ready to ask Massachusetts General Hospital senior surgeon John Collins Warren if he would let him demonstrate his discovery of ether insensibility. His request was granted, and Morton now had to be certain that everything would work satisfactorily. Matters became urgent when he received a letter, dated October 14, 1846, from Dr. Charles F. Heywood, Dr. Warren's house surgeon, requesting his presence at the Massachusetts General Hospital on Friday, October 16, at ten o'clock.[158] Needing reassurance and final words of advice, Morton consulted Dr. Augustus Gould, a Boston physician with whom he had boarded once. Gould stayed up the night before Morton's appointment, recommending that a different valve system be used. Early next morning, Morton persuaded Chamberlain to make a further modification. This delayed his arrival. With Dr. Warren poised to operate without the use of ether, Morton was ready to use his inhaler (see fig. 7.1) by 10:25 a.m. All went well.

The patient, Gilbert Abbott, was sufficiently insensible to allow his surgeon to excise the vascular tumor in his neck. Later, he said that though he felt some scraping, he had felt no pain.

This event was truly remarkable, standing historically alongside vaccination and, later, antisepsis and antbiotic therapy. It was reported the next day in the Boston newspapers and then in newspapers across America. Many people could not believe that someone could be made insensible, undergo an operation without knowing it, and then wake up.

Morton's use of ether was one of those revolutions in medicine that changed the way people thought and practiced. As John Collins Warren wrote in 1848, "a new era" had opened on the operating surgeon. He said that the surgeon's "visitations on the most delicate parts are performed, not only without the agonizing screams he has been accustomed to hear, but sometimes in a state of perfect insensibility, and, occasionally, even with an expression of pleasure on the part of the patient." Warren imagined that any senior surgeon must surely wish he had been able to work "under the new auspices." If famous surgical figures like Paré and Louis and Dessault, and Cheselden and Hunter and Cooper could see what Warren daily witnessed, surely they would long to be alive to perform their exploits once more.[159]

However, a single operation under the "new auspices" was not enough to convince, so other minor operations followed. In that way, Henry Bigelow and senior surgeons Warren and Hayward helped convince the world that ether did all it was said to do. They also knew that to be truly convincing, ether must be administered to a patient undergoing a *major*, or capital, operation. This was done first on November 6, again by Morton. Next day, a young woman scheduled for an above-knee operation was given ether, also successfully. It was claimed that "Morton was the hero of the hour."[160]

Now in the latter two months of 1846, the history of anesthesia separated into two streams. One was formed by the spread of the news around the world; the other, by the controversy that was generated in the United States by the various claims for priority of the discovery of anesthesia.

The News Spreads Beyond the United States

A key witness of Morton's demonstration, besides John Collins Warren, was Henry Jacob Bigelow. Early in November, he described ether "insensibility" to the American Academy of Arts and Sciences and, more fully, to the Boston Society for Medical Improvement. Henry's father, Professor Jacob Bigelow, and Edward Everett, the academy vice president and president of Harvard University,[161] heard Henry's talk. Everett wished to spread the word, and on November 14, he wrote to the fashionable London physician Dr. Henry Holland. His letter was probably carried by the *Britannia*; it sailed for Boston on November 16, arrived in London on December 1, and reached Holland on December 2. Holland seemed to be less excited by Everett's news than expected, but he was medically less impressive than socially and did nothing to publicize what Everett had termed "a real promising discovery."[162] In his place, Jacob Bigelow is credited with spreading the news about ether from Boston to London.

Henry Bigelow's lecture to the Boston Society of Medical Improvement was published on November 18, 1846, in the *Boston Medical and Surgical Journal*.[163] Because the lecture was considered so newsworthy, it was reprinted in the November 19 issue of the *Boston Daily Advertiser*.[164] Jacob Bigelow sent a copy of it, along with a letter, to his friend in London, Dr. Francis Boott. His letter was dated November 28, in time to catch the steamship *Acadia*, which departed for Liverpool via Halifax, Nova Scotia, on December 1.[165] Boott, in contrast to Holland, acted swiftly: he told the British medical press, informed surgeon Robert Liston, and, on December 19, 1846, organized a trial of ether for a dental extraction with his dentist friend James Robinson. Liston witnessed this, and he too acted swiftly. On December 19, he asked William Squire to give ether so that he could perform an amputation of a leg at University College Hospital. All went well, and Liston declared that ether was "no Yankee dodge."[166] Robinson went on to write a short treatise on ether, which was published in March 1847 as the first book on ether.[167]

A variation on the story of the transatlantic spread was told by Thomas Baillie.[168] He attributed the first ether anesthetic for a surgical operation to Dr. William Scott, who heard about ether from Dr. William Fraser on or about December 18, 1846, and performed an amputation on a patient under ether on December 19. Fraser, a Scotsman, had met Morton in Boston, and arrived back in Liverpool on the mail ship *Acadia* on December 16. He was bound for Dumfries, Scotland, to see his mother, who was lonesome, having just lost her son James and a daughter, with William as the sole survivor of eight siblings. The historical interest of the Dumfries operation lies in the fact that it was performed two days before Liston's operation, it had no influence on the spread of the news either to England or Europe or beyond.

World use of ether followed swiftly. It was used for the first time in Paris on December 22, 1846;[169] in Saint John, Canada, on January 18, 1847;[170] in Munich[171] and Vienna on January 25, 1847;[172] and in faraway Sydney, Australia, toward the end of May 1847.[173] The news of this innovation in medicine, later to become a specialty, spread quickly, indeed.

The Ether Controversy

Initially, and perhaps surprisingly, the use of ether in surgery was controversial. Most surgeons accepted it readily, but some thought that pain was beneficial, even stimulating, "reparative action" in the tissues.[174] Some people, lay and medical, thought that abolishing pain was against God's will, and that pain was a punishment for earthly sins. Some of the objections to anesthesia for labor stemmed from the interpretation of the biblical words stating that women should bring forth children "in sorrow."[175] This was smartly refuted by the scholarly James Young Simpson, who argued that the Hebrew translation for the word *sorrow* actually denoted effort.[176] Eventually, though, anesthesia proved a boon. Patients themselves, in submitting themselves to surgery and not feeling pain, knew this.

The use of ether was also controversial for other reasons. These may be considered under the rubric of the so-called ether controversy, which concerns Morton's claim to priority for the use of ether and others contesting it.[177] Countless individuals were involved, and much time, energy, and money was expended. One group of individuals comprised the principal claimants to the title of discoverer of anesthesia: Morton himself, who sought remuneration as well as praise, his nemesis Charles Jackson, Crawford Long, and Horace Wells, as well as their medical supporters. Another group included the members of the U.S. Congress and Senate, who had to hear and assess these claims. The third group included the press. The ether controversy served no one well, and Morton least of all. It did not affect the use of ether, but the story is part of the history of ether in the United States.

Several factors stoked the ether controversy. One was Morton's personality and his strident, even obsessional, belief that he was the sole discoverer of ether anesthesia. Realizing that his discovery was potentially a source of income, he patented it without delay. His persistent—and for some people, tiresome—petitions to Congress from 1846 to 1862, submitted in a fruitless search for confirmation as the discoverer (and remuneration to the tune of $100, 000), continually fanned the flames of the controversy.

Other factors were the claims of Charles Jackson, Horace Wells, and Crawford Long. As for Jackson, his personality worked for good and ill. Urbane and well educated, Jackson was respected for his scientific achievements and stood in contrast to the unpolished and poorly educated Morton. But Jackson had flaws: an inflated opinion of his own importance as an inventor, including that of ether anesthesia; his irritation at losing his other priority claims, such as that relating to the electric telegraph; and his obsessional nature. All this stirred the pot and kept Jackson in the forefront as Morton continued to press Congress. The battle between the ambitious Morton and the prickly Jackson in the middle years of the nineteenth century was the central feature of the ether controversy.

Yet a third factor was the entry of the representatives of Horace Wells and Crawford Long, whose claims Congress also heard. The ether controversy was never settled; indeed, the debate continues to this day, illustrating the interest and the tensions that are frequently generated when attempts are made to settle claims to priority for a scientific discovery.

Morton's secretiveness antagonized people and prevented some from acknowledging his desire for acceptance. Hospital senior surgeons withheld permission for Morton to use ether until he informed them what his so-called Letheon was.[178] (It was just sulfuric ether with some flavoring added.) Only then could Morton rely on the support of his surgical colleagues that he realized he needed. Yet Morton remained ambitious and possessive of what he regarded as *his* discovery; he feared that "another, with better opportunities for experimenting, availing himself of . . . [Morton's] hints and labors, might take the prize."[179]

Morton thought that ether, if patented, would bring him a large income, but his decision to patent a drug that was universally beneficial was resented. It also fueled an increasingly bitter struggle with Jackson. Having decided to take out a patent for ether, Morton consulted a lawyer, though the lawyer, R. H. Eddy, happened to be a friend of Jackson's. However, within a week of Morton's first demonstration at the hospital, Jackson, who was familiar by then with Morton's success, gave Eddy his side of the story. Jackson, aware of the potential value of the ever-widening use of ether, knew there could be something in it for him too. Besides, this time, he was determined not to lose out on a discovery that he believed he really had a claim to. Eddy was sympathetic to Jackson's claim that he had given Morton the *idea* of the surgical use of ether, but he found himself in a conflict of interest, for Morton had promised him 25 percent of the proceeds of the projected sales of ether under patent.[180]

Eddy, therefore, had to satisfy two clients. He reasoned as follows: From what Jackson had told him, the discovery was a joint one, made by both Morton and Jackson. It was Jackson's idea, though Morton had performed the crucial experiment. Legally, a joint discovery meant that a patent, if applied for, should have the names of both individuals. Morton did not agree that Jackson had a claim to the discovery, but Eddy told him that Jackson's chemical science would improve the patented product and that his association with Morton would give an "immediate character" to the discovery. Morton agreed to pay 10 percent of the licensing sales to Jackson, to a total of $500, though later, Eddy persuaded Morton to pay 10 percent of all licence sales.[181] Papers for the execution of the patent were drawn up on October 27, 1846. On November 12, 1846, Letter Patent 4848 was issued to Morton and Jackson.

Jackson, the apparently upright and open scientist, was upset by Morton's approach to patenting the use of ether, for his name was then linked to accusations of patent medicines and quackery.[182] He tried to put himself in a better light. Some of this antagonized Morton, and the flames of the ether controversy flickered higher. On November 13, 1846, Jackson wrote to Elie de Beaumont, whom he had met during his educational stay in Paris in 1832. Jackson told him that he had induced a dentist to administer ether vapor to patients for dental extractions and had urged him to give ether at the Massachusetts General Hospital to an individual who was about to undergo major surgery; he omitted to say anything about Morton by name. In this letter, sealed and placed inside a covering letter that was mailed on December 1, 1846, he asked that *his* discovery be communicated to the Academy of Sciences in Paris.[183]

On March 1, 1847, Jackson wrote an article in the Boston *Daily Advertiser* under the title of "Antidote to Physical Suffering."[184] He gave the impression that this was a paper that he had presented to the Academy of Arts and Sciences, but this impression was misleading, for his paper was not presented until the next day; the academy did not publish the paper and disclaimed responsibility for it. Jackson also sent copies of the newspaper to Europe, thus buttressing his claim there as the discoverer. If Morton was secretive, Jackson was cunning.

The *Daily Advertiser* article annoyed Morton. He published a note in the March 5, 1847, issue titled "The Discovery of Letheon,"[185] while a friend, Edward Warren, also published, in the same issue, an article titled "Dr. Jackson and Dr. Morton—Letheon."[186] Warren gave Morton's side of the story and tried to correct the erroneous impressions that Jackson was creating.

Although Morton would from now on claim that *he* was the sole discoverer— just as Jackson was doing—his case was weakened by his having acknowledged Jackson's significant contributions. Thus, Don Pedro Wilson, who had started work as Morton's dental assistant on November 1, 1846, testified that Morton had attributed etherization to Jackson.[187] And in his own memoir, which Edward Warren presented to the academy in Paris in the late summer of 1847, Morton admitted that he was indebted to Jackson on several points about ether.[188]

Jackson's case was also presented in a pamphlet that Martin Gay wrote in May 1847 under the title, here abbreviated, of *A Statement of the Claims of Charles T. Jackson, M.D.*[189] This appeared to do more to strengthen Jackson's case, but for those in Congress who would soon have to clarify the complex issues, it was one more paper to read and digest. Publication of Gay's pamphlet may have been a tactic in a wider strategy: it came when Jackson melodramatically destroyed the bond that had united Jackson with Morton on the patent—and with a meeting of the Massachusetts Medical Society that was held on May 26, 1847. During the society's dinner that evening, Jackson, then professor of pathological anatomy at Harvard, told his medical colleagues that he was indeed the sole discoverer of etherization, that he had been "swindled" into a joint patent with Morton, and that, in destroying the bond, he was making the use of ether "free to all mankind." Jackson was applauded; Morton's name was greeted with hisses.[190]

In his pamphlet, Gay referred to Wells' claim, in March 1847, in his own document on the discovery of anesthesia.[191] Jackson dismissed Wells' pretensions as to the effects of nitrous oxide as being absurd.[192] Wells had claimed that he who had discovered the anesthetic property of an inhaled gas should be accredited as the discoverer of anesthesia; Jackson discounted the significance of the use of nitrous oxide. From then on, and even after his death in 1848, Wells' claim would be one more consideration in the ether controversy.

While these interchanges simmered on the front burner, Morton's several efforts to have the U.S. Congress and Senate recognize his claim kept the controversy simmering on the back one. In April 1854, Georgia senator William Dawson introduced Long's claim.[193] However, because the proposed appropriations bill then being debated did not pass, Long's claim, which, interestingly, was supported by Jackson, was dropped. But like any claim that might be made for Wells, Long's was one more that had to be taken into account. Those two claims, as well as Jackson's, further diluted the strength of Morton's claim.

In deciding to patent the use of ether and persisting in his pleas to the Congress and Senate, Morton was his own worst enemy. During this time, he had to swallow the many bitter pills that were administered by the medical and dental community. The most bitter, perhaps, was his being censured by the American Medical Association on June 24, 1864. Having failed to obtain the support in Washington, Morton sued the New York Eye and Ear Infirmary for infringement of his patent. He lost. The words of the American Medical Association must have come as a peculiarly painful blow:

> Whereas, The said Dr. Morton, by suits brought against charitable medical institutions for infringements of an alleged patent covering all anesthetic agents, not claiming sulfuric ether only, but the state of anesthesia, however produced, as his invention, has by this act put himself beyond the pale of an honorable profession and of true labors in the cause of science and humanity, therefore Resolved, That the American Medical Association enter their protest against any appropriation to Dr. Morton, on the ground of his unworthy conduct.[194]

*   *   *

Who, then, should be accorded priority in the discovery of anesthesia? Long? He did use ether on March 30, 1842, but he did not deem this important enough to publish his experience immediately; however, Long has many supporters. Wells? He did recognize the significance of nitrous oxide when Colton demonstrated it on December 10, 1844, and he was the first on the following day to apply the principle of inhalation of a gas in inducing insensibility for the benefit of surgical patients. Wells also appears to have used ether in October 1844, though he preferred nitrous oxide. Jackson? He had an undoubted role in passing information to Morton, but he never experimented with ether, either in patients or in animals. Or Morton? He had the nerve, the entrepreneurial motive, even the recklessness, to bear the brunt of making someone unconscious in order to endure surgery without pain. Or should we go back to Hickman? For he had the vision of using a gas to bring about pain-free surgery, and he researched it in experiments. Or should we go back to Davy, who was the first to suggest a surgical use for nitrous oxide?

The question as to priority is open-ended. Many people have given answers in the past, and many do still. Sir William Osler chose Morton because it was he who convinced the world,[195] and certainly, the practice of surgery was altered on that day, to say nothing of the benefits for countless patients thenceforth. On the other hand, rare is the discovery that has been made in the absence of assistance and knowledge provided by others. If one concludes, first, that it is valid to talk in terms of a *discoverer*, then Long and Wells stand in the forefront; and if one thinks, rather, of the *introduction* of anesthesia, then Morton stands in the forefront. To what extent does awarding credit to only one individual negate the claims of others? As Wolfe argues, taking Osler's line of argument means that one neglects the critical assistance that Morton received from Wells and Jackson.[196]

Three other points may be noted. First, a correspondent signing himself "A" in the *Boston Medical and Surgical Journal* of May 12, 1847, noted that Jackson had suggested to Morton the use of ether, which was generally known to produce insensibility.[197] A stated that no one had "dared" use ether in this way for a surgical purpose, and he argued that the credit of bringing ether to the notice of the public was due to Morton, on account of what is not usually considered a virtue: recklessness.

The second point was made by John Fulton in 1946: the discovery of anesthesia was made by individuals who were all young. Davy was twenty-one; Hickman, twenty-three; Clarke, twenty-two; Long, twenty-seven; Wells, twenty-eight; Jackson, thirty-six; and Morton, twenty-seven. As the title of his article indicates, Fulton noted that they all had "the vision and daring of youth."[198] The introduction of anesthesia is indeed a tribute to the potency of youth.

Finally, A made another point. He said of the discovery of anesthesia that "intellectual ability and scientific attainments suggested it, recklessness brought it into use." A's conclusion is fitting: "The organist cannot perform without the blower; one superintends the scientific department, the other 'raises the wind.' What is true in this, is true in most other things, especially is it so with the ether."[199]

Chapter 3

Laying a Foundation of Anesthetic Practice:1846-1896

By demonstrating ether anesthesia on October 16, 1846, William Thomas Green Morton inaugurated a brand-new field of medicine. In its sudden appearance advent and in its novelty, anesthesia was quite different from the older specialties of medicine, surgery, and obstetrics, which had evolved over centuries. On October 15, 1846, anesthesia did not exist as a clinical entity; on October 16, it did. What did this mean?

The very novelty of anesthesia had several implications. What these were, how they affected the development of anesthesia in its first half century, and how the foundation was laid when anesthesia was essentially a craft, are discussed in this chapter.

Initial Implications of a New Field of Medicine

What were these implications? One was semantic: a specific term was needed to denote the new medical field. *Narcosis*, *analgesia*, and *etherization* were rejected in favor of *anaesthesia*. That term was suggested by Oliver Wendell Holmes.[1] In time, the precise form and usage of the terms varied in different parts of the world, as is evident in the derivations *anesthesia* and *anesthesiology* in the United States compared, for example, with *anaesthesia* in the United Kingdom, Canada, and Australia. In this book, the term *anesthesia* is used primarily as the rubric that covers all aspects of both the art and the science of anesthesia, particularly in relation to its historical context.

There are other semantic wrinkles. In the United States, before anesthesia became a specialty in the latter 1930s, practitioners were known as *anesthetists*.

This changed after anesthesia was recognized as a specialty: physicians who were certified and so classed as specialists began to be known as *anesthesiologists*, while nurse anesthetists were often termed *anesthetists*; and the term *anesthesiology* was used with respect to both the science and practice, as well as to more general aspects of the field as a whole. In the United Kingdom, Canada, and Australia, all practitioners of anesthesia are physicians, and the terms *anaesthetist* and *anaesthesia* are used. (See the definitions in the glossary in appendix B.)

A second implication of the inception of anesthesia as an entirely new medical field was cognitive. Practitioners of the new medical field needed a body of knowledge and of administration techniques that was specific to anesthesia. Some of this was created by physiologists and pharmacologists, who built on the foundations of science laid by natural scientists in the seventeenth and eighteenth centuries. But much was created by anesthesia practitioners themselves, albeit at a measured pace and at times only gradually, and what they achieved between 1846 and 1896 was of fundamental importance for the consolidation of anesthesia as a new form of medical practice.

A third implication of the innovative nature of anesthesia concerned the practice of medicine. The introduction of anesthesia brought nothing less than a sea change. Internal medicine itself was not greatly affected, though in the early years patients with conditions such as tetanus and even hydrocephalus were treated with anesthesia,[2] just as in the twentieth century, anesthesia and anesthetic techniques were used in critical care and in pain medicine. The practice of obstetrics was, however, affected significantly, as the pain of childbirth was relieved and as obstetricians could perform operations more readily. But it was the practice of surgery that was affected most.

Even so, the practice of surgery, however, was not immediately affected greatly by the advent of anesthesia. In the year following the introduction of anesthesia, for example, a little under one-half the number of operations, other than those on a limb or a breast, were performed *without* anesthesia.[3] There were several reasons for this. The age and the beliefs of the surgeon, the gender of the patient, and the geographic region of the hospital were some of the factors.[4] Others stemmed from the conviction of some surgeons that pain had positive value in healing[5] and of others that the innovative nature of anesthesia made it "fraught with danger."[6] Except at the Massachusetts General Hospital, anesthesia was untried, and so, at a distance, it seemed to be just another anodyne—like hypnosis, for example—and maybe not as effective as the standbys of opium and alcohol.

What limited the widespread use of anesthesia most, however, was the continuing and serious danger of infection, particularly following intra-abdominal and limb operations. This had always been a problem for surgeons, and it would continue to vex them (and so often kill their patients) for another two decades. Only after Scottish surgeon Joseph Lister introduced antisepsis—in

1865 with dressings soaked in carbolic acid dressings[7] and in 1870 with a carbolic acid spray[8]—were surgeons emboldened to perform many more procedures on limbs and superficial parts of the body and, eventually, within body cavities. Only then did they no longer dread the onset of postoperative sepsis. Only then could they make use of the true advantages of anesthesia.[9]

Anesthesia as a Craft: Its Early Development in England

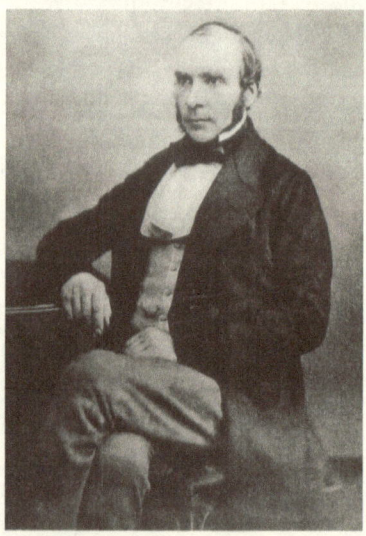

Fig. 3.1. John Snow (1813-1858)
John Snow was born in the English city of York. He served as an apprentice in the North of England before walking to London in 1836 and studying medicine and graduating there. A fine clinician and experienced general practitioner, Snow was incomparable as a researcher and educator, as well as a clinician and epidemiologist. He rose to the top of his profession, anesthetizing Queen Victoria in 1853 and 1857 and becoming president of the Medical Society of London in 1855. Snow wrote two classic texts in anesthesia and was the doyen of English anesthesia until he died prematurely in 1858. His unusual accomplishments—he was a leader in epidemiology as well as anesthesia, solving the problem of the transmission of cholera in 1855—are explained on the basis of his familiarity with the basic sciences, his ability to conduct basic and clinical research in order to understand the fundamental aspects of anesthesia, and his adeptness in integrating this basic knowledge into the clinical practice of anesthesia. Snow was always ready to instruct others in the art of anesthesia, but his own singular research also did much to lay the foundation of the new field of anesthesia. Just as it was said of Claude Bernard that he was physiology, so it could be said of Snow that he was anesthesia.

Although anesthesia was introduced in the United States, the art and science of anesthesia was developed initially in Great Britain. The leading figure was London anaesthetist and epidemiologist John Snow (fig. 3.1), who had a masterly understanding of both the art and science of anesthesia.[10] His work was of seminal importance, but he died prematurely in 1858, and so his contributions were but a fragment of what might have otherwise been an even more significant contribution to the understanding of anesthesia in its earliest years. Other work on anesthesia in the nineteenth century was carried out by London physicians Joseph Clover, Dudley Buxton, and Frederic Hewitt, who gave what was a craft some of the fundamentals of a specific body of knowledge. Clover[11] did much to maintain a high level of clinical anesthesia, though neither he nor Hewitt,[12] Clover's principal successor, had the breadth and depth of the investigations that had been made by Snow. By 1896, Hewitt himself had to admit that "the present state of our knowledge leaves much to be desired."[13] Even so, Clover and Hewitt, and Buxton to a lesser extent, did lay a sound basis for the practice of anesthesia, besides confirming the tradition of physician-anesthesia in the United Kingdom. Hewitt, in particular, paved the way for anesthesia to emerge from craft to discipline.

Building a Foundation for Anesthesia

In suggesting in 1896 that much was to be desired, Hewitt identified a central problem in the early days, when anesthesia was a craft. A body of knowledge was essential if the new field was to develop. A first step was to elucidate the nature of anesthesia and to agree on how to administer it, even though much of the knowledge was purely empirical, and even anecdotal. Because anesthesia was so new a medical field, practitioners had to answer the basic question: *what was anesthesia?* This could be answered only as knowledge was created and techniques fashioned so that ether and nitrous oxide, and chloroform from the end of 1847, could be given correctly and safely. An edifice had to built from the ground up, but many practitioners were for some time unfamiliar with the knowledge and techniques that were the building blocks. Learning about them and how to administer them was the main task for the next few decades.

In some respects, that was a huge task. The central goal was to do what had not been done before: to deliberately put a patient in a coma, let a surgeon operate, and then reverse the iatrogenic coma so that the patient would return to a normal state. This phenomenon was unique to anesthesia. A patient's body was plied with smelly chemical agents that had uncertain effects yet had to be understood; and at the same time, the body's physiological systems, especially the respiration and the circulation, had to be protected from any harm that anesthesia might inflict. Yet in that first era, all a practitioner could rely on in protecting a patient were the five senses and the intellect. That is, the practitioner had no access to any artificial monitoring methods. The essence of the approach in those days is illustrated in figure 3.2, which shows one of Clover's contributions to this new dimension of medical care. With one hand, to the patient's face he applies a mask, which is connected by rubber tubing to a portable source of anesthetic agent; with the other, he feels the pulse. In addition, his eyes observe the color of the skin and the breathing pattern. In every way, when anesthesia was a craft, the entire approach was simple and minimal.

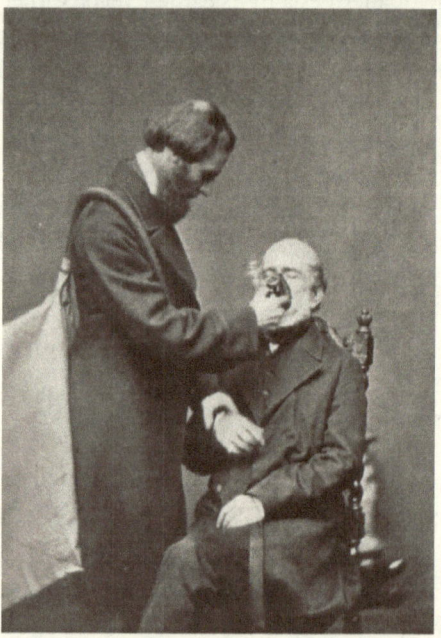

Fig. 3.2. Joseph Thomas Clover (1825-1882)
Joseph Clover was born in Aylesham, England. At age sixteen, he was apprenticed to local surgeon Charles Gibson, and at nineteen, he enrolled in University College Hospital, London, for formal medical studies, graduating in 1846. He practiced surgery full-time for some seven years and, from 1853, part-time, combining the practice of general medicine, urology, and anesthesia. Clover had begun to give anesthetics earlier, as resident medical officer at University College Hospital. Anesthesia was more to his liking than his other work, and he was appointed to Westminster Hospital and the London Dental, as well as to his own alma mater. He ascended to the pinnacle of London anesthesia left by the death of John Snow in 1858. Clover was in great demand as an anaesthetist and anesthetized a number of socially prominent individuals. He invented several pieces of anesthesia apparatus, including a chloroform bag, ether and nitrous oxide—ether inhalers, a rebreathing bag for nitrous oxide administration, and a nose-cap. His results speak for his skill: only one person out of 11,000 whom he anesthetized died as a result of anesthesia. Clover fully merited the many tributes that were paid him. It was said of him, for example, that he became the companion of leading surgeons at some of their most important operations.

The knowledge that was necessary for practitioners to administer anesthesia in the first fifty years was acquired only gradually. Most was gained only empirically, because initially, there was no science of anesthesia except for what Snow created in the decade before his death in 1858. For virtually all of its first half century, therefore, anesthesia remained an empirical craft, evolving only slowly, and at times, seemingly not at all.

In that period, anesthesia meant primarily general, inhalation anesthesia. Though two other approaches to anesthesia were developed—intravenous anesthesia in 1872 (see chapter 5) and "local" anesthesia in 1884 (see chapter 4)—anesthetists did not make use of them until well into the twentieth century, and thus neither influenced the evolution of anesthesia in the nineteenth century. They were, rather, the preserve of surgeons. Moreover, intravenous anesthesia with chloral hydrate was thought too dangerous, and local anesthesia with cocaine, too, was not free of danger. So the craft of anesthesia was centered around the three agents—ether, nitrous oxide, and chloroform.

Learning the Craft of Anesthesia

Hewitt's statement in 1896 about knowledge implied that all was not well with anesthesia. He and his colleagues knew that practitioners must be educated, but how was this to be done in the absence then of any systematic basis for education?

A knowledge of anesthesia, which had to be learned from scratch, was gained in two ways. One was to learn on the job. One was thrown in the water and had to swim, albeit with luck, with a coach giving moral support from the edge of the pool. Or if one was fortunate, one might be apprenticed to a Snow or a Clover or a Hewitt. Learning from a physician who had experience of anesthesia was easier in England than in the United States. In England, a smaller and more densely populated country, the tradition of physicians becoming interested in anesthesia had been established by Snow, who worked at several London hospitals from 1847 onward,[14] in addition to frequently giving anesthesia in patients' homes. Another physician with a hospital practice was Patrick Black, who was appointed chloroformist to St. Bartholomew's Hospital as early as 1852.[15] In the geographically much larger and less densely populated United States, however, the proportion of physicians to population was smaller than in England; and as a result, nurses, usually under the direction of surgeons, did much of the work. Too, they favored the safer ether over the more dangerous chloroform. Whatever the circumstances, individuals wishing to learn anesthesia did so partly by learning from others, as apprentices. Even so, those others might or might not be intimately familiar with the inhalational agents, the early pieces of anesthesia apparatus, how the body reacted to anesthesia, and dealing with common problems such as obstruction of the airway and depression of the circulation.

The second way of learning anesthesia was to read books by acknowledged authorities. London dentist James Robinson published a short book on ether in March 1847,[16] Snow published a fuller text in 1847[17] and a more comprehensive book on anesthesia posthumously in 1858,[18] and Buxton[19] and Hewitt[20] were other authorities who wrote books.

Administering the Raw Materials of Anesthesia

Practitioners initially had three raw elements to work with: ether and nitrous oxide and, beginning late in 1847, chloroform. The oldest was ether, which physicians had known for some time for its beneficial effects on the lungs (see chapter 2), and which the lay public, as a cartoon of 1847 suggests (fig. 3.3), knew for its euphoric effects. In the early years, ether certainly predominated, partly because anesthesia was identified with Morton and etherization and partly because of Horace Wells' apparent failure with it in 1845 (see chapter 2), and also partly because, as is discussed later, chloroform was not as safe as ether.

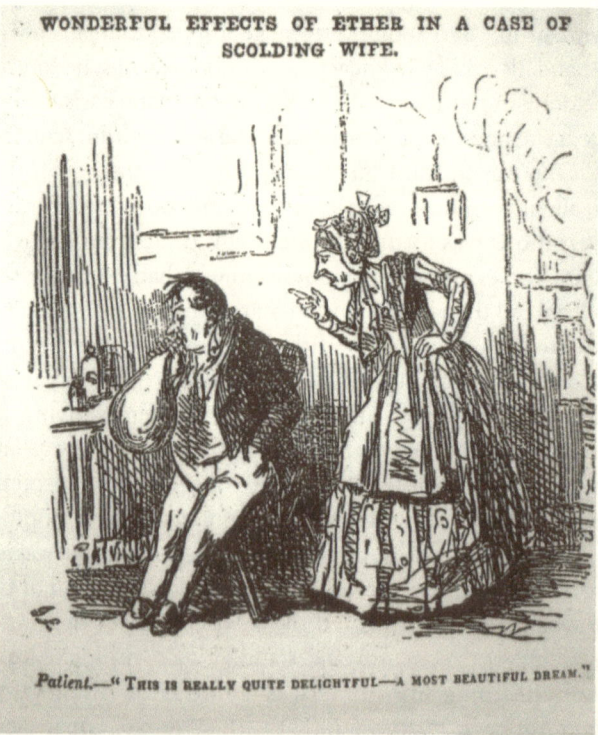

Fig. 3.3. *Punch* cartoon of 1847 indicating one aspect of public's appreciation of ether. (Source: *British Medical Bulletin* 1946-1947; 4:161.)

How to administer ether was explained most clearly and concisely by Snow. He first saw ether being given on December 28, 1846, when Robinson performed a dental procedure under ether anesthesia. Snow wasted no time in elaborating a sound basis for the practice of this new field of medicine, formulating a theoretical and a practical basis for the administration of ether. By June 1847, he had designed his own ether inhaler[21] (fig. 3.4); and by September 1847, he had written his own book on ether anesthesia, specifically with other practitioners in mind. (Strictly speaking, Snow's inhaler was a vaporizer, since it converted a liquid into a gas or vapor.)

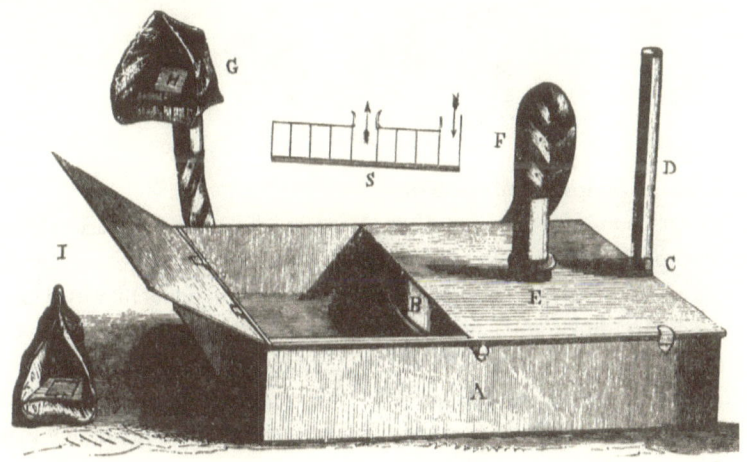

Fig. 3.4. Snow's ether inhaler (1847). (Source: J. Snow, *On the Inhalation of the Vapour of Ether* . . . [London: John Churchill, 1847], p. 17.

The second anesthetic agent was nitrous oxide. However, its use was held in abeyance until the summer of 1862—when itinerant chemistry lecturer Gardner Quincy Colton, in New Britain, Connecticut, gave a woman the gas so that a Dr. Dunham could extract some teeth[22]—when interest in it was reawakened. Interest was reinforced beginning in 1863, when it became possible to make nitrous oxide available in metal containers,[23] and in 1868, when it became possible to store it in metal cylinders.[24] After that, nitrous oxide was used widely, especially in dental practice.

The third anesthetic agent was chloroform. This was first used by James Young Simpson (fig. 3.5), the Edinburgh obstetrics professor, on November 8, 1847.[25] Chloroform was of more recent vintage than ether and nitrous oxide, having been discovered in 1831 by three individuals independently: New York natural scientist Samuel Guthrie[26], Paris pharmacy professor Eugene Soubeiran,[27] and Giessen chemistry professor Justus von Liebig.[28]

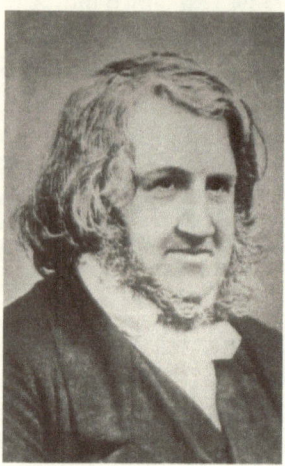

Fig. 3.5. James Simpson (1811-1870)

James Young Simpson's birthplace was Bathgate, near Edinburgh. At the age of fourteen, Simpson enrolled in the University of Edinburgh, where he studied Greek, Latin, and mathematics. This classical education gave him the background for his varied interests in later life, including the study of antiquities. However, he felt that his vocation was medicine, and he became a student of medicine, graduating in 1830. A short period in general practice was followed by a time as a pathologist, writing a thesis on inflammation. Simpson obtained the MD degree in 1832 and made a European study trip in 1835. His main interest in obstetrics and gynecology soon became evident, and he campaigned for the Edinburgh chair of midwifery in 1840. He won the coveted post by only one vote at the age of twenty-nine. Simpson was an able lecturer, but it was his charm, energy, conscientiousness, and aggressiveness also that propelled him upward to his appointment as one of the Queen's physicians in Scotland and the introduction of anesthesia for childbirth, both in 1847. Although Simpson was an obstetrician, his influence on anesthesia was profound, especially in defending the use of anesthesia in obstetrics. Together with John Snow, he was a key figure in shaping the development of anesthesia as the domain of physicians in Great Britain.

How Simpson learned about the potency of chloroform is the stuff of comedy and is always worth telling. His friend, David Waldie, a doctor who had researched chloroform in Liverpool, suggested to Simpson its possible use in anesthesia, the new field that had interested Simpson ever since he had given ether to a woman in labor on January 19, 1847.[29] (Waldie's role is analogous to Charles Jackson's in relation to Morton [see chapter 2].) On November 4, 1847, Simpson invited his assistants James Duncan and George Keith and some others, including a Ms. Petrie, to dinner. After dinner, Simpson offered his guests some elixirs to sniff, among them chloroform. According to legend, the chloroform put all the dinner guests to sleep under the dining table, Ms. Petrie believing she was an angel.[30] Simpson was entirely satisfied, and he tried chloroform on a woman in labor the very next day—no animal studies, no clinical trials, no federal approval, just a professor's authority! Simpson told his professional colleagues in Edinburgh about it on November 10, 1847, and the wider audience of the *Lancet* on November 20.[31]

Simpson customarily gets the credit for being the first to use chloroform, but he may not have been the first. In February 1847, Jacob Bell reported that chloroform, as chloric ether, had been used in the Middlesex Hospital in London.[32] And St. Bartholomew's Hospital surgeon William Lawrence may have used the same substance during the summer of 1847.[33]

It was around ether especially and, to some degree chloroform, then, that the principles and practice of anesthesia were formulated in the first fifty years of this new field. But for three reasons, anesthesia for many practitioners meant etherization. One was that many people thought of the introduction of anesthesia in terms of the introduction of ether, which, after all, was the first agent that was shown to be efficacious and reliable. The second reason was that it was relatively safe, and certainly less associated with serious problems than chloroform; thus the consensus grew that ether was the safer agent. The third reason was that until the 1870s, storage of nitrous oxide made that agent's use unreliable, apart from the aura of failure that stemmed from Wells' abortive demonstration. So it was ether that was most often expected to satisfy all the anesthetist's needs and the surgeon's demands. It was relied on to induce and maintain sleep, to secure freedom from pain during surgery, and to obtain relaxation of muscles.

The only other agent that had potential value in anesthesia was morphine. That had been available since Friedrich Serturner had synthesized and described it in 1805.[34] However, it was not used as an anesthetic agent *per se* in the nineteenth century, though in the 1860s, French physiologist Claude Bernard showed it could be used in laboratory work to potentiate, and so lessen the required dose of, chloroform.[35] Bernard's use of morphine presaged two other uses of morphine in later years: for premedication, which, however, was not introduced clinically in anesthesia until early in the twentieth century, and for the much later practice of using morphine as a primary component of anesthesia.[36]

In addition to the anesthetic agents, anesthetic apparatus constituted some of the raw materials of anesthesia. (See also chapter 7.) As with the need, starting in October 1846, for specific knowledge of anesthesia where none had existed before, so there was a need for apparatus designed specifically for anesthesia. In England, the first ether inhalers were adapted from those that had been designed for other purposes. An example is Nooth's inhaler (fig. 3.6), which was originally used to infuse carbon dioxide into water[37] and which medical student William Squire adapted when he gave ether while Robert Liston performed an amputation in London on December 21, 1846.[38] A similar inhaler was Hooper's, which dentist Robinson used two days earlier in London.[39]

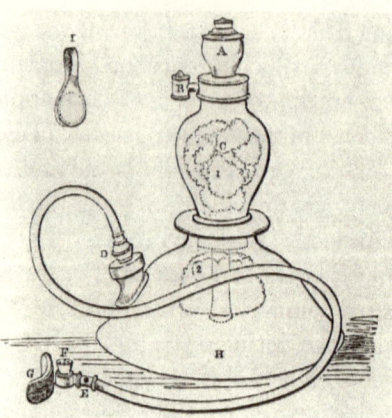

Fig. 3.6. Modified Nooth inhaler, as used by William Squire, 21 December 1846, in administering anesthesia for Robert Liston. (Source: B. Duncum, *The Development of Inhalation Anaesthesia With Special Reference to the Years 1846 to 1900* [London: Wellcome Historical Museum, 1947], p. 133.)

Because the Nooth and the Hooper had not been designed specifically for anesthesia, it was necessary to design special devices to vaporize ether and chloroform. (Nitrous oxide, a gas, had to be made on the spot and delivered from a crude tank and a face mask attached to a reservoir bag.) The first to be designed using scientific principled applicable to anesthesia was Snow's.

John Snow and His Contributions to Anesthesia

Much of the knowledge foundation of anesthesia, in relation to both basic science and clinical aspects, was established by Snow in the first decade of anesthesia. So significant was his work that it must be discussed, even if briefly.

Much of Snow's research in anesthesia anticipated much later work, such as that of precise control of anesthetic agents administered, the significance of saturated vapor pressure, blood-gas solubility, minimum alveolar concentration, and carbon dioxide absorption techniques.[40] He investigated many volatile hydrocarbon compounds in addition to ether and chloroform such as amylene and ethidine dichloride; he studied aspects such as the solubility of anesthetic agents in and the uptake of anesthetic agents by the blood; he investigated carbon dioxide production and absorption methods; and he pondered the nature of anesthesia and the difference, for example, between asphyxia and anesthesia. Clinically, he clarified the way anesthetic agents should be administered and the signs and stages of anesthetic depth, and he invented some of the very first pieces of anesthesia apparatus.

Snow was introduced to anesthesia on December 28, 1846, when Robinson extracted a tooth from a patient who received ether. Thinking about inhalers like the Nooth made Snow see how inefficient a glass inhaler was, for it would not prevent ether from cooling and losing potency. This insight was the beginning of his profound understanding of anesthesia and what was necessary to its effective administration. He realized that the temperature of the ether had to be controlled if the concentration inhaled was to be regulated accurately.[41] As early as January 16, 1847, Snow explained to the Westminster Medical Society one of the main problems of early anesthesia. He pointed out that "the operators did not at present know the quantity of vapour that they were exhibiting in the air . . . it would vary immensely according to the temperature of the air."[42] Most practitioners did not realize that after ether was placed in a glass vessel, it cooled as it vaporized, so that a lower concentration of ether was inhaled. Controlling the temperature of the ether was the way to accurately regulate the concentration of ether inhaled.[43] Snow had done all the necessary calculations; practitioners could act on his data.[44]

Though temperature control was the main feature of the Snow inhaler, two others were the adequacy of the area of exposure to ether and of the caliber of the tubing through which patients inhaled the ether so that there was no resistance to breathing.[45]

Another problem that Snow helped practitioners overcome was their ignorance of how much ether to give so as to induce and maintain anesthesia. Hence the opening of his book on ether: "The point requiring most skill and care in the administration of the vapour of ether is, undoubtedly, to determine when it has been carried far enough."[46] Snow classified anesthesia depth into stages, or degrees (table 3.1), each of which was correlated with clinical signs that practitioners could easily observe. In the third degree, for example, when anesthesia was deep enough to allow a patient to tolerate the surgical incision, the patient was quiet, breathed regularly, did not utter articulate sounds, and felt no pain. This stage could be recognized readily by looking at the eyes: the eyelids contracted when lifted up, and the eyeballs were stationary.[47]

Snow was adept as a clinical anesthetist. His approach was simple and straightforward, yet highly intelligent. It was simple in that, unlike Simpson in Scotland, Snow insisted that the practitioner feel the pulse *throughout* an anesthetic.[48] And it was Snow as a clinician that surgeons saw him; through him, they formed an image of what anesthesia could and should accomplish. He was highly regarded by the surgeons he worked with, such as William Fergusson and Caesar Hawkins, who themselves were leaders of London surgery. Snow showed surgeons, as well as other practitioners in anesthesia, what anesthesia was about: its scientific basis and how it should be practiced and what it was capable of accomplishing. In practical terms, he showed that there was a right way and a wrong way to give anesthesia. His results attested to that. Out of roughly four thousand patients whom Snow anesthetized, possibly one died due to chloroform,[49] and two died while anesthetized with amylene.[50, 51] Snow's record was unrivalled. As Caton observed, Snow's results shaped the approach other physicians took to anesthesia.[52] This made him an authority on anesthesia, and a role model for other practitioners.

Table 3.1. Snow's stages ("degrees") of ether anesthesia*

Degree	Clinical Sign
First	Awareness present
	Sometimes excitement, struggling
	Sensations in ears, struggling
	Moderate analgesia
Second	Semiconsciousness
	Voluntary movement (eyes, limbs)
	Resistance, disordered movement on surgical stimulus
Third	Lack of voluntary movement (eyes, limbs)
	Retention of eyelid movement
	Respiration "equable and regular"
	Partial absence of response to surgical stimulus
Fourth	Relaxation of all muscles
	Complete absence of response to surgical stimulus
	Breathing deep, sometimes stertorous
Fifth	Total flaccidity
	Respiration irregular, laborious, feeble; ceases

*Source: Ether-Snow, 1847, pp. 3-13; chloroform—Snow, 1858, pp. 35-48.

Snow used ether at first, but he preferred chloroform. He invented an inhaler for its use,[53] though when he anesthetized Queen Victoria in 1853[54] and 1857, he poured drops of chloroform on a handkerchief.[55] Snow, of course, always knew what he was doing; it has been said that "his approach was both bold and prudent—bold in its confidence and prudent in the way it controlled the dosage."[56] His teaching was influential, and his advocacy of chloroform influenced many other anesthetists in England, though fewer in Scotland. Snow and others liked chloroform because it was less pungent than ether and induced anesthesia more rapidly. For Snow, the benefits of chloroform outweighed the dangers, and he preferred it to the safer ether; it seemed more practical. As he told Benjamin Ward Richardson, Snow's friend and first biographer, "I use chloroform for the same reason that you use phosphorous matches instead of the tinder box. An occasional risk never stands in the way of ready applicability."[57]

Snow knew a great deal about chloroform. While it soon became clearer that chloroform was indeed more dangerous than ether, and while the unexpected death of fifteen-year-old Hannah Greener on January 28, 1848, was a setback, Snow took the opportunity to conduct research into chloroform and other anesthetics. He wrote about it, first in February 1848.[58] And three months later, he launched a series of eighty-three experiments into hydrocarbons with anesthetic potential, continuing until December 1851.[59] This was an important step, not only in Snow's own career, but for the development of anesthesia as a whole. It honed the research talents that Snow would demonstrate in his epidemiological investigations into cholera in London in 1849[60] and 1854,[61] and into the first fifty cases of anesthesia-related cardiac arrest.[62] In anesthesia, Snow's research enabled him to formulate the principles of anesthesia,[63] some of which are relevant today. The most important of those principles are listed in table 3.2. They helped put anesthesia on a scientific footing. At this early stage of anesthesia, Snow also clarified the distinction between asphyxia and anesthesia, which Hickman had pondered earlier (see chapter 2).

Table 3.2. Principles derived from Snow's research*

Relationship between agent temperature and vaporization
Accuracy of vaporizing devices in control of vapor strength
Significance of saturated vapor pressure
Apparatus effects on respiration, airway resistance,
including anatomical and airway dead space
Blood-gas solubility coefficients, pharmacokinetics
Anesthetic effect and blood-gas solubility: inverse relationship
Anesthesia dose and depth: direct relationship
Anesthesia depth preventing response to surgical stimulus (*cf. MAC***)
Carbon-dioxide production, absorption in anesthesia
Control of decrease in body temperature
Biotransformation of anesthesia agents
Anesthesia and asphyxia as distinct entities

*Source: R. Ellis (ed). *On Narcotism by the Inhalation of Vapours by John Snow MD* (London: Royal Society of Medicine Services, Ltd., 1991 [facsimile edition]), pp. xvi-xx.

**Minimum alveolar concentration.

Leaving Snow's preference for chloroform aside, the experience of others with chloroform justified the preference for ether in the United States and France. The various commissions that analyzed the results of chloroform anesthesia in the United Kingdom (*vide infra*) consistently supported the use of ether. To take one example, the British Medical Association committee that examined the data relating to the 25, 920 anesthetics that were given in Britain in 1892 reported that the "danger rate" of chloroform was eight times that of ether.[64] But by then, Snow had long been gone.

Snow, then, gave a decade of serious attention to the study and practice of anesthesia. How may his influence on the evolution of anesthesia be summarized?

As Richard Ellis noted, "Virtually alone amongst the earliest anesthetists Snow appreciated that the subject had a scientific basis which was important to understand and to apply."[65] He reached that point by deliberately educating himself to become the "compleat physician."[66] Here, he built on his knowledge of the basic sciences, particularly physics and chemistry. Early on, Snow had read widely, including texts by scientists like Joseph-Louis Gay-Lussac,[67] John Dalton,[68] and Andrew Ure.[69] In medicine, from 1836 to 1844, he went from being an apprentice in the North of England to a medical student to a physician who was not satisfied until he obtained the highest degrees that London could award him. So he became an exemplar for other physicians taking up the practice of anesthesia in England, and this is one of the reasons why anesthesia in the United Kingdom is still practiced only by physicians.

By incorporating scientific principles into clinical practice, Snow married the art and science of anesthesia. He initiated the process that would ultimately, though not for many years after his death, move anesthesia on the path of evolution from a rag-and-bottle practice to one that was based on scientific knowledge. Two anesthesiologists have succinctly summarized Snow's significance to anesthesia. Donald Caton observed that Snow was able to show doctors how they could administer better and more safely.[70] Ellis observed that Snow had a vision of what anesthesia could, or should, be.[71] In short, he was not only an authority but a representation of the ideal in anesthesia. The art and the science of anesthesia merged. His professionalism did much to set anesthesia on the path that would lead from craft to specialty.

Not all Snow's contributions to anesthesia were valued or understood in his day, any more than his contributions to the prevention of cholera were. However, they did help to lay the foundation for the practice of anesthesia, both in the short term and in the long term; and his influence on anesthesia in this formative period, and on other anesthetists, was immense.

The Influence of Clover, Buxton, and Hewitt

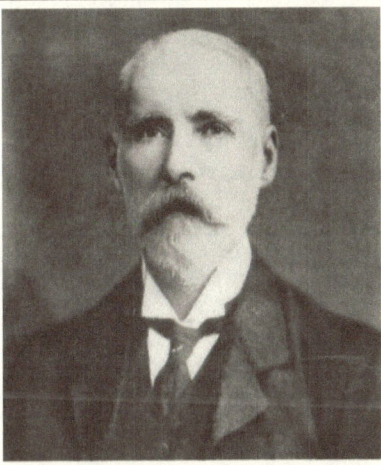

Fig. 3.7. Dudley Buxton (1855-1931)
Dudley Wilmot Buxton, a Londoner, was educated in London, at University College, and then at University College Hospital. He graduated in 1882 and obtained the MD degree in 1883. His initial work was in pharmacology, and he studied the actions of drugs on the heart. From 1885, he restricted his practice to that of anesthesia. Historically, Buxton's influence was overshadowed by Frederick Hewitt's, but the two men both filled the gap that was left by the death of Joseph Clover in 1882. Like Hewitt, Buxton stressed the need for education, believing that every doctor should have a working knowledge of anesthesia; the teaching of medical students was, therefore, important. He pointed out that anesthesia had failed to attract the attention of scientific elements in the medical profession. Together with Hewitt, Buxton did much to improve the standard and methods of anesthesia in England in the latter part of the nineteenth century and in the first two decades of the twentieth. His textbook on anesthesia of 1888 is one aspect of Buxton's influence. Buxton was also prominent in efforts to reduce the mortality associated with anesthesia mortality, and he was a member of three chloroform commissions. Their reports indicated that chloroform was significantly more likely than ether to be associated with death. Not surprisingly, Buxton used ether or gas and ether in his own practice.

Like Snow, Clover, Buxton (fig. 3.7), and Hewitt (fig. 3.8) all practiced in London. They kept an interest in anesthesia alive among physicians, and from them grew the English tradition of physician-anesthesia. That countered to some extent the custom in most hospitals of asking virtually anyone, experienced or not, to "pour ether," from the most junior of doctors to nurses to relatives and friends of patients and to hospital porters, which is one reason why anesthesia made relatively little progress in the nineteenth century. It was in a state of limbo; it was a craft that was decried by many individuals as being no more than "dropping ether" or "passing gas." Only later in the nineteenth century would anesthesia begin to emerge from a craft (in the sense of an occupation) to become a discipline, as a specific field of study that was based on scientific principles (see chapter 8). In England, the way for this transition was paved by Clover, Buxton, and Hewitt, all of whom knew that empirical knowledge was not enough when anesthetic agents were potentially dangerous, and they regularly informed other practitioners of that point.

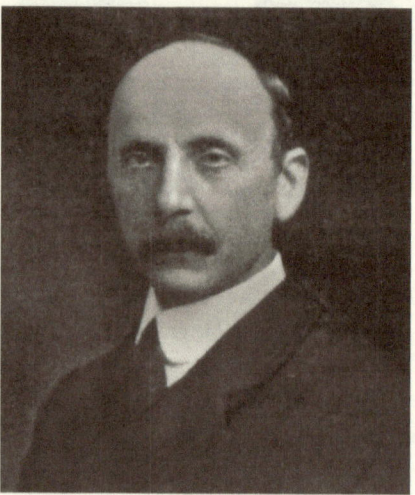

Fig.3.8. Frederick Hewitt (1857-1916)
Frederick William Hewitt was a Londoner. He was educated at Cambridge, and then St. George's Hospital in London. He obtained the Cambridge MD in 1886. His intention of taking up internal medicine was negated by poor eyesight; he opted for anesthesia. His natural intelligence and ability gained him appointments in anesthesia at Charing Cross Hospital (1884) and as a lecturer in anesthesia at the London Hospital (1886). A member of the staff of the National Dental Hospital (1885), Hewitt became interested in the use of oxygen with nitrous oxide. His studies stimulated his inventive mind, and the stopcock that allowed him to regulate the concentrations of oxygen and nitrous oxide was a result of his studies. Hewitt also invented an oral airway and modified the Junker and Clover inhalers. He stressed the need for education in anesthesia, and he did his part in this respect by lecturing and by writing three textbooks, particularly his *Anaesthetics and Their Administration*, which was first published in 1897 and went through several editions. Like Snow and Clover, Hewitt maintained the tradition of physician-anesthesia in England. Like them too, Hewitt anesthetized socially prominent individuals, most notably King Edward VII in 1902, just before the coronation was due to take place. For this, he was knighted; and in this, he differed from both Snow and Clover.

Clover, a qualified surgeon, was a highly competent anaesthetist who did much to advance anesthesia in the post-Snow era. He had a talent for invention,[72] and he emphasized the need for accuracy in the administration of anesthesia. In 1862, for example, he attached a large bag holding 4.5% chloroform in air (and not more) to a length of tubing that he slung over a shoulder and that was connected at the other end to a valved face mask.[73] (See fig. 3.2.) In 1876, he designed an apparatus that enabled him to induce anesthesia with nitrous oxide before giving the more pungent and irritating ether.[74] He followed this in 1877 with a portable regulating ether inhaler.[75] This was an improvement on other inhalers, for one could control the concentration of ether given, which made induction easier. Clover's inventiveness was an important step in the long process toward safer and more certain anesthesia.[76]

Hewitt too wished to make anesthesia safer and more effective.[77] Beginning in 1885, he carried out research into nitrous oxide anesthesia with the idea of adding oxygen to nitrous oxide. This had previously been done only by Edmund Andrews, the Chicago surgeon who had advocated it in 1868,[78] and by Paul Bert in France, who wrote about the gas-oxygen mixture in 1879, urging that the mixture be administered under pressure to get the full advantage of the analgesic property of nitrous oxide.[79] Hewitt's own solution was to incorporate a regulating device by which oxygen could pass through a controllable number of small holes to enrich the nitrous oxide with a varying proportion of oxygen. This nitrous oxide-oxygen stopcock he described in 1892 when he discussed the results of eight hundred cases of nitrous oxide-oxygen anesthesia.[80] Hewitt also designed an ether inhaler[81] to solve the problem of anoxia that was sometimes associated by Clover's ether inhaler. Another invention was the oral airway of 1908,[82] a device that is no anachronism today.

Hewitt's work was highly significant in the evolution of anesthesia. It facilitated the emergence of anesthesia from a craft, typified by the skill of the artisan, into a discipline, as characterized by a branch of learning. Hewitt combined clinical excellence, inventive ability, emphasis on education, and authorship. He took anesthesia as a branch of learning—as discipline—far beyond the skill and dexterity and empirical knowledge that characterized crafthood. Hewitt provided a link to the further development of anesthesia as a discipline that occurred particularly in the United States in the period before World War I. Hewitt understood the need for adequate respiratory exchange and efficient oxygenation, emphasized efficiency and safety in anesthesia apparatus, and worked in a manner that was always "painstaking, extensive and very fruitful."[83] All these were characteristics of Americans such as Walter Boothby, Karl Connell, and James Tayloe Gwathmey, who were, as related in chapter 7, all active in the twentieth century before World War I.

Hewitt's work, then, represented learning that moved anesthesia away from a craft. As with Snow, his learning came from his own investigations, which enabled him to discuss general points concerning nitrous oxide anesthesia, such as the position of the patient, the signs of anesthesia, and aids to anesthesia such as mouth props. He incorporated some of his knowledge into his writings such as *Select*

Methods in the Administration of Nitrous Oxide and Ether, published in 1888,[84] and *The Administration of Nitrous Oxide and Oxygen for Dental Operations*, published in 1897.[85] Like Snow, he was a master of the art and the science of anesthesia; like Snow, who anesthetized Queen Victoria when she was in labor in 1853 and 1857, Hewitt was a royal anesthetist, for he anesthetized King Edward VII in 1902.

Compared with Clover and Hewitt, Buxton lacked the *cachet* of the other two, but he did contribute to the gradual improvement of the status of anesthesia in this era.[86] Besides publishing a textbook in 1888,[87] he was an excellent clinical anaesthetist who advocated premedication and modified the Junker chloroform inhaler. He emphasized education in anesthesia and the importance and the methodology of teaching. He was a member of the British Medical Association committee that investigated the safety of anesthetics in England in 1892, and he wrote the report that was published in 1900. Buxton was also treasurer of the Society of Anaesthetists on its founding in 1893.

Clover, Buxton, and Hewitt, like Snow, were all physicians; and if in any sense they constituted a "school," it was one that was physician oriented. In this manner, the practice of anesthesia in England is distinguished, in ways both large and small, from practice, particularly in the United States. Other national differences may be discerned as the development of anesthesia in Scotland, France, the United States, and Germany is discussed.

Anesthesia in Scotland

Snow in London, Simpson in Edinburgh: a tale of two cities separated by a few hundred miles, but by significant differences in their approach to anesthesia. Those differences resided in their personalities and their approach to work. Snow was a general practitioner who came to specialize in anesthesia, as well as being, by force of circumstance, a diligent epidemiologist; Simpson was primarily an obstetrician who held a prestigious chair in an ancient university of great distinction, and whose interest in anesthesia was not his primary one. Snow was modest. His approach to anesthesia was careful and methodical, and he was aware of the need for restraint and for research. Simpson was outgoing and flamboyant. He was unconcerned with backing up his statements about chloroform and labor, for example, with adequate documentation.[88]

The Scottish approach to chloroform was identified with Simpson, who had introduced it in November 1847. Snow was ready to criticize the Scottish methods; Simpson was equally ready to criticize the English. Snow inferred from remarks by Professor James Miller, of Edinburgh, that chloroform in Scotland was given in a "somewhat slovenly, and not very cleanly manner."[89] According to Miller, "anything that will admit of chloroform in vapour being brought fully in contact with the mouth and nostrils" would do, whether a handkerchief, a towel, or a worsted glove; the Scottish method was than to "produce insensibility as completely and as *soon* [*sic*]" as is possible, whether this required fifty drops or five hundred. As far as Simpson was concerned, Londoners did not give enough chloroform; he told Charles Kidd that "you are too much afraid of it."[90] Lister, of carbolic acid fame, when still in Scotland, gives us another look at Scottish anesthesia practice. He wrote that "the very prevalent opinion that the pulse is the most important symptom in the administration of chloroform is certainly a most serious mistake." He even said that the pulse should be disregarded "altogether," and that instead, the attention should be on the breathing. Neither Snow nor Clover would agree with that; Clover's practice is clearly illustrated in figure 3.2.

Simpson is remembered for carrying the pro-chloroform banner in support of anesthesia to relieve the pain of labor (see chapter 14). Simpson made his own influence on anesthesia felt, and like Snow, he shaped the practice of anesthesia that others could follow as they wished. The English tended to prefer the scientific and the technological approach, while the Scots favored a minimalist approach. It is gently ironic that Snow, who developed two inhalers, is remembered as an anesthetist for his handkerchief technique *a la reine*[91] in anesthetizing Queen Victoria.

Anesthesia in France: Contributions of Physiologists

Some research into anesthesia was conducted in France, but primarily by physiologists. They were interested in the basic science aspects of anesthesia in the laboratory, not in clinical anesthesia, which none of them practiced. They studied anesthesia so they could immobilize their experimental animals; Claude Bernard is a notable example. They passed on information to surgeons, but they would apply this knowledge as they saw fit.

In this setting, clinical anesthesia was controlled by surgeons; French anesthetists barely existed. Among these surgeons were Joseph Francois Malgaigne, Philibert Joseph Roux, and J. E. Petriquet.[92] Another, Louis Velpeau, a professor of surgery in Paris, stated that pain relief in the form of what became known as anesthesia could never come about, though the evidence that anesthesia was a fact did later convert him. French surgeons failed to advance the cause of anesthesia. According to one M. Giraldes, some surgeons, even as late as 1868, would not make use of anesthetics at all.[93] Though concerned with clinical work, surgeons had even less impact on anesthesia than physiologists.

Physiologists at least conducted basic research. A prominent one was Marie-Jean-Pierre Flourens. He investigated aspects of chloroform and ethyl chloride while studying the physiology of the nervous system.[94] Even more prominent was Bernard. Trained in medicine, he became the exemplar of the experimental approach in physiology and medicine.[95] Though he worked on animals, he conducted basic research into the actions of anesthetics, concluding, albeit incorrectly, that they caused a reversible "semi-coagulation of the nerve-cell."[96] As noted in chapter 5, Bernard is better known in anesthesia for his study of the action of curare on the neuromuscular junction.[97]

Bernard's animal work led him to explain anesthesia as being the result of reversible semi-coagulation of nerve cells, though this was less fruitful than Snow's concept of anesthetic agents diminishing oxidation in the body.[98] More significant were Bernard's observations on morphine, which reduced the required dose of chloroform.[99] Like his seminal work on curare, which is discussed in chapter 5, years would elapse before morphine became an integral part of clinical anesthesia.

Bert also enhanced the theoretical understanding of anesthesia. He studied the physiological effects of high atmospheric pressure, and in 1878, he recommended that anesthetic gases be administered at high atmospheric pressure. The gas would be efficacious and asphyxia avoided.[100] This was theoretically sound, but difficult to apply, since a special mobile cast-iron chamber was required. Because the logistical difficulties could not be overcome in hospitals outside Paris,[101] Bert's technique was impractical.

Anesthesia in the United States

Anesthesia practice also had it own character in the United States in the second half of the nineteenth century, largely because the New World was huge and sparsely populated. The standard of medical education varied. Training in anesthesia lacked any formality, though the availability of the textbooks by J. F. B. Flagg (1851,[102] the first American textbook), Laurence Turnbull (1870),[103] and Henry Lyman (1881)[104] helped. Ether was widely used in the pioneering environment of the United States, though in cities, nitrous oxide was used also. Ether was considered safer and more practical than chloroform. Anesthesia was frequently given by nurses, under the eyes of surgeons.

Nitrous oxide, which had been used for the first time as an anesthetic in the United States, lay fallow after Wells' abortive efforts in encouraging its use as an anesthetic in 1845, and after while, Morton's own demonstration of ether established its merit. However, its resurgence also occurred in the United States, as a result of Colton's enthusiasm beginning in 1862 and its ready availability in cylinders later. Interest in nitrous oxide then stimulated the development of anesthesia machines, in England as well as the United States, though the growth of nitrous oxide anesthesia is best considered in the United States.

Colton's contribution to nitrous oxide anesthesia[105] is one of many examples of the variety of individuals and the conjunction of circumstances that make the history of anesthesia fascinating. As noted in chapter 2, it was Colton who, as a peripatetic chemistry lecturer, had stimulated Horace Wells' interest in nitrous oxide. For his part, Colton continued going about his business of lecturing, and he was doing so one day in the summer of 1862, back in Connecticut, this time in New Britain. Colton then told of having worked with Wells, and a woman in the audience asked him if he would give her gas while a dentist extracted some of her teeth. Colton did so, and at the same time showed the dentist, a Dr. Dunham, how to make the gas.

Colton returned to New Britain a year later, when the dentist told him that he had given the gas to hundreds of his patients. Colton concluded that giving gas might be better than being a peripatetic lecturer; and so in 1863, he set up the Colton Dental Association specifically to administer nitrous oxide. His efforts were facilitated by A. W. Sprague's having developed a new method of preparation of the gas from ammonium nitrate in 1863.[106] And from 1864 to 1897, more than 193, 800 patients were said to have received nitrous oxide in the office of the Colton Dental Association, evidently without a fatality.

Edmund Andrews, a Chicago surgeon, was also interested in nitrous oxide. He experimented with it in animals, and he gave it to four patients. He recommended the addition of 25% oxygen to the nitrous oxide as an alert to the danger of asphyxia.[107] He concluded that "there was strong reason to think that it will prove the safest, and by far the pleasantest, anaesthetic known." Sound though Andrews's idea of adding oxygen was, it had little impact beyond his native Chicago for many years. For example, Clover designed an apparatus for the administration of ether and nitrous oxide, which he described in 1876,[108] but it had no provision for oxygen as opposed to air. Not until 1886, when Hewitt began adding holes for oxygen in his inhaler,[109] was there any thought in England about the addition of oxygen.

Nitrous oxide was used in dental practice, while ether and chloroform were the main agents in general surgery and obstetrics. Though not perfect, unlike nitrous oxide, they could be given over long periods; they could also be given in the field and in people's homes. However, complications occurred. The most serious was death, which was more commonly associated with chloroform. (By 1863, in all countries, 123 deaths were attributed to chloroform anesthesia,[110] though this is likely not accurate since some cases would have gone unreported.) In this respect, nitrous oxide occupied a somewhat-different position from ether and chloroform. Though it did not have the obvious side effects of ether and chloroform, and was efficacious in operations lasting a few minutes, it was not safe in longer procedures. (In England, the Odontological Society's nitrous oxide committee reported in 1872 that it induced anesthesia by "preventing oxidation."[111]) Even when given with air, the amount of oxygen was so limited that asphyxia and anoxia were always possible—Bert's thinking was thus sound—though their more subtle manifestations might not be evident. This was not understood in the 1840s, when Wells used it, but then nitrous oxide was overshadowed by the advent of ether, and then chloroform, which could be used for lengthy surgical procedures. But for short surgical and dental procedures, nitrous oxide was an attractive alternative to ether and chloroform.

Other factors besides Colton's business and the Sprague manufacturing process maintained an interest in nitrous oxide. One was the demonstration and exhibition of gas apparatus in different cities. In 1867, Colton showed the apparatus in Paris, where American expatriate dentist Thomas Wiltberger Evans learned the technique of administration from Colton. The following year, Evans, in turn, demonstrated nitrous oxide in London,[112] where two influential individuals took up gas anesthesia. One was Clover, who modified his apparatus for chloroform anesthesia by attaching a supplemental reservoir bag to the face mask.[113] The other was the English dentist Alfred Coleman, who was the first person after Snow to use carbon dioxide absorption, incorporating "slaked lime" into his apparatus.[114] As Clover had in the 1860s,[115] Coleman used a nosepiece for nasal administration.[116]

The increasing use of nitrous oxide in the United States soon led to the development of machines for its administration. (See also chapter 7.) A prominent manufacturer was the S. S. White Company, which had produced cylinders for liquefied nitrous oxide in 1872 and for compressed oxygen in 1888.[117] The manufacture of apparatus for anesthesia with nitrous oxide was a logical step, and in the next few years, the company manufactured machines for the administration of nitrous oxide and, influenced by Hewitt's work in England, of oxygen.[118]

Anesthesia in Germany and Austria

Although in Germany what surgeons thought and said ruled the day, the first studies on the volatile anesthetic agent ethyl chloride were carried out there in the latter 1840s. Its ether-like action was studied by Ernst von Bibra and Emil Harless,[119] who confirmed Flourens' suggestion that it induced unconsciousness. Erlangen surgeon Johann Ferdinand Heyfelder then tested it in three patients in 1848,[120] with some success, though its volatility and its price militated against its use.[121] Like nitrous oxide, ethyl chloride was not used in anesthesia again until the 1860s, when, in 1866, Benjamin Richardson initiated its use as a local anesthetic by making use of the spray form to freeze local areas of skin.[122] Then in 1890, Camille Redard, in France, found that in spray form, it induced refrigeration local anesthesia of the gum.[123] And in 1894, H. Carlson, a Swedish dentist, was surprised to find that it accidentally induced general anesthesia in two patients.[124] One Thiesing, another dentist, had a similar experience in 1895.[125] Others confirmed the anesthetic properties of ethyl chloride, which then joined ether, chloroform, and nitrous oxide as an anesthetic agent, remaining in use for the next sixty years.

The work of Austrian F. E. Junker also is notable.[126] He graduated from Vienna in 1854 and became a member of the Royal College of Surgeons of England in 1860. He practiced in England, served in Germany during the Franco-Prussian War, and then became chief surgeon at the German Hospital in Saarbrucken. He continued to roam, moving to Japan in 1873 and back to England in 1882. In anesthesia, Junker is associated with the inhaler that bears his name[127] (fig. 7.5). He invented it in 1867, in order to limit the quantity of chloroform that could be inhaled. Though it was used in England, Switzerland, and Germany, it was not entirely safe: the attached hand pump and the possibility made the inhaled concentration vary. Even so, tributes to its value were paid in the form of the many modifications that were made, including those by Buxton and Hewitt in England as a chloroform inhaler.

Selection of Anesthetic Agent: Preferences and Mortality

Selection of the Anesthetic Agent

By the 1870s, both ether and chloroform were in wide use. They were efficacious, and they could be used for all types of surgery. In contrast, nitrous oxide, though efficacious and apparently safe, especially if given with oxygen, was considered suitable only for short procedures, especially as it did not provide muscle relaxation. Commonly, therefore, the choice was between ether and chloroform. But chloroform had the reputation of being the more dangerous, and deaths did seem to occur not uncommonly with it. Therefore, two questions were asked in the last three decades of the nineteenth century. One was whether to use ether or chloroform; the other, how dangerous chloroform actually was.

What governed the choice of ether versus chloroform? For major surgery, either might be used; though regional, national, and also personal preferences often ruled. In the lightly populated United States, ether, regarded as a Boston "discovery," was preferred over chloroform, which was used more frequently in the warmer south. However, chloroform seemed to be more dangerous than ether, and because relatively few physicians practiced anesthesia full-time, even fewer physicians were comfortably familiar with chloroform. The situation in England was different. Though both ether and chloroform were used there, the well-established tradition of physician-anesthesia that had begun with chloroform advocate Snow was associated with personal preferences for that agent. Moreover, the nonflammable chloroform did have the significant advantage of being safer for domiciliary practice in homes that were heated by open fires. Chloroform was also favored in Scotland and in Europe.

Other regional differences had an impact. In Europe, anesthesia was under the thumb of surgeons, and physician-anesthesia was slow to develop. In the United States, while in New York some physicians gave anesthetics, the country as a whole was still being developed; and much of medicine, including anesthesia, was imbued with the pioneer spirit. Even late in the nineteenth century, in both the United States and Europe, anesthesia was not thought to require physicians. In leading centers such as the Mayo Clinic, nurses shouldered much of the burden of anesthesia as they administered the preferred ether drop by drop onto gauze-covered masks. Between 1890 and 1920, nurse anesthetists Dinah and Edith Graham (the latter became Mrs. Charles Mayo), Alice Magaw, and Florence Henderson became highly skilled and greatly respected,[128] so that when Dr. Isabella Herb (later of ethylene fame[129]) joined the Mayo Clinic in 1899 as the first physician anesthetist, she found that her path had been forged by those remarkable nurses.

Studies of Anesthesia Mortality

Though practitioners became more familiar with anesthesia, its dangers were ever present. The 1863 report heightened the anxiety about chloroform. One problem in assessing anesthesia mortality is the difficulty of obtaining reliable data, but the German Surgical Society's statistics for 1890 were, and are, representative. The data for Germany, Austria, Russia, Sweden, Holland, and Belgium showed that among 24, 625 anesthetics, six were fatal, and that the chloroform mortality was one in 3776, in contrast to zero for ether given alone.[130]

The mortality associated with chloroform also concerned physicians in Great Britain and British India, where eight committees reported between 1864 and 1901. Though they provided little information that was unknown and that changed the pattern of practice, they did point to current concerns, and their recommendations are of historical interest.

The Chloroform Committee of London's Royal Medical and Chirurgical Society reported in 1864.[131] One conclusion was already familiar: chloroform depressed the heart, and the committee reminded practitioners that the use of a mixture of 2% to 4% in 98% or 96% of air incurred "little or no risk to life." A new recommendation was for the "ACE" mixture, which George Harley had concocted out of one part of alcohol, two parts of chloroform, and three parts of ether. Ether itself was thought to be "inconvenient." According to Duncum, this report marks the end of the supremacy of chloroform.[132]

Nitrous oxide replaced chloroform for dental procedures in England beginning in 1868, and the first report of the Odontological Society's nitrous oxide committee, published in that year, furthered interest in the gas.[133] Its second report, in 1872, warned that "nitrous oxide induced anaesthesia by preventing oxidation."[134] Evidently, nitrous oxide was also dangerous. Anesthesia was still far from perfection.

In 1875, a *British Medical Journal* census provided information about the choice and usage of anesthetic agents.[135] Chloroform was being used less often, being replaced by ether. Of note was Clover's sequential technique of administering nitrous oxide to induce sleep and ether then providing and maintaining surgical anesthesia. Chloroform, however, seemed useful in certain circumstances: operations around the head and neck, fracture work, obstetrics, and in the very young and the elderly.

In 1875 also, the British Medical Association struck the Glasgow Committee.[136] The same refrain—the "special danger" of chloroform and ether's "disadvantage" of a lengthy induction—was heard; and the committee, perhaps wishing to provide a different song, unexpectedly recommended that ethidine dichloride, investigated by Snow and favored by Clover, be preferred to ether and chloroform. Like so many committee reports, the Glasgow Committee's report, published in 1880, was ignored, and the nature of practice remained generally unchanged.

Two other commissions studied anesthesia outcome in India, assessing the dangers of chloroform in 1888 and 1889.[137] The interest in chloroform of Edward Lawrie, principal of the Hyderabad Medical School, led the Nizam of Hyderabad to form one commission. Lawrie claimed to have superintended forty thousand or even fifty thousand chloroform anesthetics with not one incident of heart damage or other dangerous event. The commission's method was to examine no fewer than 128 "full-grown pariah dogs,"[138] but this curious approach was too much for the *Lancet*, which opined that the findings were "utterly at variance with the experience alike of experiment and practice as carried out in Europe."[139] The *Lancet* challenged Lawrie to repeat the experiments, and pharmacologist Lauder Brunton represented the journal in Hyderabad. This time, experiments were carried out on "four hundred and ninety dogs, horses, monkeys, goats, cats, and rabbits." Surprisingly, in view of his earlier statement that chloroform killed by "stoppage of the heart,"[140] Brunton now cabled from India that the Lawrie experiments revealed that "danger from chloroform is asphyxia or overdose; none whatever heart direct."[141]

The *Lancet* remained skeptical. Supervised by Dudley Buxton, an investigation studied the effects of chloroform in human beings. A questionnaire was sent to physicians in Great Britain and to hospitals in Europe, the "Colonies," the United States, and India. The findings, collected by the end of 1891 and reported in 1893, differed from those of the Hyderabad commissions: deaths did result from heart failure.[142] The findings also confirmed those of the earlier chloroform committee reports of 1864 and 1880. The consensus in all these investigations was that chloroform was more likely than ether to cause death. Hewitt, however, pointed out in 1912 that statistics relating to death under anesthesia should be interpreted cautiously, since some deaths attributed to anesthesia should have been attributed to other factors. Even so, he estimated that ether was six times safer than chloroform and that in "ordinary" practice, ether was suitable for longer operations, and nitrous oxide for shorter operations.[143]

The various investigations into mortality may or may not have modified practice, but concerns about chloroform did have two positive consequences. The first was a definitive explanation for the effect of chloroform on the heart. Research provided two sets of answers. Research was conducted by J. A. MacWilliam, in Aberdeen, and W. H. Gaskell and L. E. Shore, in Cambridge. McWilliam's work was significant partly because, in 1889, he identified ventricular fibrillation as a cause of the heart failure and sudden death rather, not standstill of the heart in diastole.[144] That work was followed by A. Goodman Levy's finding in 1911 that ventricular fibrillation developed when cats were anesthetized with quite *light* concentrations of chloroform.[145] The second positive consequence was noted by Duncum: according to her, "the Report of the Second Hyderabad Commission . . . startled anaesthetists out of their lethargy and set them arguing . . . and observing and testing their observations."[146] The decline in anesthesia that had been taking place in the post-Snow years was halted. The greater understanding of problems such as anesthesia mortality that developed in the Buxton and Hewitt era generated a revival of interest and endeavor in the practice of anesthesia. It was another indication that anesthesia was evolving.

One other committee report of note is the British Medical Association's, formed in 1891. All anesthetics given in 1892 were scrutinized. Though its report did not appear until 1901, it did provide information that was still current.[147] It noted "the *cases of danger (including deaths) considered to be due entirely to the anaesthetic.*" Two important conclusions were, first, that chloroform, by itself or in combination, was six times more dangerous (in terms of death or potentially fatal complications) than ether, and second, that the rate for chloroform alone was more than eight times that of ether alone.[148] Specific death rates for anesthetic agents had, in fact, been given in 1888 by Buxton, as follows: for chloroform, one in 2500-3000; for ether, one in 23, 204; and for nitrous oxide, one in 100,000.[149]

*   *   *

The first half century of anesthesia was a formative one. The basis was initially laid by John Snow, who built up a specific body of knowledge and an understanding of anesthesia itself before he died in 1858. Joseph Clover, Dudley Buxton, and Frederic Hewitt, and French physiologist Claude Bernard added to the knowledge and understanding of anesthesia in the nineteenth century.

In general, however, from the late 1850s to the late 1880s, anesthesia evolved only slowly. This is not surprising: it was a brand-new field; few piercing minds were focused on it; and besides, medicine itself did not become a science until 1900, when an intellectual and scientific ferment redirected medical thought.[150] Hewitt summed it up well when he said in 1896 that the state of knowledge in anesthesia left much to be desired.[151] Yet in this period, a partial foundation for the practice of anesthesia was laid, even though the principles and practice of administering anesthetic agents and their effects on the body had to be learned, the function and operation of anesthetic apparatus to be understood, and the care of the temporarily unconscious patient to be mastered. There were other obstacles too: anesthesia had to appeal to physicians, the responsibilities of administering an anesthetic had to be appreciated, and the practice whereby so many unskilled individuals gave anesthetics had to cease; moreover, the mortality associated with anesthesia remained disturbingly high.

Anesthesia in this period was essentially a craft. The clinical aspect of practice developed as a result of empirical learning, formal education was lacking and, in the post-Snow era, research was absent. As a result, anesthesia failed to attain the status of a discipline in the nineteenth century, though the work of Hewitt in England in the 1880s and 1890s provided a basis for the evolution of anesthesia to the stage of a discipline—a transition that would not come until early in the twentieth century.

Chapter 4

A New Approach:
Local Anesthesia

Up to September 1884, only general anesthesia could prevent the pain of a surgical operation, though hypnotism, cold, and acupuncture were also used, much less frequently, in the Western world. All this changed on September 11, 1884, when Carl Koller (fig. 4.1) placed drops of cocaine in a patient's eye and operated on it without causing any pain. Koller did not just turn a new page in the history of anesthesia: he opened a new chapter.

Koller was an ophthalmology resident at Vienna's Allgemeines Krankenhaus, and so he was not high enough in the medical hierarchy to do what should be done next: to tell more senior physicians that he had made an amazing discovery. To satisfy protocol, and to obtain credibility, Koller asked Dr. Josef Brettauer to report his discovery to the German Ophthalmological Society that was scheduled to meet in Heidelberg on September 15, 1884.[1] The society thus learned of an approach to pain prevention and relief in surgery that was entirely new in now reliably making just one part of the body insensible rather than all of it as with general anesthesia. Koller's discovery of the powers of cocaine—a seemingly magical substance that, like curare, was obtained from a South American plant—was groundbreaking, in surgery at first and in anesthesia later.

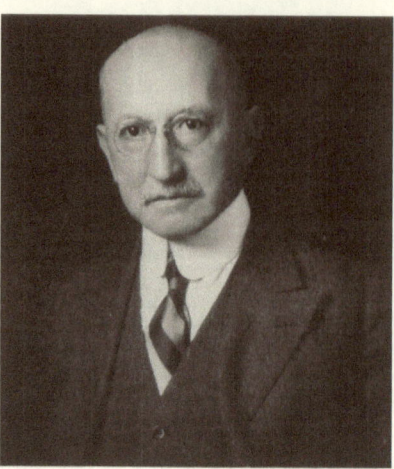

Fig. 4.1. Carl Koller (1857-1944)

Carl Koller was born in Schuttenhofen, Bohemia. He trained in medicine at the University of Vienna, graduating in 1882. Koller then studied ophthalmology under Carl von Arlt. While at Vienna's Allgemeine Krankenhaus, he knew Sigmund Freud, who wished to use cocaine as an addiction treatment for a morphine-addicted colleague. Koller's earlier research in embryology interested Freud, who thought that it would help him in his investigation of cocaine. Freud and Koller worked on cocaine together in 1884, though, while Freud absented himself to visit his fiancée, Koller continued the work on his own. It was then that Koller observed that his tongue became numb after it came into contact with some cocaine. Koller's association with von Arlt had made him aware that a substitute for general anesthesia might lessen the risk of eye-endangering complications such as nausea and vomiting, and he decided to see whether cocaine would numb the eye as well as the tongue. Experiments on animals, on himself, and on others showed Koller that it did. This finding was obviously worth reporting, and on September 15, 1884, Dr. Josef Brettauer reported to the German Ophthalmological Society on Koller's behalf. Cocaine immediately became of enormous value as a local anesthetic in ophthalmology. Koller had made a name for himself, and after he migrated to the United States, he built up a highly successful practice in New York.

This chapter, which is concerned with the early history of local anesthesia, focuses on two connected aspects of the subject. One is the introduction of cocaine in 1884 and of some of the drugs that replaced it beginning in 1904, including stovaine, procaine, dibucaine, tetracaine, and lidocaine. (Those that were developed after 1946 are considered in chapter 12.) The second is the way those drugs were administered, as in local infiltration or in nerve blocks, which constitute the practice of local, or regional, anesthesia. The context is that of two periods: the cocaine era and the post-cocaine era.

The Cocaine Era

Though the use of cocaine was new, the principle of local anesthesia was not. For hundreds of years people had known that cold would numb parts of the body, while compressing the nerves of limbs to abolish the circulation to them was also known to obtund feeling. English surgeon John Moore had described nerve compression in 1784,[2] and soon after that Baron Dominique Larrey, one of Napoleon's military surgeons, supposedly had used cold as an analgesic in amputations, though there appears to be no firm evidence for this.[3] London anesthetist John Snow in England also used cold with some success,[4] and ether and ethyl chloride sprayed on areas of the body froze and numbed the sprayed area as the spray evaporated.[5, 6] The ether spray was used in attempts to facilitate major abdominal operations such as ovariotomy[7] and Cesarean section,[8] but it acted only topically, and its effect was only transient. It sometimes had to be complemented with a general anesthetic. Though in these ways the principle of local anesthesia was established, the efficacy of the various techniques was not. Cocaine was infinitely superior.

Local anesthesia with cocaine was a great step forward because of its inherent anesthetic effect and because it clearly had many advantages over general anesthesia. In general anesthesia, a patient had to be made unconscious, and various aftereffects often followed recovery of consciousness. In contrast, cocaine could simply be applied to the surface of the eye or injected into the tissue under the skin, and absolute and long-lasting anesthesia resulted; and if it was used carefully, there were no side effects.

Physicians recognized the value of cocaine at once. One of those physicians was S. Ormond Goldan, of New York, who was active in anesthesia at the turn of the century and was the first anesthetist anywhere to use cocaine to induce local anesthesia. Goldan, who was also the first physician to suggest that anesthetists be recognized as "a distinct class,"[9] wrote two papers on cocaine given by intraspinal injection.[10, 11] However, he later switched to gynecology and gave up anesthesia.

Although other physicians—such as James Tayloe Gwathmey, the first president of the New York Association of Anesthetists; Adolph Erdmann, the founder-president of the Long Island Society of Anesthetists; and Providence physician Albert Miller—were prominent in anesthesia at this time, neither they nor their colleagues elsewhere incorporated cocaine into anesthetic practice in the early years of local anesthesia. It was not anesthetists but surgeons who made the greatest use of local anesthesia. They knew that general anesthesia, which could provide muscle relaxation only when very deep and which caused problems such as nausea and vomiting and even jaundice following surgery, did not satisfy all their operative needs, so they seized on this new drug. As they read about cocaine, many were fascinated by its history.

The Discovery of Cocaine

The history of cocaine is indeed fascinating: the story of the discovery of cocaine is as interesting as any in anesthesia. Its prehistory stretches back for centuries before it was ever used as a local anesthetic, and the story is full of adventure. Moreover, there are intriguing similarities between the prehistory of local anesthesia and that of general anesthesia. In each, the manner of the discovery offers interesting lessons in history. In 1934, after an extensive experience of both general and local anesthesia, Rudolph Matas, a New Orleans surgeon, reached this conclusion about the discovery of cocaine:

> Every epochal innovation has had its precursors and has been preceded by a more or less long period of intellectual and material preparation during which isolated observations and seemingly unrelated facts and experiences have remained latent and sterile for years and even ages, until some superior mind endowed with greater vision has risen out of the multitude to grasp the significance of the unrelated facts or phenomena and give them the character of a revelation.[12]

These comments are true of other discoveries in anesthesia, such as nitrous oxide and ether and curare. In discovering the effect of cocaine, Koller was preceded by others who had come close to realizing its significance earlier, and who broke the ground for later work. The same is true of the history of general anesthesia: ground was broken by Vesalius, Harvey, Boyle, Priestley, Beddoes, Davy, and Hickman, even though they themselves were not directly the instruments by which anesthesia was finally established by Wells and then Morton. Matas' comments illustrate other aspects of the elements of seminal progress: the raw material from which the discovery is made, the spirit of enterprise, imagination, capacity for logical and convincing demonstration, tenacity of purpose, and conviction in the face of opposition.

The history of cocaine is indeed a long one. It was obtained from the leaf of the shrub genus *Erythroxylum*. This plant, which grows in South America (as do the plants from which curare and similar substances are derived), may have been cultivated more than five thousand years ago.[13] The actual species from which cocaine is obtained in high concentration is *Erythroxylum coca*.

The coca leaf had long had meaning for the earliest peoples in the regions that the Incas came to occupy. Coca leaves were found beside mummies of Indians buried as early as the sixth century AD.[14] Many myths arose around coca. Before coca was a shrub, it was believed to have been a beautiful woman who was executed for adultery, cut in two, and buried, after which the coca plant grew from one part of her, blossomed, and was eaten by men in her memory. Later, coca leaves were offered to the Incas' gods to ensure safe passage of voyagers through the Andes and also in hopes of health being restored to the sick. Initially, coca had religious significance, and the leaves were eaten only by the upper classes. Later, laborers in public works projects and the military were allowed to chew coca leaves, because it seemed to maintain their energy. The local anesthetic properties of coca leaves were known in early times as well; the saliva issuing from chewed leaves was evidently dribbled over trepanotomy wounds.[15]

Much of our knowledge of the coca leaf comes from the Spanish occupants of South America.[16] In 1539, Vicente de Valverde, bishop of Cuzco, stated that chewing coca leaves sustained and refreshed the Indians; and in 1635, Bernabé Cobo noted that chewing coca leaves relieved a toothache. The addictive danger was known as early as 1582, when Francisco Falcon referred to the difficulty of freeing oneself of the "custom" of using coca. Accounts from many indigenous peoples indicate that primitive lore is often sound, and the history of cocaine illustrates that. For example, the validity of the ancient practice of chewing coca together with powdered chalk or shell ash was verified only recently, when it was shown that calcium carbonate enhances the absorption from the mouth of cocaine and its euphoric effects.[17]

Interest in coca was maintained, but attempts to isolate the active principle of the coca leaf could not be made until laboratory methods were developed. Then in 1860, the German chemist Albert Niemann isolated what he named cocaine.[18] Its molecule contained carbon, hydrogen, and oxygen atoms and a single nitrogen atom, a grouping that foreshadowed the interest to come concerning the relationship of the chemical structure of other local anesthetics, volatile general anesthetics, and muscle relaxants to their activity[19]—an increasingly important aspect of the understanding of anesthesia.

Niemann noticed that cocaine numbed the tongue, as did Wilhelm Lossen in 1865[20] and the Russian Basil von Anrep, who had been performing animal experiments in the same year.[21] Von Anrep and Tomes Moreno y Maiz in 1868[22] also suggested that cocaine might have use as a local anesthetic. But their suggestions, like Humphry Davy's of 1800 regarding nitrous oxide,[23] were ignored. They were not taken up for another decade and a half, when psychiatrist-to-be Sigmund Freud strode onto the stage.

In the early 1880s, Freud was working in Vienna's Allgemeines Krankenhaus, where a colleague, Ernest von Fleischl-Marxow, who was plagued by pain from a neuroma, became addicted to morphine. Freud, who sought to help Marxow beat the addiction, was familiar with the current opinion that cocaine aided patients in withdrawing patients from morphine addiction,[24] and he pursued his interest in this.[25] He was interested in the report by von Anrep[26] and one by Theodor Aschenbrandt on the uplifting effects of cocaine,[27] and he himself wrote a monograph on cocaine. He listed seven possible therapeutic uses for cocaine; one was its effect on morphine addiction, and another its value as a local anesthetic.[28]

Sometime in the summer of 1884, Freud was joined in his research by ophthalmology intern Carl Koller. Freud thought that Koller's earlier experience of laboratory experimentation in embryology[29] would be helpful in the study of cocaine, and so the two worked together. Taking it by mouth, they observed the effect of cocaine on their muscular strength and fatigue. Freud, however, had to absent himself for a while to visit his fiancée in Hamburg, and so Koller carried on alone.

Koller repeated the earlier discovery that cocaine numbed the tongue. In realizing the significance of this rediscovery, he went farther than other experimenters had by acting on it. Two circumstances led him to do this. First, he knew that his chief, Professor von Arlt, was always irritated by the nausea and vomiting that followed general anesthesia, since this jeopardized the outcome of his delicate eye surgery. An alternative to general anesthesia was clearly desirable. Second, Koller wished to produce a creditable piece of research that would earn him a position in the hierarchy of ophthalmology.

Cocaine's anesthetizing the tongue immediately impressed Koller. As he wrote, "I realized that I had in my possession the local anesthetic I had been previously searching for."[30] He went to the laboratory, instilled a drop of cocaine into a frog's eye and then into a guinea pig's. A eureka moment followed: the conjunctiva and the cornea were anesthetic. He did the same thing to himself, colleagues, and patients. The first eye operation under cocaine (for glaucoma) followed on September 11, 1884. Coca-Koller, as Freud called him,[31] had made one of the great discoveries in medicine. It ranks with Jenner's vaccination and Morton's use of ether and, later, with Pasteur's and Lister's work on microbial growth and its prevention and with Fleming's with antibiosis. It would transform anesthesia and surgery.

The news of Koller's discovery spread as rapidly as the news of ether had. Brettauer's reading of Koller's first paper, on local anesthesia on the eye, before German ophthalmologists on September 15, 1884,[32] was heard by New York ophthalmologist Henry D. Noyes, who promptly wrote to the *New York Medical Record*. His report was published on October 11, 1884.[33] Noyes thus scooped Koller because the New York report was the very first publication on the clinical use of cocaine to appear in the medical literature. Koller's second paper, which he gave himself to the Vienna Medical Society, was not published until October 25.[34] In any event, the response by the medical profession was immediate. As Seattle anesthesiologist Ray Fink remarked, "Everyone rushed to test the wonder drug on mucous surfaces,"[35] including the mouth and throat and the genital tract.

Cocaine and Early Nerve Blocks

New Orleans surgeon Rudolph Matas was one of those surgeons who realized that cocaine inaugurated a new era in surgery.[36] When used judiciously, cocaine was efficacious and safe. It was painted in glowing terms. It was "a marvel," "a miracle,"[37] and "a wonder drug."[38] The discovery was an "epochal finding," "a sensation,"[39] and "a prodigious achievement."[40] Certainly it was versatile; it could be used topically, in drops, or it could be injected into various parts of the body so that, like in the eye, they could be made analgesic. It was a splendid alternative to general anesthesia.

But cocaine had a down side, for it was not free of danger. Between 1884 and 1891, there were reports of thirteen deaths and two hundred cases of systemic intoxication that were attributed to the use of cocaine; sometimes it was given too freely in concentrations as strong as strong as 10% to 30%.[41] Therefore, cocaine had to be used judiciously.

A large part of the attraction of cocaine was that it could be given not only topically to numb the eye but also by injection, to numb areas of the body that were innervated by the cocaine-frozen nerves. Initially, the term that was used to denote this broader use of cocaine was *local anesthesia*, a term that was introduced by Edinburgh obstetrician James Young Simpson in 1848.[42] However, within a couple of months of Koller's discovery, cocaine was given in a number of different ways so that its numbing effects were local (when injected by infiltration of tissues) or regional (when injected in the vicinity of nerves or the spinal cord, that term itself being coined by neurosurgeon Harvey Cushing in 1902[43]).

By injecting cocaine into different parts of the body, surgeons—and much later anesthetists—were able to greatly expand its reach. Five techniques of injecting cocaine and its descendants were developed. One was to infiltrate a limited area of tissue under the skin around the proposed incision—the *infiltration* technique. Another was to inject the local anesthetic near large nerves, such as those of the arm or leg, to induce *regional anesthesia* in the part innervated by a single nerve (e.g., the ulnar) or of a nerve plexus (e.g., the brachial). A third technique was to insert a needle between the vertebrae, penetrating the space enclosing the spinal cord, and to inject cocaine into it. This technique, which was termed *subarachnoid anesthesia*, made the lower parts of the body numb since the nerves issuing from the cord were anesthetized. A fourth way was similar, though the path of the needle stopped short of the subarachnoid space. Known as *epidural anesthesia*, it was achieved by injecting cocaine so that it would be placed into the negative-pressure territory known as the epidural space, which lies closer to the skin than the subarachnoid space and from which it would be taken by the circulation to the larger nerves. The fifth technique was to inject cocaine into a limb vein, or *intravenous regional* anesthesia, which caused the limb nerves to become ischemic and in time affected with local anesthetic to a limited degree.

How early surgeons and, later, anesthestists used cocaine may be learned by considering the ways the nerves and the spinal cord were anesthetized using various nerve blocks.

Halsted and Nerve Blocks. Although the first to write about cocaine as a local anesthetic in the United States was William Burke, who injected 5 minims of a 2% solution into the right hand of a man with a bullet wound to block the ulnar area,[44] Richard Hall and William Halsted, in New York City, were the first to seriously study this form of anesthesia. Halsted realized that cocaine would block nerves and, with Hall, experimented with various techniques to do this. On November 26, some six weeks after Noyes' letter appeared, Hall published a report of nerve blocks in his own arm and leg and of the area around the infraorbital foramen for dental work.[45] Halsted followed this with a paper on cocaine in over one thousand minor surgical operations. He suggested that cocaine "probably produces anaesthesia . . . only when made into or very near a nerve-filament or nerve-trunk."[46] One of these procedures was *brachial plexus block*, which he was the first to perform. He did so by surgically exposing the nerve plexus that runs under the clavicle to the arm, and then injecting cocaine.[47] Halsted very quickly laid the basis for the practice of local anesthesia in the formative period from 1884 to 1904.

The evolution of local anesthesia can be thought of in terms of individuals, drugs, and techniques. Among the *individuals*, those who made seminal contributions, besides Koller, Halsted, and Bier, included the following: In the United States, the pioneers were Leonard Corning, Dudley Tait and Guido Caglieri, Matas, and Goldan; in Germany, Heinrich Braun, Alfred Einhorn, Heinrich Quincke, and Carl Schleich; and in France, Theodore Tuffier, Paul Reclus, Jean-Athanase Sicard, and Fernand Cathelin. The *drugs*, in addition to cocaine, were procaine (novocaine), stovaine, and Alypin. The *techniques*, besides peripheral nerve anesthesia, consisted of sacral epidural anesthesia, subarachnoid anesthesia, infiltration anesthesia, and intravenous regional anesthesia.

Corning, Quincke, Bier and "Spinal" Anesthesia. Corning, a New York neurologist, reasoned that a drug like strychnine acted on the spinal cord not directly but through the local blood vessels as the intermediary.[48] On October 27, 1885, he wrote that injection in the "vicinity" of the cord of a "minimum quantity of a medicinal substance" would produce "the most immediate, direct, and powerful effects," and that injection of cocaine would induce such effects after the circulation had taken it to the cord. Corning injected 5 minims of a 2% solution of cocaine "into the space situated between the spinous processes of two of the inferior dorsal vertebrae" of a dog, after which the hind legs appeared to become anesthetic. In a man, he injected 30 minims of 3% "between the spinous processes of the eleventh and twelfth dorsal vertebrae," and again after six or eight minutes had elapsed. These two injections impaired the sensibility of the lower half of the body for "an hour or more."

Although Corning was the first to think of placing cocaine in the vicinity of the spinal cord, he probably injected it in the epidural space rather than near the spinal cord in the subarachnoid space. His concept was that of an indirect rather than a direct effect of cocaine on the cord, by depositing the solution in the area of the *venae spinosae*. Corning never referred to the subarachnoid space, which is filled with cerebrospinal fluid, or to the presence of such fluid when he inserted the needle. That is why it is thought that he was actually inducing epidural rather than subarachnoid anesthesia. Even so, in his initiative lies the origin of the approach, developed much later, of *neuraxial* (subarachnoid or epidural) anesthesia.

Anatomical knowledge of the subarachnoid space, which encloses the spinal cord, and of the liquid that bathes the cord, is essential whenever a drug—whether a local anesthetic or a drug like an antibiotic—has to be placed very close to the spinal cord. That the spinal cord is bathed in cerebrospinal fluid (CSF) was known to Dominico Cotugno in 1764,[49] and Quincke understood its significance in 1891, when he drew off some of the fluid by lumbar puncture to reduce the increased pressure in patients with hydrocephalus.[50] This technique had been described earlier by Essex Wynter, who used a Southey tube,[51] but Quincke made the point that the lumbar puncture needle would not impinge on the spinal cord if it was inserted below the second lumbar vertebra in adults and the third in children. Quincke is therefore credited with the first use of lumbar puncture.

Bier was the first to actually inject cocaine in the subarachnoid space in order to induce local anesthesia. A colleague of Quincke's, he realized that cocaine when given by infiltration anesthesia had limited value as an alternative to general anesthesia for major surgery, and Schleich himself, in 1895, described its use only in minor operations.[52] Bier concluded that it was better to inject "extraordinarily small amounts of cocaine (0.005 gm.)" into the CSF, so that it would spread to affect not only the spinal cord but also unmyelinated nerves.[53] As he put it, "large areas of the body can be made insensitive to pain and major operations can be performed within these areas." Bier reported his experience in six patients whom he anesthetized between August 16 and 27, 1898. This was an enormous step forward, though it was initially only a faltering step, for vomiting and headache marred the postoperative course. Bier therefore decided, in the honorable tradition of self-experimentation, to submit himself to lumbar puncture and the injection of cocaine. Dr. Hildebrandt, Bier's assistant, performed the lumbar puncture, injecting 0.005 grams of cocaine. However, the needle did not fit the Pravaz syringe, and "much" CSF was lost, so the experiment was unsuccessful. Hildebrandt—no doubt feeling abashed, if not ashamed—then volunteered to be the guinea pig. This time, no CSF was lost, and anesthesia was induced. Even so, both Bier and Hildebrandt noticed that they had a headache. That was a lesson, and Bier thought that the headache in their case was in part due to their being too active after the experiment—drinking wine, smoking cigars, and walking and working the next day—and also due to the loss of CSF. Bier concluded his article with the following words: "The escape of cerebrospinal fluid should be avoided, if possible."

Bier's courageous initiative not only laid the basis for future practice but accurately presaged it. As Harvard anesthesiologist Leroy Vandam put it in 1989, "every detail of spinal anesthetic technique as we practice it today was known [then] except for minor details regarding apparatus and drugs, and with a beginning awareness of the immediate and delayed complications."[54] Cocainization of the spinal cord (subarachnoid anesthesia) became a standard technique, and a great deal of surgery was performed, as it still is, under subarachnoid block. The two great advantages of this type of block are its providing complete analgesia in one part of the body and excellent muscle relaxation—relaxation that was difficult to provide with ether or chloroform except when large amounts of these agents were given. Among those surgeons who followed Bier's initiative were the following: In the United States, Tait and Caglieri, in San Francisco, performed subarachnoid block on October 26, 1899, [55, 56] and Matas, in New Orleans, did so on November 10, 1899.[57, 58] In France, subarachnoid anesthesia was popularized by Tuffier, who gave his first spinal anesthetic on November 9, 1899.[59]

Schleich and Infiltration Anesthesia. Even though Bier had pointed out the defects of the simpler technique of injecting cocaine under the skin so as to infiltrate the tissues in the operative field, the technique had much practical value for surgeons. The technique had been suggested by Halsted, as he pointed out to Sir William Osler, when he first began using cocaine.[60] Beginning in 1890, other surgeons began practicing infiltration anesthesia. In France, Reclus realized that deaths associated with cocaine resulted from use of high concentrations, and he thought that lower concentrations, such as 0.05%, would prevent absorption of cocaine in toxic amounts.[61] Pernice and Kummer, in France, also used cocaine to infiltrate the tissues,[62] but the most notable proponent of infiltration anesthesia was Schleich in Germany.[63] He used an even more dilute solution of 0.02%, thinking that a 0.02% solution of salt would come halfway between the water that Halsted had used and the "normal" salt solution of 0.6%. Braun, however, regarded Schleich's ideas as unphysiological, holding that the infiltrative solution should be of the same osmotic pressure as body fluids.[64]

Sicard and Cathelin and Sacral-Epidural Anesthesia. Epidural anesthesia was achieved in 1901, when Sicard echoed Bier's observation that cocainization of the spinal cord was sometimes attended with "certain difficulties."[65] After experimenting in dogs, he injected a cocaine solution into the sacral canal, which is anatomically an extension of the epidural, in nine patients with neuralgic pain of the lumbar region. The pain was immediately relieved. Since this technique appeared to be "absolutely innocuous," Sicard recommended that sacral injection replace subarachnoid injection. Independently and simultaneously, Cathelin, also of Paris, came to the same conclusion.[66]

Bier and Intravenous Regional Anesthesia. Bier also conceived of the technique of local anesthesia that he termed "direct vein anesthesia," known today as intravenous regional anesthesia. Describing his technique in 1908,[67] he used procaine, its lower toxicity being compatible with injection into veins. He exsanguinated an area in the arm or leg by placing two tight bands around the arm and injected procaine so that it would be distributed throughout the bloodless area. This area became anesthetized within fifteen minutes, remained so as long as the proximal band was left in place, and regained normal sensation soon after the band was released.

The Post-Cocaine Era

The toxicity of cocaine necessitated a search for replacements. Procaine, which was described in 1905 by Braun, of Germany,[68] met many of the needs, and it remained the standard local anesthetic for another four decades. Bier's use of it for intravenous regional anesthesia in 1908 illustrates its value. (Stovaine, introduced in 1903, was also widely used for a while.) After the First World War, dibucaine (Nupercaine), introduced in 1925, and tetracaine (Amethocaine, Pontocaine), introduced in 1928, were added to the list of local anesthetics. The new drugs were all amino esters and had that in common with cocaine. However, none of these cocaine replacements was ideal. Procaine was not particularly potent; and the potential, and sometimes actual, toxicity of dibucaine and tetracaine when given in large volumes in practice limited their use to subarachnoid anesthesia.

The replacements for cocaine became available when anesthesia was undergoing great changes. They augmented the progress that was being made in this era when anesthesia was a discipline, and together with the development of nerve blocks, anesthetic practice was greatly enhanced. Some facets of this aspect of the development of anesthesia and of an enhanced understanding of local and regional anesthesia merit brief discussion here.

Subarachnoid Block: Research and Usage

When Bier introduced subarachnoid anesthesia in 1898, he had no way of realizing that it would frequently lower the blood pressure, because the pressure in surgical patients was not measured until Harvey Cushing described sphygmomanometry in 1902.[69] The problem of low blood pressure, or hypotension, was not investigated until 1912, when H. T. Gray and L. Parsons, in England, did so.[70] They attributed hypotension during subarachnoid anesthesia, which froze the thoracic, as well as the lumbar nerves, to paralysis of the abdominal and thoracic muscles, which in turn decreased the negative intrathoracic pressure during inspiration. In 1915, G. S. Smith and W. T. Porter examined the blood pressure variations in cats that had been subjected to subarachnoid block.[71] They concluded that the volume, rather than the concentration, of the anesthetic was an important factor and that hypotension resulted from paralysis of the vasomotor fibers that regulate the tonus of the splanchnic vessels. A third view was that of Gaston Labat, who suggested in 1927 that it's not the fall in blood pressure itself as the resulting depression of the circulation to the brain.[72]

Two solutions for this problem were proposed. One was to inject ephedrine subcutaneously before the local anesthetic could have an effect, which became standard practice for many years. The other solution was to control the flow of the anesthetic agent in the CSF. Arthur Barker, a London surgeon, proposed this in 1907.[73] Using stovaine, he found that baricity (or specific gravity) of the local anesthetic agent and position of the patient influenced the spread of the stovaine. To help him visualize the spread of the anesthetic agent, Barker designed a glass model of the spinal canal. He made the specific gravity of the local anesthetic heavier than that of the CSF (i.e., hyperbaric) by adding glucose to the solution, positioned his patients carefully, recommended puncture in the midline so as to ensure even spread of the anesthetic agent, and stressed the need to see that the CSF flowed satisfactorily before the agent was injected. Barker's careful approach to subarachnoid block is an example of the fact that, as Vandam observed, the essentials of the technique of subarachnoid anesthesia was laid down in the earliest years.[74]

In contrast, hypobaricity was proposed by W. W. Babcock in 1912.[75] Like Barker, Babcock used stovaine, and with 10% alcohol, he created a solution with a specific gravity of 1.000, which was lower than the 1.0065 for CSF. Babcock's technique seems cavalier today: his patient was seated during the injection phase, he was quite happy to operate on the stovaine-anesthetized head and neck, and he evidently combined the duties—as was common practice in those surgeon-oriented days—of surgeon and anesthetist. On the other hand, he knew what he was doing and, in particular, was concerned about adequate resuscitation should the need arise.

Surgeons liked subarachnoid anesthesia because it provided excellent anesthesia and because the mortality was not high. As noted in chapter 3, general anesthesia, especially chloroform, continued to be associated with disturbingly high death rates, though they varied from hospital to hospital, and from report to report over the years, so that the data are impossible to validate. However, those rates did appear to be much higher than those associated with subarachnoid anesthesia. Matas, for example, referring to the experience at the Charity Hospital in New Orleans from 1899 to 1926, when 7,322 subarachnoid anesthetics had been given, stated that there were only thirty-four postoperative deaths, none being attributed to the anesthesia.[76] Even if mortality was attached to subarachnoid anesthesia, particularly if a "total spinal" and hypotension were not recognized and so not treated, many surgeons preferred subarachnoid to general anesthesia.

Matas was not the only surgeon who opted for subarachnoid block as the anesthesia of choice for a variety of operations. T. Jonnesco, in 1909,[77] and

H. Koster, of New York, in 1928,[78] favored subarachnoid anesthesia for many surgical procedures, including those above the torso such as thyroidectomy and tracheoplasty. Like Matas, they considered that high subarachnoid block was safe, even for operations well above the diaphragm. Obviously, operations lower in the body would seem more suitable, and so subarachnoid block was a natural choice for some in obstetrics. As early as 1900, Otto Kreis, in Switzerland,[79] and S. Marx, in the United States,[80] injected cocaine intrathecally to relieve childbirth pain.

Several other problems existed besides hypotension with subarachnoid block. A common one was headache afterward, as Bier had found out in 1898.[81] In the 1920s, as many as half the patients complained of headache. One recommendation was for the patient to drink plenty. Tait and Caglieri believed that increased intracranial pressure caused the headache; the flow of CSF through the lumbar puncture needle appeared to be greater if saline was given intravenously,[82] which was consistent with the advocacy of fluids in abundance. However, the caliber of the needle turned out to be the most important factor. Lincoln Sise, of Boston, used an introducer that allowed a narrower needle to pass through the tough tissues on its way to pierce the dura, which lessened the likelihood of CSF leak.[83] Sise also was concerned with the mortality of subarachnoid block, which in some hands was as high as one in one hundred patients in the 1920s.[84] Sise helped to reduce this to less than one in one thousand, in part by controlling the fall in blood pressure by injecting ephedrine subcutaneously.[85]

A different problem was the duration of anesthesia, which might be too short for some operations and too long for others. William Lemmon, of Philadelphia, was concerned with anesthesia that was too brief, and to overcome this, in 1940, he developed what he termed "continuous spinal anesthesia."[86] He inserted a malleable needle into the subarachnoid space, bent it so that it could be made to lie flush with the skin, attached rubber tubing to the hub of the needle, and then injected 1 ml to 2 ml of a solution of 600 mg of procaine with 6 ml CSF when required.

Growth of the Practice of Regional Anesthesia

The 1920s and 1930s were in many ways a fruitful period in anesthesia, and progress in the use of local anesthetics contributed to it. Anesthetists began to show increasing interest in administering nerve blocks, both to patients undergoing surgical operations and to those with chronic pain. Instrumental in these respects was Gaston Labat (fig. 4.2). A French surgeon whom Mayo Clinic surgeon Charles Mayo invited to Rochester, Minnesota, to teach regional anesthesia at the Mayo Clinic, Labat worked there in 1920 and 1921. In addition to teaching, he wrote his influential textbook on regional anesthesia.[87] His legacy launched, Labat moved to New York,[88] where he continued to publicize the value of regional anesthesia both in his book and in his involvement with the American Society of Regional Anesthesia, of which he was founding president in 1923.[89]

After Labat left, John Lundy oversaw regional anesthesia at the Mayo Clinic. Later head of anesthesia there, Lundy greatly benefited from Labat's earlier presence in Rochester, and he in turn influenced others, notably Ralph Waters. In 1927, Waters moved to Madison, Wisconsin, and set up a department and a residency program and taught local anesthesia to a myriad others,[90] who, as "Aqualumni," spread the word. Anesthetists began to use local anesthetics increasingly. Labat's influence thus reached far.

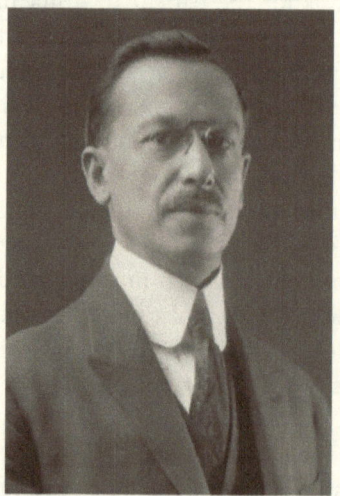

Fig. 4.2. Gaston Labat (1877-1934)

Gaston Labat, a native of the Seychelles, was educated in Mauritius, where he worked as a legal clerk. He also had a job constructing machinery that was used in the sugar business. He was thirty-eight before he began to study medicine in Montpellier in France in 1914. He interned in Paris and shared an interest in regional anesthesia with leading French surgeon Victor Pauchet. He became skilled in regional anesthesia as a result, paravertebral block being a special area of expertise. In 1920, Labat's skill in regional anesthesia was noted by Charles Mayo, who was visiting Paris, and Mayo invited Labat to move to the Mayo Clinic in order to teach regional anesthesia there. He remained in Rochester for a year, and then moved to New York, where he built a successful career in anesthesia. He wrote his celebrated textbook on regional anesthesia in 1922, was appointed clinical professor of surgery (anesthesia) at Columbia in the same year, and was elected founding president of the original American Society of Regional Anesthesia in 1923. He performed his clinical work in anesthesia at Bellevue Hospital in New York City.

Local Anesthesia as a Component of Balanced Anesthesia

It was at this time that Lundy conceived the concept of balanced anesthesia,[91] a concept that logically embraced local anesthesia. It illustrates what anesthetists were trying to do in the second half century of anesthesia. Originally, anesthesia was induced and maintained by ether or chloroform, which was given in blunderbuss fashion to provide all the components of the triad of unconsciousness, analgesia, and muscle relaxation. Later, they were achieved to a varying degree by different drugs. Nitrous oxide would be used with ether; or ethyl chloride might be given to induce anesthesia, which was anesthesia by ether or chloroform; or the ACE mixture of alcohol, chloroform, and ether might be administered. The idea behind balanced anesthesia was to deliver smaller doses of each, so that the best features of each drug could be relied on and the worst features minimized. In Lundy's day, a hypnotic was given before operation, local or regional anesthesia induced with a drug like procaine, and general anesthesia induced with an inhalational agent. Relatively small amounts of each drug lessened the unpleasant untoward results of anesthesia. The concept of balanced anesthesia remained valid even when other drugs were introduced in later years.

Local anesthesia thus added a new dimension to anesthetic practice. If the advent of the general anesthetics in the 1840s was one revolution, that of cocaine and other local anesthetics by anesthetists in the 1920s was another. Local anesthesia gave anesthetists greater opportunities to provide pain relief in patients in operating rooms and, in time, in patients in other areas such as the labor suite and pain clinics.

Development of Other Nerve Blocks

The prototype of nerve block was *brachial plexus block*, as practiced originally by Halsted in 1884, though he exposed the plexus surgically first. Of more interest to anesthetists, who did not expose nerves surgically, were Hirschel's description of the percutaneous approach via the axilla and Kulenkampff's of the supraclavicular, both in 1911.[92] Their techniques were later modified, but the basis for brachial plexus was laid quite early in the twentieth century. Blocks of other nerve plexuses were also described early: paravertebral by Sellheim in 1906,[93] celiac by Braun in the same year,[94] cervical by Rovenstine and Wertheim in 1912, and stellate by Labat in 1930.[95]

Caudal block, the basis of which had been established in 1901 by Cathelin[96] and Sicard,[97] became popular in obstetrics beginning in 1909 with the work of W. Stoeckel, a German gynecologist. Cathelin, a urologist, only had available the potentially toxic cocaine, which he thought unwise to give to women in childbirth. Stoeckel, however, was familiar with the less toxic procaine, which he used with some success in caudal blocks.[98] He was careful to warn that labor might be slowed if the analgesic effect was great.

In 1942, Waldo Edwards and Robert Hingson, of Cleveland, Ohio, refined the caudal technique by adding the element of continuity to the block. They injected metycaine through a malleable needle at intervals, thus providing a continuous block.[99] They provided more details in a fuller account in 1943, which was based on reports of 10, 000 cases managed in North American medical schools and teaching hospitals, as well as an analysis of 1, 050 cases of their own.[100] Yet Edwards and Hingson failed to acknowledge what S. A. Manalan had done, at much the same time, in introducing a ureteral catheter through a needle and leaving it in place until analgesia was required.[101] However, the Manalan technique was not truly continuous. Caudal block was also advocated for use in general surgery, Arthur Lawen doing so in 1910.[102]

The basis for the closely related *epidural block* was also laid at the beginning of the twentieth century. The epidural approach, with the needle placed most frequently in the lumbar region rather than the sacral, was described by the Spaniard Fidel Pages in 1921.[103] Acknowledging the caudal technique as used by Cathelin, Sicard, and Tuffier, and Kappis' observation of 1912 that liquids injected into the paravertebral space did spread into the epidural space, in 1920 Pages conceived the idea of "detaining" a needle inserted intraspinally within the spinal canal, but before it pierced the dura. He found that an injection of 375 mg of novocaine in 25 ml of physiologic serum through a cannula produced hypesthesia that permitted an inguinal hernia to be repaired "without the least discomfort to the patient." He described his results in forty-three patients, in only two of whom the block was unsuccessful. Pages's article is admirably detailed and illustrated, and it says much for his work as an individual investigator, who was then a *capitan medical* in the military. Pages was followed in 1931 by Archile Mario Dogliotti, in Italy, who benefited from the recent discovery that the pressure in the epidural space was negative.[104] The following year, Eugene Aburel, of Romania, inserted a ureteral catheter to provide continuous block in labor.[105] And Alberto Gutierrez, in Argentina, described the hanging drop technique to identify the epidural space.[106]

The Introduction of Lidocaine

The search for local anesthetic agents continued in the first half of the twentieth century, and the synthesis in 1943 of lidocaine was a milestone in this quest. Its synthesis is another example of the contributions that chemists have made to anesthesia and, in particular, of the part that an understanding of the relationship between chemical structure and pharmacological activity plays in those contributions. Lidocaine differs from the earlier local anesthetics in being an amide compound. The new drug was found to be relatively safe, stable, and of longer duration than procaine. From 1946 on, lidocaine greatly expanded the scope of local anesthesia.

The synthesis of lidocaine is another of the many human endeavors that make the development of anesthesia fascinating.[107, 108] The story starts in the early 1940s in Sweden with B. A. F. Erdtman's finding that gramine, an alkaloid, numbed the tongue. In contrast to the history of cocaine, there was now no delay between an observation and intensive research. Research on aniline derivatives was conducted by Nils Lofgren and Bengt Lundqvist between 1943 and 1946. Lidocaine was actually synthesized in 1943, but its stability and resistance to the high temperatures of resterilization warranted further study. Studies included Lundqvist's using lidocaine on himself, even by subarachnoid administration. There was some delay in selling the rights to a commercial company, but these were purchased by Astra Laboratories in September 1943.

Clinical testing was done by anesthesiologist Torsten Gordh and his physician wife, whose subjects included students. Remuneration was the equivalent of sixty cents for nonstudents: either Gordh's 1945 thesis or a package of American cigarettes. Naturally, the latter, being difficult to obtain in wartime, were preferred. Gordh presented the results to the Swedish Anesthesia Club in 1947 and published them in 1948,[109] as was Lofgren's thesis on lidocaine.[110] Thereafter, this new wonder drug, with its high tissue penetrance and low systemic toxicity, was used increasingly widely and replaced procaine as the standard local anesthetic.

The release of lidocaine, with its lower toxicity, allowed anesthesiologists to use it for any of the standard local anesthetic techniques, such as peripheral nerve blocks, infiltration anesthesia, subarachnoid anesthesia, caudal epidural anesthesia, and intravenous regional block. This was similar to the situation in general anesthesia: those anesthesiologists working in the 1940s were the beneficiaries of all the painstaking and challenging work that their predecessors had done and so laid a path to a smoother present. In local anesthesia, as in general anesthesia, the period from 1896 to 1946 was one of consolidation.

* * *

The evolution of local anesthesia is similar to the evolution of general anesthesia in that suggestions of the potential value of an agent—in this case, cocaine—were made long before it was used clinically. But it differs too, for much of the knowledge and techniques of local and regional anesthesia was laid down relatively soon after the discovery of the anesthetic property of cocaine. As Vandam observed in 1989, "By the year 1900, some 16 years after the advent of cocaine use for anesthesia, practically all that we now hold true about the technique and complications of spinal anesthesia was made known."[111] The historical significance of those who forged a path from 1884 to 1989 in particular is all the more remarkable.

Chapter 5

Developments in General Anesthesia in the First Half of the Twentieth Century

During the first three decades of the twentieth century, anesthesia passed beyond the initial stage of a craft to that of a discipline. Several factors gave anesthesia a new look. One was the acquisition of a body of knowledge that was specific to anesthesia. That had begun in England earlier with John Snow and then Frederic Hewitt. Both understood the importance of anesthesia-oriented research in building knowledge, Hewitt's own investigation of optimal flows of oxygen during anesthesia with nitrous oxide to make it safer[1] being an example of this. In the United States, in the first two decades of the twentieth century, Hewitt's counterparts included Walter Boothby and Dennis Jackson, who, as noted in chapter 7, revolutionized the design of anesthesia machines. In the work of Hewitt and Boothby and Jackson and other inventive individuals, one can discern the beginning of a new and more disciplined look in the practice of anesthesia, and of a concern with improving the administration of anesthesia.

Basic physiological research also yielded knowledge. Examples of research include studies on respiration by Samuel Meltzer and John Auer and on the circulation by A. Goodman Levy. Meltzer and Auer, in 1909, showed that respiratory movements in themselves are not essential to respiration,[2] as long as oxygen is insufflated into the lungs via a narrow tube in the trachea. This established the basis for the insufflation technique of anesthesia that was popular immediately before and during World War I. (See also chapter 6.) Their work was followed two years later by Levy's demonstrating that light chloroform anesthesia and adrenalin secretion could combine to cause ventricular fibrillation and sudden death,[3] which explained in part some of the deaths that were all too frequent with chloroform. Those two bricks in the edifice of knowledge confirmed the need for, and the value of, research in the growing field of anesthesia.

Yet another advance early in the twentieth century provides evidence that anesthetists were interested in taking a more objective approach to anesthesia—the kind of approach that Snow had taken so many years earlier. That was the sphygmomanometer, which the American neurosurgeon Harvey Cushing introduced in 1903,[4] and which enabled anesthetists to measure the blood pressure of surgical patients and so make anesthesia safer. The sphygmomanometer was an advance in anesthesia because it provided anesthetists with an early warning of deterioration in a patient's condition so that corrective action could be taken promptly. As the first artificial monitor, the sphygmomanometer was the first in a long line of monitors that, in themselves, would create mini-revolutions in the practice of anesthesia in the twentieth century (see chapter 10).

Thus, by the outbreak of the First World War in 1914, the state of anesthesia was characterized by progress when compared with the somewhat stagnant years of the last few decades of the nineteenth century. After the turn of the century, anesthesia was shaped increasingly by a more objective, and even scientific, approach. This was even more evident after the war, when three other lines of progress became apparent.

One line of progress was technical. An example was the modification that two English anaesthetists, Ivan Magill and Stanley Rowbotham, made to the Meltzer and Auer technique of insufflation anesthesia. As noted in chapter 6, they developed true endotracheal anesthesia by using wider tracheal tubes.[5] That led to improved care of the airway, and it facilitated the use of innovations such as ventilators and of a generation of new inhalational and intravenous agents that were developed in the 1920s and 1930s. It is unlikely that heart and lung surgery would have developed without such progress.

The second line of progress is evident in the development of new anesthetic agents, some of which were introduced as a result of research by anesthetists themselves. Included among the inhalational agents are ethylene, cyclopropane, and divinyl ether; among the intravenous agents, hexobarbital, thiopental, meperidine, and curare. Use of these agents gave greater flexibility to the administration of anesthesia, and it began the process whereby the standbys of ether and chloroform were eventually replaced. How these new agents were developed and used are considered at some length in this chapter.

A third, though less obvious, indication of progress was the growing interest among anesthetists in regional anesthesia and the treatment of pain with nerve blocks. Though this interest was not fully developed until after the Second World War (see chapters 4 and 12), its beginning can be traced to the 1920s.

Two other aspects of anesthesia should also be borne in mind as this period of the evolution of anesthesia is considered. One is the perennial quest—at times a holy grail but more obviously a mirage—for the ideal anesthetic agent. Though that quest was never successful, a great deal of effort was expended by anesthesiologists themselves, pharmacologists, and those pharmaceutical companies that developed and marketed them.[6] Between the lines of this chapter, therefore, must be read those innumerable efforts that were not so much a failure as a continuing search for the ideal anesthetic agent.

Underlying all the foregoing, however, was the presence of a second quest: that of recognition of anesthesia as a specialty. As is noted in chapter 8, this quest occupied the attention of a number of anesthetists in the 1920s and 1930s. They knew full well that among those physicians who would reject or accept anesthetists' request for specialty recognition were their surgical peers. In this period, therefore, *how* those anesthetists used anesthetic agents and techniques affected the way in which anesthetists were viewed and, in particular, whether the practice of anesthesia had matured to the extent that it might be seen to merit the label of specialty.

Progress in Inhalational Anesthesia

Table 5.1. Comparison of inhalational agents,* 1900-1950, with theoretically ideal agent**

Variable	Agent				
	EC	Ethylene	Cyclo	DVE	Trilene
Potency	++	++	+++	+++	+
Stability	+	++	+++	+++	++
Safety	+/-	++	++	++	++
Fast action, recovery	++	++	+++	++	+
CNS action-specific	+	+	++	++	++
Nonflammability Nonexplosiveness	++	+++	++	+++	++++
Odorlessness	+	++	+++	++	+++
Muscle relax'n	+	++	+++	++	+
Nontoxic: body in postop stage little biotransformation	+	++	+	++	+

*EC=ethyl chloride; cyclo=cyclopropane; DVE=divinyl ether
**Ideal agent given ranking of +++++

The new inhalational agents to a large extent supplanted the older ether and chloroform and, to some extent, nitrous oxide. Various aspects of these agents, including their rating with respect to the theoretical ideal agent, are summarized in table 5.1. As the table indicates, none was an ideal anesthetic agent; each was used until a better agent was introduced.

It is not surprising that so many volatile agents were introduced in this era. Organic chemistry had steadily advanced from its beginnings in the nineteenth century, and the chemical and pharmaceutical industries were able to synthesize innumerable useful products. Chloroform had been synthesized in 1831, choral hydrate in 1862, and barbituric acid in 1863.[7] How they were introduced into

anesthesia varied. Ethyl chloride, which was used as a local anesthetic spray in the
nineteenth century, was serendipitously found to have general anesthetic properties
when sprayed in the mouth during dental surgery. Ethylene was also developed as
a result of a chance observation, in relation to the marketing of carnations. Divinyl
ether was investigated following pharmacological conjecture on its chemical
structure and the likelihood that it might serve as an anesthetic. Cyclopropane
was studied after an isomer of a substance with purported anesthetic potential
was found to be toxic. And trichloroethylene was enrolled as an anesthetic when
industrial use showed that it affected the nerves of workers. These agents were used
widely in anesthesia up to the 1950s, and were not replaced until the advantages
of halothane, introduced in 1956, became clear. In the mean time, they further
exemplified the transition of anesthesia to the stage of a discipline.

Ethyl Chloride

Although the introduction of ethyl chloride is more fully discussed in chapter 3,
it is noted briefly here because while it was known in the nineteenth century, its
impact was felt in the twentieth. Therefore, it is necessary only to recapitulate
the main points here.

The anesthetic action of ethyl chloride was known as early as 1847, and it was first
used clinically in 1848. However, obtaining it was difficult and costly, and so it was not
used as a general anesthetic until toward the end of the nineteenth century, though it
was used to induce local anesthesia as a freeze-producing spray. In fact, that was how
it came to be reintroduced as a general anesthetic toward the end of the nineteenth
century, for it followed the chance observation that spraying ethyl chloride as a topical
spray in a dental operation induced unconsciousness in a dental patient. Ethyl chloride
was then used to induce general anesthesia for the next fifty years, though it was not
free of danger. Its use ceased as fluorinated agents became available.

Ethylene

Ethylene, known in the eighteenth century as olefiant gas, was studied for its
anesthetic properties in England in 1849 by Thomas Nunneley. He found it
less satisfactory than ethylene dichloride,[8] a compound that was also used by
James Young Simpson in Edinburgh.[9]

The story of ethylene in anesthesia illustrates two aspects that lend
fascination to the specialty. One is the serendipitous nature of its discovery;
the other, its illustrating the fact that work on an anesthetic agent is sometimes
conducted and published by several groups simultaneously—a not-uncommon
occurrence in many different scientific fields.

In 1908, carnation growers noticed that their flowers were "going to sleep" in
greenhouses; since the buds failed to open, the flowers were unmarketable. The cause
lay in the illuminating gas; some 4% of the gas was ethylene.[10] Study of the anesthetic

and analgesic properties of a mixture of 80% ethylene and 20% oxygen confirmed an anesthetic action.[11] After World War I, studies were resumed. The earlier-unpublished data were confirmed, and the research was extended to animals and twelve humans, including researchers Arno Luckhardt and J. B. Carter themselves. Though none of the humans underwent surgery, Luckhardt and Carter concluded in 1923 that "deep surgical anesthesia can be rapidly induced by ethylene without any sense of asphyxia," and even that it produced "complete muscular flaccidity."[12] They demonstrated their findings to doctors, including anesthesiologists at the University of Chicago, among whom was Isabella Herb. She began using ethylene clinically on March 14, 1923. In 505 operations, ethylene anesthesia was found to be superior to nitrous oxide. Muscular relaxation was more noticeable, and tissue oxygenation was greater since a higher concentration of oxygen could be administered.[13]

Canadians had also been studying ethylene. In 1917, J. H. Cotton reported that ethylenated ether had anesthetic and analgesic properties.[14] Toronto anesthesiologist William Easson Brown also studied ethylene. Without knowing of the work of Luckhardt and his colleagues, Brown published the results of his work in March 1923[15]—the same month in which Luckhardt and Carter published their paper but before Herb published hers.

Though ethylene was efficacious, its disdvantage was flammability. At the end of the 1920s, research was beginning on the more potent cyclopropane, which replaced ethylene. Yet ethylene was widely used in its day, and its interesting story was told with charm by Luckhardt himself later.[16]

Acetylene

Like ethylene, acetylene is an unsaturated hydrocarbon. Snow had used amylene, another unsaturated hydrocarbon, but he reported two deaths with it,[17] and its use was discontinued. Others of this group that are known to have anesthetic properties include propylene and butylene.

Acetylene, as Narcylen, was commonly used in Germany, where it was introduced in 1923.[18] Its introduction was reported by Langton Hewer.[19] Induction of—as well as recovery from—anesthesia was rapid, muscle relaxation was adequate, and the agent was odorless. These advantages also characterized cyclopropane, which was preferred in the United States.

Cyclopropane

The introduction of cyclopropane as an anesthetic was also serendipitous. When August Freund discovered it in 1882,[20] he noticed that an isomer, propylene, was present as an impurity. In view of the narcotic properties of alcohol, propylene seemed possibly more potent an anesthetic than ethylene. In 1924, Easson Brown reported that propylene did have anesthetic properties,[21] but heart rhythm abnormalities were of concern.

Seeking the cause of the cardiac problem, Toronto pharmacologists George H. W. Lucas and Velyien E. Henderson studied the isomer cyclopropane. In 1929, they reported that it was not toxic but anesthetic: two kittens who breathed the gas in a jar slept peacefully and awoke quite normally.[22] The work continued,[23] and several individuals were anesthetized with cyclopropane, including Henderson, Lucas, and Frederick Banting, of insulin fame. Brown was now ready to anesthetize a patient with it, but, as Lucas wrote later, "At this particular time our luck changed." Previously, three patients had died after receiving ethyl chloride, which generated unfavorable publicity. The head of anesthesia in Toronto, Samuel Johnston, did see Banting being anesthetized, but the ethyl chloride deaths led him to ban the use of cyclopropane in humans.[24]

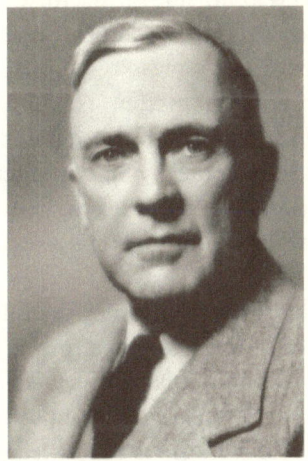

Fig.5.1. Ralph Waters (1883-1979)

Ralph Waters was born in North Bloomfield in Ohio, took his early education at Western Reserve University in Cleveland, and graduated in medicine in 1912. General practice in Sioux City, Iowa, followed. Waters was especially interested in obstetrics and anesthesia. In that era, Waters was self-trained, learning from what worked and what did not. He was influenced by the quarterly anesthesia supplement of the *American Journal of Surgery*, by Elmer McKesson and his writings and his anesthesia, and by the ideas of Dennis Jackson on carbon dioxide absorption, the last of which contributed to the design of his own to-and-fro apparatus. In 1923, Waters moved to Kansas City, where he specialized in anesthesia and managed a clinic specifically for anesthesia. In 1927, he was appointed to head up anesthesia in the new state hospital, with an academic position. He had a clear vision of the integration of education and research with clinical practice, and inaugurated a residency training program in 1930, many of his "Aqualumni" going on to head up programs elsewhere. Appointed to a university chair in 1933, he made Madison the mecca of North American anesthesia and an anesthesia center of international renown. In the United States, Waters profoundly shaped all aspects of anesthesia and did much to expedite the recognition of anesthesia as a specialty.

Ralph Waters (fig. 5.1) and his colleagues at the University of Wisconsin then took over the research. Waters had heard Lucas talk on cyclopropane on June 21, 1929. He then obtained a ten-gallon tank of cyclopropane from the Ohio Chemical Company and tested the gas on a dog for "forty minutes." He was "satisfied" that he would not "harm the patients," and so gave it to three surgical patients.[25] (In this era, it was not necessary to conduct exhaustive studies and obtain federal approval before a drug could be released for general use.) Its pharmacologic actions were investigated by M. H. Seevers and others, including anesthesiologists Emery A. Rovenstine and J. A. Stiles.[26] In 1933, Waters demonstrated the results of his group's work, and the first clinical report on the use of cyclopropane as a general anesthetic agent in 447 cases followed.[27] The Madison team found cyclopropane satisfactory, that it could be given with plenty of oxygen, that it relaxed muscle, and that it could be administered it in Brian Sword's circle system.[28]

The definitive clinical study of cyclopropane in more than two thousand anesthetics was published in 1934.[29] It confirmed the advantages of cyclopropane: rapid induction, acceptable odor, potency, and conducive to tracheal intubation, use of 100% oxygen, and good relaxation. It was, however, flammable. But used carefully, it remained in use, even for some time after halothane appeared as the next semi-ideal agent in 1956.

Waters' work on cyclopropane illustrates the qualities that made him so influential in anesthesia as it was evolving from a discipline to a specialty. He had his own vision for anesthesia. He valued research with laboratory scientists as well as anesthetists; he seized the opportunity to conduct research on cyclopropane, for example, because the knowledge it yielded advanced the practice of anesthesia. Waters always sought to serve his patients better, and his work on cyclopropane, in combination with his own to-and-fro carbon dioxide absorber, was an example of this. He strove to teach his students as well as possible and to encourage and guide his own peers in anesthesia; and in these ways, he communicated his natural interest in anesthesia, his inborn curiosity as a medical scientist, and his teaching ability to other anesthetists. Waters was an admirable colleague for the surgeons whom he worked with, and he was able to gain their support in when he sought to have anesthesia recognized as a specialty. He set a fine example for other anesthetists to follow. In his time and afterward, Waters was the representative of anesthesia par excellence, who showed why anesthesia justified recognition as a specialty.

Divinyl Ether

The introduction of divinyl ether is one of many contributions that pharmacologists have made to anesthesia. The pharmacologist who developed divinyl ether was Chauncey Leake, of Madison and then San Francisco. He studied divinyl ether and introduced it as an anesthetic agent in 1933,[30] as a result of logical conjecture concerning the relationship between chemical structure and activity, as opposed to serendipity. Aware of the possible relationship between chemical constitution and biological action, Leake and his colleagues wondered whether the characteristic unsaturated carbon atom of ethylene would enhance the anesthetic properties of ether if it was part of the ether molecule. Leake and Clarence Muehlberger obtained divinyl ether for study, Randolph Major synthesizing more because, though it was said to have been isolated by Friedrich Semmler in 1887,[31] it was not clear whether it had been isolated or synthesized. Following Major's synthesis,[32] Leake, Mei-yu Chen,[33] physician P. K. Knoefel, and Indiana anesthesiologist Arthur E. Guedel, initiated studies of the unsaturated ethers in animals.

In Alberta, Canada, Samuel Gelfan, a physiologist and pharmacologist, having a sample of the agent from Leake, asked his internist colleague, Irving Bell, to administer divinyl ether to him. This he did "very lightly and cautiously." After nine minutes, Gelfan was "completely unconscious" and showed evidence of complete muscular relaxation. He recovered promptly and subjected himself to the same treatment two days later, together with a second individual. Gelfan and Bell concluded that divinyl oxide was worthy of clinical trial and evaluation.[34] Through Leake's good offices, their paper on divinyl ether was published in the same issue of the January 1933 journal that contained the paper on the pharmacology of the agent by Leake, Knoefel, and Guedel.[35]

Divinyl ether (Vinesthene) was administered as an anesthetic over the next two decades. It was used in short procedures in which rapid induction was desirable and for induction prior to ether anesthesia. It was given by the drop method and from a special vaporizer, such as Victor Goldman's. That vaporizer foreshadowed the inhaler that was designed for use with halothane (see chapter 9), the agent that came to replace vinyl ether and the older volatile agents.

Trichloroethylene

The introduction of trichloroethylene (Trilene) into anesthesia was fortuitous, just as ethyl chloride and ethylene had been. Discovered by Emil Fischer, of Jena, Germany, in 1864,[36] it is, like chloroform, a hydrocarbon of the fatty series. Used in industry as a fat solvent and cleaner, from 1916, it was known to cause sensory loss in the trigeminal nerve.[37, 38, 39, 40, 41]Hence its use in treating trigeminal neuralgia.[42, 43, 44, 45]A logical question followed: if trichlorethylene had an effect on the trigeminal nerve, might it have other effects on the central nervous system? Anesthetic effects had been described in 1911,[46] and it was used as a general anesthetic in the United States after being administered to 304 patients in 1935 by Dennis Jackson and his colleagues in Cincinnati,[47] who reviewed the literature. In England, Hewer and Hadfield published a report on it in 1941.[48]

Trilene was suitable as a general anesthetic for short procedures, together with nitrous oxide, but once again, disadvantages limited the use of a seemingly promising agent. Heart rhythm disturbances occurred when it sensitized the myocardium to adrenaline; dichloracetylene was produced when Trilene was used in a closed circuit with soda lime, causing cranial nerve damage. Even deaths were reported. The by-product also decomposed into phosgene and hydrochloric acid when heated during cautery. Even so, the analgesic properties gave Trilene a place in the labor suite for self-administration to provide women in labor a means of controlling uterine pain.

Progress in Intravenous Anesthesia

An even wider variety of anesthetic agents were developed for intravenous use in this period. They radically changed the practice of anesthesia in the first half of the twentieth century. In contrast to the inhalational agents, they induced separate aspects of the triad of hypnosis, analgesia, and muscle relaxation that constitutes anesthesia. That greater specificity of action was the main advantage, for ideally, drugs should induce specific and controllable effects on the nervous system rather than the blunderbuss all-in-one effects of the inhalational agents. The intravenous agents of this period are listed in table 5.2, which sets each against the ideal agent.

Table 5.2. Comparison of intravenous agents, 1900-1950, with theoretically ideal agent*

Variable	Agent			
	Hedonal	Barbiturates	Opioids	Curare
Potency	+	++++	++++	++++
Stability	+	+++	++++	+++
Safety	+	+	++	++
Ease of use	+	+	++	++
Fast action, Recovery	+	++++	++	++
Nontoxic: body in postop stage; little biotransformation	+	++	++	++
Lack of allergy	0	+	+	++
Drug compatibility	+	+	++	+
Main action	Hypnosis	Hypnosis	Analgesia	Muscle relaxation

*Given ranking of +++++

In a sense, use of the intravenous agents updated the concept of balanced anesthesia, introduced originally in 1926 by Mayo Clinic anesthetist John Lundy[49] (fig. 5.2). One drug (a barbiturate) would induce hypnosis; another (curare), muscle relaxation; and the third (e.g., meperidine), analgesia. Drugs in each of the three classes, each tailored to a specific action, would replace the nonspecific and gunshot effect of anesthetics like ether and chloroform, which had to be given in relatively large amounts in order to achieve the triad of effects that could now be obtained by small doses of the newer agents.

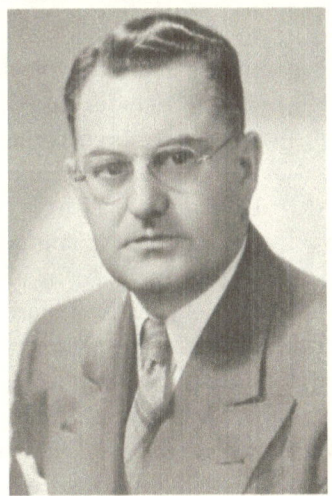

Fig. 5.2. John Lundy (1894-1973)

John Lundy was born in Seattle. He graduated from Rush Medical College in Chicago in 1920, then moved back to Seattle and began giving anesthetics immediately, using a Gwathmey machine. In 1924, Dr. William Mayo passed through Seattle and was sufficiently impressed by Lundy's personal stature to invite him to join the Mayo Clinic. Lundy did, initially being responsible for regional anesthesia, since general anesthesia was in the hands of some eighteen nurse anesthetists. Dr. Charles McCluskey joined Lundy at the beginning of 1925, and arrangements were soon being made to establish a Section of Anesthesia, together with a postgraduate-degree-granting university program. A formal residency program was started in 1935. Lundy was therefore at the center of a new sphere of influence in anesthesia, and he contributed a great deal to anesthesia at the Mayo Clinic in particular, and to American anesthesia in general. His emphasis on the value of regional nerve blocks, his concept of balanced anesthesia, his early work on sodium thiopental, his instituting the first blood bank in the United States in 1935 and the first American recovery room in 1942, together with the publication of *Clinical Anesthesia* also in 1942, were some of Lundy's many obvious accomplishments. But also, like Ralph Waters, Lundy worked tirelessly in order to ensure that anesthesia be recognized as a specialty.

Antecedents: Opium, Chloral Hydrate, and Hedonal

Before drugs could be given intravenously, the fact that blood circulates round the body had to be proved. This was done, as discussed in chapter 1, by William Harvey in 1628 in a work that still repays attention.[50] A second key step was to show that pharmaceutical substances could act when injected into the blood; that was done in 1665 by the natural scientist, astronomer, and architect Christopher Wren, of Oxford and London. After ligating a vein in the neck and introducing a quill attached to a bladder, Wren injected a solution of opium into a "large Dogg," which was soon "stupefied."[51]

Opium. Opium was the first drug to be given by vein, though neither opium nor morphine, its derivative, was used to induce anesthesia until the twentieth century.[52] Wren, however, may not have been the first to inject opium. He referred to "Books, printed beyond the Seas, treating of the Way of Injecting liquors into Veines," and two Germans may have preceded Wren: Johann Sigismund Elsholtz, who evidently attempted to induce anesthesia by injecting an opiate in 1665,[53] and Daniel Johann Major in 1667, or perhaps earlier.[54] However, the technique of intravenous injection had to be developed further, and two hundred years passed before the next step was taken.

That step was the invention and development of the piston-and-barrel syringe and the hollow needle in the 1840s and 1850s. Francis Rynd, Charles Pravaz, and Alexander Wood are commonly linked to these inventions. Rynd's claim to priority has, however, been discounted, for Wood, who used an "elegant little syringe" that had been made by a Mr. Ferguson, of London, has been regarded as the facilitator.[55] The syringe allowed doctors to inject, through a hollow needle, perchloride of iron into nevi that were to be sclerosed. Though the identity of the inventor or inventors of the syringe and the needle remains unknown, countless anesthesiologists—and patients—benefited from this small but immensely significant step. Another step was the recognition of the principle of sterility of equipment, following the nineteenth century work of Louis Pasteur in France[56] and Joseph Lister in England.[57] Infection from procedures and equipment was preventable, and drugs could now be given intravenously without fear of infection.

That Other antecedents of intravenous anesthesia were ether, chloral hydrate, and hedonal. Ether had been given intravenously to dogs in 1847 by Nikolai Pirogoff, of St. Petersburg, Russia,[58] but many of them died, and ether was not used that way clinically. However, Pirogoff did confirm that intravenous medicinals could induce anesthesia. He then took another tack, administering ether by rectal injection.[59] This was more successful, and others, notably James Tayloe Gwathmey, made use of it early in the twentieth century.[60]

Chloral hydrate. This was a popular sedative[61] that was injected in dogs by Bordeaux surgeon Pierre-Cyprien Oré in 1872.[62] He gave it to a human on February 9, 1874.[63] Oré believed it was innocuous and efficacious in a small dose, but he was overly optimistic. He was criticized for stating that chloral was superior to chloroform, and he lost his job as a surgeon.[64] Chloral hydrate is excreted slowly from the body, which likely led to respiratory complications. Deaths associated with its use led to its discontinuation in anesthesia. Chloral hydrate, however, continued to be used by physicians as a sedative.

Hedonal. Hedonal (methylpropyl carbinol urethane) was more effective as an intravenous anesthetic. Urethane compounds were studied in Germany by Oswald Schmiedeberg beginning in 1855,[65] and hedonal was the first to induce anesthesia. While potent, it was not, however, entirely safe.[66] Nicholas Krakow, a St. Petersburg pharmacologist, began investigating it in 1901, and described its use prior to chloroform inhalation in 1903.[67] His surgical colleague, Sergei Fedoroff, then became interested.[68] Hedonal was first given by mouth to surgical patients before they received chloroform or ether. Though it was poorly soluble in water, A. P. Jeremitsch, in Krakow's laboratory, showed that it could be given intravenously to dogs. He used it clinically on December 7, 1909.[69] Though his apparatus was cumbersome, the results seemed acceptable. Hedonal was used before World War I, first in Russia—as one of that country's contributions to anesthesia[70]—and then in England. Charles Page, a London surgeon, cited Fedoroff's work when he reported his own use of hedonal in London in two hundred cases in 1912.[71]

However, low solubility, slow onset, and long duration made hedonal impractical, though it continued to be used until about 1930. Once again, a better agent was needed. Substances that were tested include paraldehyde (in 1913),[72] magnesium sulfate (1916),[73] and ethyl alcohol (1921).[74] Meanwhile, another substance that was neither an inhalational nor an intravenous agent that was used in this period was tribromethyl alcohol (Avertin),[75] though this was given by rectum and it was discarded when superior anesthetics became available.

What David Davis said in 1968 was true of drugs then, earlier and later: "Many . . . intravenous agents have collapsed . . . [and] few . . . have been resuscitated."[76] Indeed, many are called, but few are chosen, and relatively few drugs have had a permanent role in the anesthesiologist's pharmacopeia. Even so, by 1920, intravenous anesthesia had reached the stage at which it could offer a practical alternative to inhalational anesthesia. That was when the barbiturates became prominent in anesthesia.

The Barbiturate Era

Barbiturates were used as anesthetics beginning in the 1920s. Barbituric acid was synthesized by Adolf von Bayer in 1863—soon after morphine, atropine, chloroform, and chloral hydrate were becoming familiar[77]—but its hypnotic effect was not noted until 1903, when Emil Fischer and Josef von Mering synthesized diethyl-malonyl urea (Veronal).[78] Even so, the early barbiturates, including phenobarbitone, were unsuitable as anesthetic agents because they were slow to act and induced long-lasting sleep.

Of greater interest was Somnifen (a mixture of diethyl—and allyl-barbituric acid), which was first used in France in 1921.[79] The first barbiturate to be considered as an intravenous anesthetic was Pernoston (the sodium salt of sec-butyl-[2-bromallyl]-barbiturate), which was made available in 1927.[80] Its action was relatively short, however. Sodium amytal followed in 1929.[81] This was used, as was Pernoston, by Ralph Waters and his group in Madison.[82] Two years later, pentobarbital (Nembutal) was used by Lundy at the Mayo Clinic.[83]

None of these barbiturates appeared to be a "true anesthetic substance,"[84] but one soon appeared: hexobarbital. This cyclohexenylmethyl derivative of barbituric acid was synthesized in 1931 and marketed as Evipal. Helmuth Weese and W. Scharpff used it clinically in 1932.[85] Metabolized rapidly, its action was very short. An improved sodium preparation became popular, but it caused excitatory reactions. It gave way to the sulfur-containing derivative of pentobarbital known as thiopental (Pentothal), which Abbott Laboratories marketed beginning in 1934. Though hexobarbital was used only for a few years, its association with Weese is notable. Weese was one of those medical scientists to link universities and industry in producing anesthetic agents.

If hexobarbital was the prototype, thiopental was the definitive barbiturate that was used in anesthesia. Sulfur-containing barbiturates had interested Donalee Tabern and Ernest Volwiler since the early 1930s,[86] for they knew that Alfred Eichorn had incorporated a sulfur atom in the barbiturate structure in 1908 to produce a 5, 5-disubstituted 2-thio derivative, though it was unstable. They did some of the early seminal work on thiopental, while it was used clinically, in a 10% solution, for the first time on March 8, 1934, by Ralph Waters in Madison.[87] He and his colleagues noted that it was a hypnotic and not an analgesic; that as a nonvolatile compound, it was "not controllable," though broken down in the body very rapidly; and that it produced "a short period of satisfactory anesthesia with a relatively prompt complete recovery." They advised that it be given by "a capable anesthetist who is equipped to cope with problems involving an oxygen and carbon dioxide balance." In other words—and words whose significance was not appreciated sufficiently during the first decade of its use—thiopental was a potent drug whose administration should not be entrusted to an inexperienced administrator.

On June 18, 1934, Lundy, at the Mayo Clinic, also gave thiopental.[88] He and Ralph Tovell referred to it again in 1935 as "barbiturate A" in April of that year.[89] Lundy later concluded that though the ideal intravenous agent had not yet been found, thiopental was "satisfactory in certain types of cases"[90]—a prediction that turned out to be accurate indeed. Because Lundy wrote more often about sodium thiopental than Waters did, he is often given priority for its initial use.

Thiopental became very popular. At first, it was erroneously regarded as a complete anesthetic, as opposed to only the hypnotic that it really was, and misunderstanding and misuse gave it a bad name. Injected in individuals who were wounded and in shock, doses that most doctors were accustomed to giving to the uninjured depressed the circulation. That notably occurred in military personnel who were injured in the Japanese bombing of the American fleet in Pearl Harbor on December 7, 1941. Few doctors knew about the adverse circulatory effect, and deaths ensued. In retrospect, this is understandable. Before the war, Evipal had been given to thousands of patients without untoward sequelae, and thiopental seemed just as safe. However, in Pearl Harbor the circumstances were quite different: few of the wounded had a normal or resilient circulation, and thiopental was the last straw. Neither the words of Waters in 1934 nor the adverse effects of seemingly normal doses in the injured were understood, for many of those who gave thiopental were not trained or experienced anesthesiologists and had only been pressed into anesthetic service. The early administrators did not understand that thiopental should not be used as the sole anesthetic, that redistribution of intravenous anesthetics in the body sensitized patients in shock to thiopental,[91] and that very small doses should be given. These dangers eventually became widely known, partly because they were publicized in two articles and in an editorial in *Anesthesiology* in 1943.[92, 93, 94]

The popularity of thiopental in particular was unchallenged for another few decades. Thialbarbital and methohexital also were used, though to a lesser extent, but they did emphasize the apparent versatility of the barbiturates as a group of very useful drugs in anesthesia.

The Opioids: Morphine and Meperidine

Uses of morphine. Opium, the parent substance of morphine, long predominated as an *anodyne* in the treatment of pain. Euphoria made it desirable for hedonists: Thomas de Quincy, for example, referred to "the marvelous agency of opium, whether for pleasure or pain."[95] Eventually, opium was replaced by morphine, which was isolated by Friedrich Serturner, in Germany, beginning in 1803.[96] Morphine then dominated as the anodyne in medicine.

In anesthesia, morphine became more commonly used as a *premedicant* in sedating patients before operation. The history of drugs in sedating patients before surgery actually extends back to the seventeenth century. In 1682, Georg Wedel, in Jena, advocated a "moderate" draught of opium on the night before operation so that a patient undergoing an amputation might "bear the cutting of the limb in a readier spirit."[97] In 1731, William Cheselden, in London, gave a "quieting draught" to help his surgical patients following lithotomy.[98] Cordials, in the form of alcohol, were used as well, to enhance the effect of opium. Even after the advent of anesthesia, alcohol continued to be prescribed. Clover, for example, gave his patients "a teaspoonful of brandy, without water," a few minutes before they were to receive chloroform.[99]

This was part of the background for the use of morphine for premedication. In the second half of the nineteenth century, the practice was more common in Continental Europe than in England. It may have been used in Turin, Italy, as early as 1850, by Lorenzo Bruno, who gave a simple injection of morphine an hour before operation to lessen psychic trauma.[100] Though it has not been verified, Bruno's alleged practice occurred three years before Wood's report of a syringe and needle. Use of morphine in premedication was furthered, as noted in chapter 3, by the advocacy of Claude Bernard, the French physiologist. He found that when he gave dogs morphine, the effects of chloroform were potentiated. Bernard never practiced medicine, but he understood the principles of clinical anesthesia, and he believed that chloroform added to morphine might be of help in surgery. He suggested giving morphine first and then chloroform, although in much smaller doses than usual. Side effects would be prevented, including agitation and also the accidents associated with large doses of chloroform.[101] The value of morphine for premedication was confirmed by many clinical reports in the nineteenth century,[102, 103, 104] so that there was a good base of support for the practice in the twentieth century.

A different approach to preventing "chloroform refractaires" was to give atropine before chloroform.[105] Yet another was to give both morphine, or a derivative, together with atropine, or an atropine-like drug. This too originated in earlier ideas. In 1858, for example, Benjamin Bell, in Edinburgh, discussed the therapeutic relationship of opium and belladonna.[106] This was consistent with the belief that morphine and atropine were mutually antagonistic. In Paris, Charles-Edouard Brown-Sequard gave the two alkaloids together whenever one of them was indicated.[107] This was not taken up immediately in anesthesia, though atropine an hour before chloroform was found to protect the heart of cats against the effects of chloroform.[108] The vagolytic effect of atropine prevented the slowing of the heart when used before chloroform[109] that sometimes caused cardiac syncope. Lyons surgeon P. Aubert took up the suggestion to give atropine and morphine before the use of chloroform,[110] claiming that this calmed patients, facilitated induction of anesthesia, made for greater safety, and decreased the incidence of side effects such as nausea and vomiting.[111]

Anesthetists eventually recognized the advantages of premedication with morphine and either atropine or scopolamine. In 1906, W. Fingland, for example, having prescribed atropine preoperatively "for many years," noted that it abolished salivation, facilitated ether induction, and decreased the incidence of postoperative nausea and vomiting.[112] Dudley Buxton, in England, also recognized the value of premedication,[113] arguing that a frightened patient after a sleepless night was in poor shape for an anesthetic and an operation, and he recommended scopolamine and morphine. By 1912, according to Bellamy Gardner, premedication was "indispensable."[114]

Though premedication was not generally accepted for years, it became an integral part of the anesthetic technique for much of the rest of the twentieth century. The combinations of drugs given for premedication varied—sedatives, tranquilizers, neuroleptics, and narcotic and non-narcotic analgesics—but the aim of giving a drug to make patients ready for anesthesia remained fast.

Later, morphine became used as an *anesthetic agent*. At first, it was accompanied by scopolamine and given intravenously. In 1900, Schneiderlin, in Germany, gave either a trial dose of 0.0003 gram of scopolamine and 0.01 gram of morphine, repeating this after one to two hours, or the first dose on the evening before surgery and a larger dose on the day of surgery.[115] Even then, further doses might be required to provide adequate anesthesia. Some thought this imprecise. The following year, Berthold Korff formulated a dosage regimen of a total of 0.001 gram scopolamine hydrobromide and 0.025 gram morphine hydrochloride (in 10 grams distilled water) in three aliquots over the two and a half hours before operation.[116] If this was not adequate for surgical purposes, it could be supplemented with "a few drops" of ether or chloroform.

A variant of morphine-scopolamine anesthesia was "twilight sleep." This was favored in surgery and in obstetrics in the first decade of the twentieth century, both in Europe and North America (see also chapter 14). In Germany, Hocheisen described the combination in 1906,[117] as did Bass in 1907.[118] In the United States, Robert Smith reported the technique in 1908 in 229 cases.[119] The technique was thought to diminish mental stress preoperatively, to shorten anesthesia time, since the patient could be prepared in the operating room before a volatile agent was given; to lessen any unpleasantness experienced by patient; and to reduce the incidence of nausea and vomiting after surgery. No ill effects occurred, but as Smith admitted, there were side effects. Patients tended to sleep for longer than after ether or chloroform given alone, respiration was often depressed, and deaths sometimes occurred. These complications, and the lack of abdominal relaxation, militated against success of the technique, which did not persist. However, morphine was used more extensively as a primary anesthetic agent beginning in the 1960s (chapter 14).

Meperidine. Morphine is beneficial in inducing analgesia, calm, and euphoria; but it may also cause nausea and vomiting, constipation, itching, addiction, and respiratory depression. Chemists and pharmacologists therefore sought drugs that had greater analgesic specificity and no adverse side effects and that could be synthesized. The first such drug was diamorphine, or heroin, which was synthesized in 1875.[120] As the product of chemical manipulation of a natural opioid—an early example of altering chemical structure to produce a desired pharmacological effect—it was a semisynthetic rather than a wholly synthetic opioid. However, it was more addictive than morphine. A better drug in anesthesia was papaveretum (Omnopon, Pantopon), a crude opium preparation that was used for premedication.

A major advance was the synthesis of meperidine (Pethidine, Demerol) by Schaumann and Eisleb in Germany in 1939.[121] Not only was this a potent analgesic, but also, it was the first completely synthetic opioid. It was a serendipitous advance also, for it was the outcome of research that had been directed to finding a substitute for atropine.

A Revolution in Anesthesia: Curare

On January 23, 1942, there occurred one of four events in the development of anesthesia that were so revolutionary that we remember their precise dates. (The introduction of ether we remember every October 16; cocaine was first used on September 11, 1884; and thiopental sodium on March 8, 1934.) On that January day in 1942, Harold Griffith (fig. 5.3), in Montreal, aided by resident Enid Johnson MacLeod, injected a drug that was chiefly known until then as a poison called "the flying death." They made history by injecting curare in a patient anesthetized with cyclopropane to achieve a greater degree of muscle relaxation during an appendectomy. This inaugurated a fourth era of anesthesia, that of the muscle relaxants. It led to revolutionary changes in anesthesia practice—and in other fields of medicine besides.

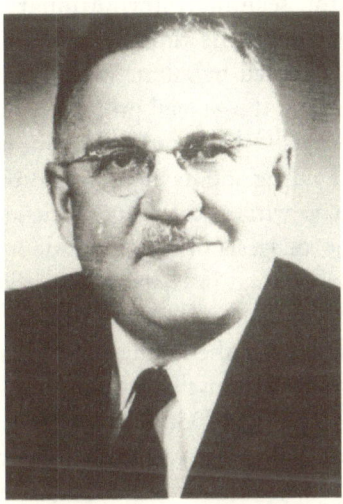

Fig. 5.3. Harold Griffith (1894-1985)
Harold Randall Griffith was born in Montreal, where he practiced except during both world wars. He fitted in one year of medical school at McGill University before serving in the military as a stretcher bearer, winning the Military Medal at Vimy Ridge. He also served in the Royal Navy as a surgeon sublieutenant. Griffith graduated in medicine in 1922, the same year he wrote his first paper on anesthesia. He gained the doctorate of homoeopathic medicine in 1923, and from 1923 to 1959, he was chief of anesthesia at Montreal Homoeopathic Hospital. His early publications were noted by Francis McMechan, Ralph Waters, and Wesley Bourne, and he was drawn into the inner circle of North American anesthetists. Griffith was interested in tracheal intubation, spinal anesthesia, and cyclopropane. In 1942, he became known internationally when he introduced curare. In World War II, he, Bourne, and Digby Leigh organized short courses in anesthesia for the military, and his appointment to the Royal Canadian Air Force put him in a select group of individuals who served in all three arms of the military. In 1943, Griffith was elected founding president of the Canadian Anaesthetists' Society. After the war, he held a professorship at McGill, and in 1955, he became founding president of the World Federation of Societies of Anaesthesiologists. Griffith's stature was therefore truly international.

The impact of curare on anesthesia. Curare had a profound impact on the practice of anesthesia. It was profound because it was now no longer necessary to give deep anesthesia with an inhalational agent in order to provide the surgeon with muscle relaxation. Curare joined thiopental and meperidine to make the third part of the anesthetic triad of hypnosis, analgesia, and, now, muscle relaxation, each part of which it was now possible to achieve with separate intravenous drugs. In this way, curare, like thiopental, wrought a truly revolutionary change in anesthesia.

However, despite the seemingly revolutionary nature of curare—or perhaps because of it—it was some time before curare and the principle of a paralyzing drug were accepted by all anesthesiologists. In this respect, the initial use of curare illustrates the general principle in medicine, and noted by anesthesiologist Ralph Waters[122] that a significant time often elapses between the discovery and first use of a drug and its incorporation in clinical practice. This is apparent in anesthesia, as witness the delay, discussed in chapter 2, between the demonstration of the analgesia of nitrous oxide in 1800 and its use as an anesthetic in 1844, and, as noted in chapter 9, the delay between laboratory experiments with succinylcholine in 1906 and its first use in 1951. In the case of curare, a further problem was the failure to fully understand the extent to which it affected the respiratory muscles, a point that was driven home by the huge study by Henry Beecher and Donald Todd in 1954.[123] That study gave the erroneous impression that curare was toxic and jeopardized recovery, and it obscured the real problem, which was the lack of knowledge about curare, especially in the United States. Anesthesiologists did not fully understand the action of curare on the respiratory muscles, the need to adequately reverse this by pharmacological means, and the importance of ensuring adequacy of ventilation before releasing patients from anesthetic supervision.

That caveat aside, curare clearly changed the object and the technique of general anesthesia. Besides making it possible to select a drug specifically to relax a patient's muscles, use of curare facilitated tracheal intubation and abolished the need for the strenuous efforts that were sometimes needed to maintain a patient's airway (see also chapter 6). But the need to assess the action of the breathing muscles until the effects of the curare had worn off meant that an anesthesiologist had to assume responsibility for a patient's breathing at all times, including postoperatively when the patient might still be partially paralyzed. (It was neglect of this second aspect of the anesthetist's respiratory responsibility that underlay part of the negative opinions about curare that were noted in the Beecher and Todd report of 1954, already cited.) Eventually, anesthetists realized that it was easy to ventilate a curarized patient, either manually by rhythmically squeezing the breathing bag attached to the anesthesia machine or by using a mechanical ventilator. Artificial respiration of the anesthetized and curarized patient then became routine.

The introduction of curare had another salutary effect. To the onlooker, anesthesia no longer had the appearance of a craft; it did, indeed, seem to be more like a medical specialty, requiring the attention of a specialist.

The impact of curare on surgery and medicine. The use of curare also benefited surgeons especially, but also internists. Surgeons could perform operations that required a patient's muscles to be relaxed more easily. Operations that followed in the 1950s, such as those on the heart, were greatly facilitated. Care of patients who were critically ill and requiring intensive care could now be done through intubation and managed on a ventilator much more easily. In medicine, the ability to paralyze a patient in whom the respiration was affected and to manage the condition with the aid of artificial ventilation was similarly facilitated. Patients whose muscles were weakened by poliomyelitis, for example, or spastic as in tetanus or rabies, were given a much greater chance of survival. As discussed in chapter 11, one consequence of the use of curare was the development of the new specialty of critical care.

The impact of curare on physiology. In the long run, perhaps the single greatest consequence of curare was the impetus to study anew the transmission of impulses from nerve to muscle. That study opened a new chapter in the work that had been launched in the nineteenth century by Claude Bernard and followed up in the twentieth century by Ramon y Cajal and other luminaries such as Charles Sherrington, Henry Dale, Otto Loewi, Wilhelm Feldberg, Bernard Katz, and Stephen Kuffler. Their work, so well related by Maxwell Cowan and Eric Kandel,[124] laid the basis for the understanding of the rational use of curare and other muscle relaxants.

Three points became clear. First, nerve impulses are transmitted to muscle by chemical not electrical means; it's a matter of soup, not sparks. Second, the chemical mediator of impulses is acetylcholine, the main ingredient of the "soup" and that is released at the neuromuscular in quanta, or discrete packets, thus initiating muscle contraction. And third, the action of curare, which results from its blocking the action of acetylcholine at receptors at the neuromuscular junction, is reversed by drugs that prevent it from competing, as it does, with acetylcholine. Some of the knowledge so gained was worked out before curare was recognized as a muscle relaxant (by Sherrington, Dale, and Lowei) and some later (by Feldberg, Katz, Kuffler), but all contributed to the understanding of the actions of curare and of its replacements, as noted in chapter 9.

The discovery and early use of curare. The history of curare is as fascinating as any aspect of the history of anesthesia. The story of its discovery, its study, its isolation, and its applications not only to anesthesia but also to other fields of medicine is engrossing.[125] Much of the story takes place far from the operating room; many of the dramatic and complex events occurred, over many years, in completely different environments.

Curare is a product of a plant that grows in the South American jungle, in Guiana and Ecuador especially, where native Indians have long used it in hunting. Botanically, it is derived from the Menispermaceae, which includes varieties of the genus *Chondrodendron*, and from the Loganaceae, which includes the genus *Strychnos*. Samples of curare lianas were taken back by early explorers to Europe for more intensive study, though the delay of the sea voyages frequently caused the samples to deteriorate.

The initial studies of curare were of relevance to medicine rather than anesthesia. In 1811, for example, Benjamin Brodie, who ventilated animals under the influence of curare, suggested that it might be used in the treatment of tetanus.[126] That was 131 years before it was finally introduced as a muscle relaxant in anesthetic practice.[127] The use of curare to treat conditions such as tetanus[128, 129] and to facilitate electroshock therapy[130] long preceded its use in anesthesia.

The history of curare illustrates several points of interest. Thus, it is one of few anesthesia agents that are obtained from a plant source, cocaine being another. Second, the history of curare is lengthy, and much longer than many other drugs in medicine, such as insulin and penicillin. And third, the use of curare highlights contributions that anesthesia has made outside anesthesia, to intensive care as well as to knowledge of the neuromuscular junction. Curare is no longer used in anesthesia, because synthetic replacements became available, but its place in the history of anesthesia is firm.

The story of curare leading up to its initial use in anesthesia in 1942 can only be summarized here. Many of those who had parts in the four-hundred-year story of its discovery, gradual elucidation, and realization of its use in medicine were intriguing, and the story is highlighted by absorbing elements of drama. The story can be told as a play in three acts.

Act I
1516-1844

As all good plays should, act I introduces fascinating characters and intriguing elements. We must envision dark and dangerous forests in South America, where natives kill silently with poisoned arrows. Entering these forests are intrepid European explorers who are lured by the romance of the unknown and who make observations about the flora and fauna in those lands. They are a motley but distinguished cast: an English admiral and general who later lost his head, a Frenchman whose travels are sponsored by the French Academy of Sciences, a German plant collector, an English physician and naturalist, an Italian anatomist and physiologist who was also an abbe, a prominent English surgeon who is interested in poisons, an eccentric country squire and naturalist who has little fear and wandered in South America before experimenting with the potent poison in the quiet English countryside, two anglicized German naturalists and travelers, and an American expatriate who is at home in the Ecuadorean jungle. As the play unfolds, we realize that the story of curare is unparalleled in anesthesia, giving the history of anesthesia its own flavor.

The story starts with Pietro d'Anghiera, a well-connected Italian member of the court of Ferdinand and Isabella of Spain in the fifteenth century. Familiar with the New World through tales told by returning travelers in Columbus' era, he retold them in *De rebus oceanicis et novo orbe* in 1516.[131] D'Anghiera described some of the people in the New World and some of their customs. He spoke of "the juice they distil from certain trees in which they dip their arrows," so that they became "poisoned arrows." D'Anghiera did not name any poisons that might or might not have contained curare. No doubt some of the tales that he and others told are the stuff of myth and legend, and we wonder if they can be relied on.

As the story unfolds, we learn the names of the cast, all of whom were bemused by the mystique of the poisoned arrows. They learned about curare and its unusual power. The most notable were Sir Walter Raleigh, Charles-Marie de la Condamine, Felix Fontana, Alexander von Humboldt, Edward Bancroft, and, later, Charles Waterton. Raleigh, according to J. A. Carman, was interested in Indians called Piaros, who had "the most strong poison on their arrows," though he never named the poison.[132] At one time a favorite of Queen Elizabeth I, Raleigh introduced tobacco and potatoes to England; later, accused on dubious grounds of piracy, he succumbed to the executioner. De la Condamine, a French scientist who spent ten years in Ecuador, got to know natives who killed animals with blow darts. He was the first to take back samples of what he called "wourali" to Europe, and in 1745, he demonstrated its lethal effects on chickens.[133] (Curare was known by several other names, including *ticunas, urari, oorali*, and *woorara*.) Abbe Fontana, an Italian naturalist, observed in 1781 that wourali destroyed the irritability of the voluntary muscles, but not the heart; injected into the jugular vein of a rabbit, the animal fell "down as dead as if it had been struck by lightning."[134] Also active participants in the collection and study of curare were Richard and Robert Schomburgk, who showed that the curare of the Macushi Indians was derived from *Strychnos toxifera*.[135] Von Humboldt's contribution is interesting because he described the effect of the curare poison on a human being: "C'est un charpentier d'une force musculaire extraordinaire. Ayant eu l'imprudence de frotter entre ses doigts le *Curare*, apres s'etre blesse legerement, il tomba par terre saisi d'un vertige qui dura pres d'un demi-heure."[136]

Edward Bancroft, son of a physician, enters the story because he supplied curare to Benjamin Brodie, the nineteenth-century English surgeon.[137] Brodie was one of the first to bring medical science to bear on the problem of curare. Interested in poisons,[138] he stated that he had curarized a rabbit and, through a tracheostomy, kept it alive for 83 minutes by rhythmically inflating its lungs.[139] Though the rabbit died, Brodie recognized the value of artificial ventilation, believing it should be carried on until the effects of the poison had worn off. Brodie repeated the experiment on a cat, who was kept alive for 160 minutes. After sleeping for another 40 minutes, the cat suddenly woke and walked away, having used up one of its lives. Brodie's research appears to be the beginning of a more serious approach to the study of curare and added to the understanding of the place of artificial respiration in resuscitation.

Meanwhile, Charles Waterton, the eccentric Yorkshire squire, set off, also in 1812, on an expedition in Guiana, where he had been managing the family-owned sugar plantation since 1804. An eclectic naturalist in an age when many educated persons called themselves naturalists, he succeeded in obtaining "a quantity of the strongest Wourali poison"[140] from the Macushi Indians in Guiana (then, Demerara). Along the way, he witnessed the deaths of a chicken and a sloth, and then a large ox. He did not resuscitate the animals—he was particularly interested in antidotes to the poison—but he referred to the suggestion that "wind introduced into the lungs by . . . a small pair of bellows" would revive a patient. By 1814, Waterton, back in England, supplied the curare that was used in an experiment performed by Brodie and veterinarian Professor Sewell, which showed that a curarized animal could be effectively resuscitated in this manner. The animal was an ass who had received wourali in the shoulder and appeared to die. The trachea was incised, and the she-ass was ventilated with the aid of bellows. She recovered completely, "neither in agitation nor pain," and is remembered as Wouralia.[141]

It was such experiments that stimulated thinking on the clinical use of curare for the treatment of hydrophobia (rabies) and tetanus. Thus, Waterton in 1838: "Our philosophers suppose that the Wourali poison will cure patients labouring under hydrophobia and the lockjaw."[142] Sewell attempted to treat two cases of equine tetanus in 1833,[143] and Francis Sibson, a physician who practiced anesthesia, hoped to treat a patient with rabies with crude curare in 1839.[144]

Act II
1844-1914

Act II begins with the entry of Claude Bernard (fig. 5.4) on the stage. His philosophy was that "we experiment to bring to birth observations which may in turn bring to birth ideas."[145] Though the work of Brodie and Waterton suggested that curare might be useful in medicine, *how* it worked was not clear. It was Bernard who showed how. From Francois Magendie, Bernard would have learned about curare, for von Humboldt had given Magendie samples of *ticunas* so that laboratory animals could be immobilized.[146] Bernard himself studied curare so he could learn more about its action on the body and thus facilitate his physiological work. In 1844, he injected curare in a frog, which became paralyzed within seven minutes. Autopsy revealed a beating heart, but more remarkable was the fact that electrical stimulation of the nerves failed to induce movement of the muscles while direct stimulation of the muscles led to their vigorous contraction. In other words, curare seemed to affect nerve rather than muscle.[147] This fundamental observation led him to determine precisely where curare acted.

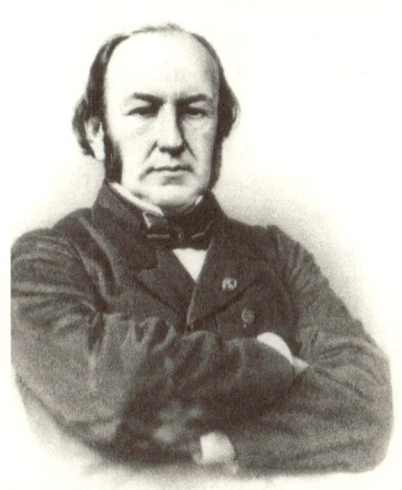

Fig. 5.4. Claude Bernard (1813-1878)
Claude Bernard was born near Villefranche, France. Before graduating as a physician in 1839 from the Sorbonne, he was a pharmacist, which perhaps explains his readiness to use drugs in his experiments. Advocacy of the experimental method in medicine is what Bernard is most widely known for; he was the exemplar of the experimental method. He sought truth for truth's sake. After graduating in medicine, he worked with Francois Magendie, which led him to become interested primarily in physiology. Bernard's achievements in physiology led to the observation that he was not just a physiologist, but that he *was* physiology. A chair in physiology was created for him at the Sorbonne in 1854, and in 1858, he was appointed to the chair in medicine at the College de France. In general, physiology Bernard conducted key studies on digestion and the vasomotor system. In anesthesia, his contributions included three important concepts: reversible intracellular coagulation to explain anesthetic action (like Snow, he did not believe anesthesia was a form of asphyxia), synergism of action of morphine and chloroform, and location of the action of curare at the neuromuscular junction.

Bernard was not short of curare, obtaining his supply from several sources: Dr. Edwards, a Brazilian; Emile Carrey, whose supply came from the Amazon; M. Rayer, who had a Venezuelan sample; M. Boussingault, who had been in Brazil; and M. Goudot, who gave a supply to M. Pelouze,[148] Bernard's assistant in some of his experiments. (As a result, the uniformity of the curare Bernard used is questionable.) In 1850, he and Pelouze extended the description of the earlier work, which confirmed the ability of that muscle to contract independently of the nerve supplying it.[149] In 1854, Bernard also showed that curare had no action on the nervous system as a whole. Leaving the sciatic nerve intact, he ligated the blood vessels of the hind leg of a frog, so that curare inserted under the skin of the back would be prevented from reaching the part of the leg below the ligature. The frog soon became immobile. Stimulation, by pinching or electric current, of the nonligated limbs failed to elicit any movement of those limbs since the curare had circulated to the leg, but stimulation of the ligated limb did evoke response in that limb, for it was not curarized. Furthermore, stimulation of the intact hind limb produced movement also in the ligated limb. These experiments suggested that only the motor nerves were affected by curarization.[150] Bernard later summarized his findings:

> The physiological conclusion which follows from these experiments is very clear: the sensitive nervous element, the motor nervous element, and the muscular elements each have their autonomy, since curare divides them and is toxic to only one of them . . . . The nervous element, sensory or voluntary, is the point of origin of the motor impulse. Next the motor element transmits this impulse to the muscle which executes it, or in other words manifests it. If only one of the preceding elements happens to be missing, the act does not occur. In poisoning by curare, sensitivity exists, as does the will to move; contractility and consequently the possibility of executing a movement exists; but just because the motor nervous element that hyphenates sensitivity with movement is destroyed by the poison, everything seems to us to be annihilated.[151]

Bernard's experiments were crucial. They gave birth to the idea that followed on from the inability of the paralyzed muscle to respond to indirect stimulation: curare acted somewhere between the nerve and the muscle. As French surgeon Edmé-Felix-Alfred Vulpian put it in 1857, "Curare paralyzes the motor nerves, particularly at the point at which they make contact with their muscles."[152] Bernard's reference to "the motor nervous element that hyphenates sensitivity with movement" is interesting because even though the concept of a motor end-plate (*plaque terminale*) was current in Bernard's day,[153] the next step in elucidation of the mode of action of curare was to learn precisely how it acted at the myoneural junction.

Precisely how curare affected the myoneural junction would not be revealed until well into the twentieth century, but in the meantime, one of the problems was that samples of curare were far from uniform, and certainly not standardized, and so the results of administration were not predictable. Rudolph Boehm, of Germany, did separate curare into *pot, gourd,* and *tube* forms in 1894, though this was not an indication of purity or potency; he is said, however, to have isolated active extracts from *calabash* (or gourd) curare in 1897[154] as curarine. However, the validity of one sample of curare against another was uncertain, which made it difficult to compare results.

By the end of the nineteenth century, despite the glimmerings of understanding that curare paralyzed muscle and might be used to overcome muscle in spasm, no one had thought of using it to overcome muscle tension during surgery. To achieve adequate abdominal relaxation, ether or chloroform were used, though they usually depressed a patient's condition. Local anesthesia, in the form of local infiltration, field blocks, or subarachnoid or epidural anesthesia, was another solution, but these were not always fully effective. Therefore, the step that was taken in 1912 by Arthur Lawen, a Leipzig surgeon, was a significant one. Understanding what was then known about neuromuscular transmission, he applied his knowledge to the problem of relaxation of the abdominal muscles. Lawen knew that curare "sets up a block between the motor end plates and the skeletal muscle," and he knew also that mice and guinea pigs whose respiratory muscles had been paralyzed with curare could be kept alive by artificial respiration. He therefore decided to use curarine, the active principle that Boehm had prepared, as a way of overcoming "the abdominal rigidity in a different way" from the use of deep anesthesia or local anesthesia.[155] Lawen administered curarine by subcutaneous or intramuscular injection, though he had the prescience to suggest that "smaller doses will be sufficient when given by intravenous injection." However, he was unable to follow through on this because his supply of curarine was insufficient.

Even so, Lawen was far ahead of his time. Apart from F. P. De Caux in England, who also used curare in anesthesia in 1928,[156] he was the only one to use curare in anesthesia long before Griffith. While he would have known about motor end plates, he would not have known about chemical transmission across the motor end plate. That only became known later when Henry Dale, in London, began to describe his work on the physiological actions of acetylcholine from 1914 onward.

Act III
1914-1942

In 1914, Dale, working at the Wellcome Physiological Research Laboratories on the autonomic nervous system, concluded that acetylcholine was closely related to the functions of the sympathetic and parasympathetic systems.[157] The suggestion of Otto Loewi that the vagus nerve could be stimulated to produce acetylcholine—and Feldberg's confirmation, with Dale, in 1934 that acetylcholine mediated the effects of the vagus nerve on the stomach—affirmed the view that transmission at the neuromuscular junction was, in fact, mediated by chemical rather than electrical means.[158]

In the Linacre Lecture in 1934, Dale further elucidated the role of acetylcholine in transmitting the effect of a motor nerve impulse to a voluntary muscle fiber.[159] That contributed to the fast-moving events that make act III of the curare drama a busy one. The roles of some anesthesiologists were among those that were important.

In 1931, J. A. Aeschlimann and M. J. Reinert synthesized curare-antagonist neostigmine methylsulphate.[160] In 1932, Ranyard West described the use of curare (purified from a sample Sherrington had once given him) for spastic disorders,[161] and in 1934, Leonard Cole used curare to treat tetanus.[162] In 1935, Harold King, in Dale's laboratory, showed that d-tubocurarine chloride was the active principle of crude curare,[163] and large-scale production of the pure alkaloid followed. In 1939, M. S. Burman treated patients with spastic and dystonic states with curare,[164] and A. E. Bennett used it to prevent fractures and dislocations resulting from metrazol convulsive therapy.[165]

Curare was used in two forms. In North America, it was Intocostrin, derived from the supply of *C. tomentosum* brought back from Ecuador by the naturalist and jungle-lover Richard Gill. Gill gave some to Bennett, which was standardized by Nebraska pharmacologist A. R. McIntyre,[166] and by H. A. Holaday, using the rabbit head-drop test. E. R. Squibb and Sons prepared it.[167] Chemists Wintersteiner and Dutcher found that pure crystalline tubocurarine contained chondocurine dimethochloride,[168] so the pure alkaloidal curariform compounds were checked for potency.[169] In England, d-tubocurarine was preferred. It was produced by Burroughs Wellcome & Company.[170]

By 1940, then, curare evidently had a number of therapeutic potentialities, yet it had not been used in anesthesia, apart from its transient use by Lawen in 1912 and De Caux in 1928. How did it finally become used in the operating room?

In 1940, a film by Bennett and McIntyre showing Intocostrin being used in shock therapy[171] was viewed by Lewis Wright, medical advisor to Squibb, who had used curare in the laboratory. An obstetrician, he knew that curare had a possible use in facilitating pelvic relaxation in mentally disturbed female patients undergoing internal examination.[172] He then conceived the idea of using curare as an adjunct to volatile agents to produce relaxation during surgery. He gave Intocostrin to anesthesiologists Emery A. Rovenstine, of New York, and Stuart C. Cullen, of Iowa City, to learn more about curare.[173] However, their trials were unsuccessful. Emanuel Papper, Rovenstine's assistant, found that curare, in etherized cats, caused bronchospasm; and respiratory paralysis developed in two patients also anesthetized with ether (in hindsight, not surprisingly). Cullen did no better than Papper. He even stated that Intocostrin could never be used in the operating room.

Wright then spoke to Griffith, a McGill University anesthesiologist in Montreal in 1941, and Griffith agreed to try curare. On January 23, 1942, he injected 5 ml Intocostrin intravenously during cyclopropane anesthesia in a twenty-year-old plumber undergoing appendectomy. Assisted by resident anesthesiologist Enid Johnson, Griffith soon collected a series of twenty-five patients, and the groundbreaking report of curare in cyclopropane anesthesia was published in July 1942.[174] That inaugurated a new era in anesthesiology. Deliberate paralysis of muscles, to please surgeons, would be a new component of anesthesia; for anesthesiologists that component was far from impractical: as Ibsen showed in 1952, during the poliomyelitis epidemic in Copenhagen, bag ventilation by hand was feasible in the critically ill.[175]

*   *   *

The evolution of anesthesia in the first half of the twentieth century reveals an appreciable degree of objectivity. Research was more evident. Early in the twentieth century, more became known about both respiration (e.g., on insufflation anesthesia, with the work of Meltzer and Auer,[176] on laryngoscopy Chevalier Jackson[177], and on carbon dioxide Yandell Henderson[178]) and circulation (e.g., Einthoven's string galvanometer electrocardiograph[179] and the relationship between light chloroform anesthesia and Levy's demonstrating the role of adrenalin and light anesthesia in the causation of ventricular fibrillation[180]). Anesthetists also had to adapt to surgical advances such as those in thoracic surgery, neurosurgery, and plastic surgery, which had developed out of World War I experiences. After World War I, new anesthetic agents, techniques such as tracheal intubation, and more sophisticated anesthesia machines and ventilators appeared.

In its second half century, anesthesia was less a service-oriented craft than practice that was more obviously influenced by a scientific approach. It was a discipline that was shaped by the application of scientific principles. In that way, the ground was prepared for anesthetists to present to their surgical and medical peers, in the 1930s, the case for recognition of anesthesia as a specialty.

Chapter 6

CARE OF THE LIFELINE
CONTROL OF THE AIRWAY

During anesthesia, a patient is no longer able to control the reflexes that normally keep the breathing passages open. If they are not kept open, neither oxygen nor inhalational agents can reach the lungs unimpeded. An important part of the anesthesiologist's responsibility, therefore, has always been to maintain the patency and integrity of the unconscious patient's respiratory tract, or airway. Over the years, much attention has been given to ensuring that the airway functions as normally as possible during an anesthetic, and that it is not blocked by spasm or secretions or liquid or solid substances, or even by the tongue falling backward in the pharynx. In this endeavor, various means have been used to preserve what is indeed a patient's lifeline. They constitute a significant aspect of the history of anesthesia, and they form the focus of this chapter.

Four points should be borne in mind while this aspect of the history of anesthesia is related. One concerns the fact that innumerable techniques and devices have been developed in order to aid the practitioner keep the airway open—the so-called artificial airway. Second, a large part of the design of anesthesia machines is concerned with the delivery of oxygen and anesthetic gases to the airway, which is only touched on here but is discussed at length in chapter 7. Third, the airway is indirectly protected by means of devices that alert the practitioner to changes in the concentrations of oxygen, carbon dioxide, and anesthetic gases as they are breathed in and out. (That is discussed under the rubric of monitoring in chapter 10.) And fourth, though the emphasis in this chapter is on the airway of the patient under inhalational anesthesia, some of the considerations also apply to the patient who is receiving purely intravenous anesthesia.

Maintaining the Airway: Dealing with Obstruction

The conscious individual naturally keeps the breathing passages intact, the normal reflexes serving to prevent obstruction of the pharynx and larynx. Secretions, blood, or food are cleared away if their presence is potentially harmful, usually by coughing or swallowing. During general anesthesia, however, those reflexes go to sleep just as the patient does; and the muscles of the pharynx and larynx become abnormally relaxed, and the natural gag and cough reflexes are depressed. The guardian of the lungs has gone absent without leave. The practitioner then has to step in.

In the first few decades of anesthetic practice, there were no artificial airways, and practitioners had to use their own hands to support a patient's jaw and so to prevent the tongue from falling backward and obstructing airflow. In the early days of anesthesia, it did not matter too much if the support was not fully adequate, nor did it matter if some blood accumulated, because surgeons operated at lightning speed and most operations lasted for a matter of minutes. (Surgeons operated speedily then, either because they were used to the absence of anesthesia or because they feared the danger of postoperative infection, especially if surgery was prolonged.) For anesthetists, speed was welcome because it meant that a serious degree of respiratory obstruction did not have time to develop. But after Glasgow surgeon Joseph Lister introduced the antiseptic carbolic acid spray in 1867,[1] surgeons began performing major operations without worrying so much about infection, and many operated more slowly and deliberately. The responsibility of anesthetists for maintaining the integrity of the patient's air passages then became all the greater.

The problem of respiratory obstruction in anesthesia was actually recognized even before the era of antisepsis by the Nottingham physician Francis Sibson. In 1847, he advised that "in the most difficult subjects it is only needful to bring both hands together, the fingers under the chin, the thumbs to each side of the nose, and the head pressed against one's own body."[2] Sibson's solution was to thrust the lower jaw forward and upward (and with it, the tongue), which is still a basic step in caring for anyone who is unconscious.

Passivity of the musculature of the upper respiratory tract could be overcome in that way, but not blockage by blood or secretions. If that was likely, some surgeons, concerned that blood might pass into the lungs, simply refrained from operating. However, tumor or infection around the mouth did make surgery necessary, and the likelihood of obstruction from the presence of blood or secretions or detritus had to be accepted. To deal with this problem, Sibson's contemporary, London anaesthetist John Snow, devised a twofold solution. He kept anesthesia light enough so the glottis retained its natural protective function, and he would "hold the head forward now and then . . . in order to allow the patient the same opportunity of breathing that he would require if he were awake."[3]

Sometimes, however, light anesthesia and manual support of the natural airway were inadequate because many conditions could cause respiratory obstruction. These included anatomical variations in the mouth and pharynx, pathological lesions of the upper respiratory tract, and poor visualization of the glottis, as well as the presence of blood, secretions, or nutriments. Anesthesia equipment could also cause obstruction. Thus, in explaining how his ether inhaler worked, Snow pointed out that the tube through which a patient breathed had to be wider than the trachea, to avoid "impediment to the most rapid inspiration," and that the width of the tube might "compensate for the resistance arising from friction of air against the interior of the tube."[4] However, neither Snow nor Sibson referred to respiratory obstruction as such.

The first person to refer specifically to respiratory obstruction was J. Heiberg. In 1874, he too recommended extending the head and thrusting the jaw forward.[5] Six years later, Benjamin Howard pointed out that it was the posterior movement of the tongue, not the downward slipping of the epiglottis, that caused respiratory obstruction.[6] It was often tiring to maintain the airway, but various devices made control of the airway easier.

Early Artificial Airways

One solution was devised in 1868 by London anesthetist Joseph Clover. For dental anesthesia, he administered nitrous oxide through a nosepiece that capped the nose and so facilitated the dentist's access to the mouth.[7] Alfred Coleman, the London dentist, also gave the gas nasally.[8] (Coleman is also known for allowing rebreathing, and for absorbing carbon dioxide in the expired air with "slaked lime." This was the first time carbon dioxide absorption was used clinically,[9] Snow having done so experimentally in 1851.[10]) In 1888, Stephen Coxon, also a dentist, put a tube in the mouth to make nitrous oxide easier to give.[11]

Further progress was made by Joseph O'Dwyer, of New York, and George Fell, of Buffalo. O'Dwyer, who looked after desperately ill children with diphtheria, stated in 1885 that he had inserted a metal tube beyond the glottis. Air did not leak around the tube because a conical tip lay at the glottis. An introducer was required because in the days before laryngoscopy and direct vision of the larynx, a tube could only be passed "blindly"; it was felt but not seen as it passed through the larynx.[12] Fell's equipment, described in 1887 as a means of forcing respiration in opium poisoning,[13] comprised a face mask, an intubation tube, an oxygen supply, and a foot bellows. Neither individual's equipment, however, was intended for use in anesthesia, but the combination, known as the Fell-O'Dwyer apparatus (fig. 6.1), was used to insufflate gas into the trachea.[14] That led to the later practice of tracheal intubation, which eventually became part of the care of some anesthetized patients, of the critically ill, and of those, later still, who needed to be resuscitated. The O'Dwyer and Fell apparatus, though not intended for use in anesthesia, was more radical than was required, and it was certainly more problematic than the later device of a short curved tube that could be placed between the teeth so that it lay over the tongue as a "supraglottic" airway. That type of tube, the oropharyngeal airway (fig. 6.2), was described in 1908 by Frederic Hewitt, another London anesthetist. He designed it to overcome the natural tendency of the tongue of the anesthetized patient to fall backward and block the oropharynx.[15] The result of a great deal of thought about respiratory obstruction,[16] Hewitt's airway was the template for others in the twentieth century.[17] A well-known one was that of Arthur Guedel, which was introduced in 1933 and became very widely used (fig. 6.3).[18] However, none of the oropharyngeal airways completely overcame the problem of respiratory obstruction, and it was necessary to return to the concept of tracheal intubation.

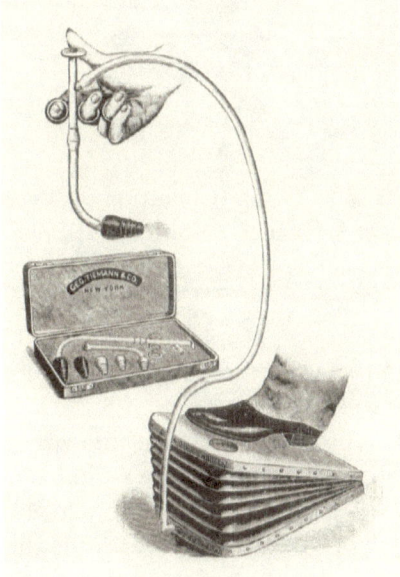

Fig. 6.1. Fell-O'Dwyer apparatus for artificial ventilation, c.1896. (Source: T. Keys, *The History of Surgical Anesthesia* [New York: Dover Publications, Inc., 1963], opposite p. 67.)

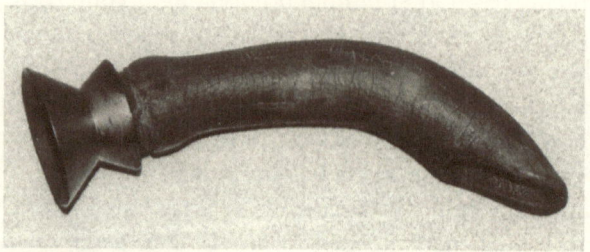

Fig. 6.2. Hewitt oral airway (1908). (Collection of Wood Library-Museum of Anesthesiology.) (Source: F. Hewitt. An artificial 'airway' for use during anaesthetization. *Lancet* 1908; 1:490-91.)

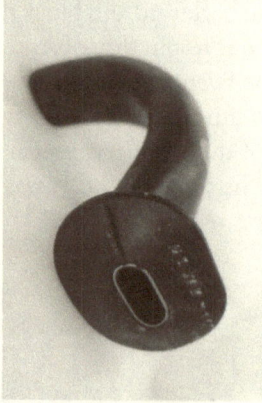

Fig. 6.3. Guedel oral airway (1933). (Collection of Wood Library-Museum of Anesthesiology.) (Source: A. Guedel. A nontraumatic pharyngeal airway. *JAMA* 1933; 100:1862.)

Tracheal Intubation and Laryngoscopy

Supraglottic airways were effective in persons without an anatomical or pathological abnormality of the upper airway, but they were of no help if such an abnormality was present in the upper part of the airway or in the trachea or the bronchi. Nor were they practical in anesthetics of long duration. The answer was to pass a long tube into the trachea, so that it lay, as an "infraglottic" airway, *below* the glottis. While a tube like O'Dwyer's could be modified for anesthesia, better were tubes that were designed specifically for use in anesthesia. That led to the next step: intubating the trachea as part of the anesthetic technique.

The Development of Tracheal Intubation

Placing a tube in the trachea was known long before the nineteenth and twentieth centuries. About AD 1000, Avicenna had intubated the trachea.[19] And in 1543, Andreas Vesalius, the great anatomist, inserted a reed in a sow's windpipe.[20] However, the medical practice of tracheal intubation was more closely related to the resuscitation of drowning victims (see also chapter 14.) Charles Kite, in London in 1788,[21] described passing a curved tube into the larynx, and Herholdt and Rafn, in Denmark in 1796, reported passing a tube blindly over fingers positioned behind the epiglottis.[22] Tracheal intubation was performed in the latter part of the eighteenth century and in the nineteenth century by physicians like O'Dwyer who were concerned with disorders such as diphtheria, croup, and edema of the glottis. Tracheal intubation was therefore not uncommon in medical practice many years before the introduction of anesthesia. Physicians who engaged in this practice include the following: James Curry (1791), Fine (1800), Dessault (1801), Chaussier (1806), Cap (1828), Depaul (1845), Horace Green and D. M. Reese (1854), Bouchet (1857), Truehead (1869), Schrotter (1876), and Wilhem Hack (1878).[23, 24]

As far as use of a tracheal tube in anesthesia is concerned, Snow reported that chloroform could be administered through a tube placed in the trachea through a tracheostomy, but this was in a rabbit.[25] Clinical use was reported by German surgeon Friedrich Trendelenburg in 1871.[26] Of greater interest in the history of anesthesia is the feat performed by William Macewen, the Glasgow surgeon, in 1878. He administered an anesthetic agent through a tube placed in the trachea deliberately for this purpose,[27] and he was the first to do so. His feat was the more remarkable because before inducing anesthesia, Macewen inserted a tracheal tube with his patient awake. He did so because his patient's tongue was deformed by cancer, and because he intubated him before local anesthesia with cocaine was introduced. Macewen learned how to do it by practicing in the autopsy room, and he thought deeply about what had to be done in such a difficult case. Administering chloroform via the endotracheal tube doubtless prevented many of the complications that might otherwise have arisen, though tracheostomy might have been an alternative.

These various initiatives led to other aspects and uses of intubation. Macewen, for example, left one tube in place for up to thirty-nine hours, which by many years antedated the later practice of inserting tracheal tubes to aid ventilation. The Fell-O'Dwyer device, besides generating the concept of endotracheal insufflation, was adapted by the New Orleans surgeon Rudolph Matas to facilitate anesthesia for thoracic surgery.[28] The tracheal tube was fitted with a plug that sealed the area around the larynx so that positive pressure could be applied through the glottis. O'Dwyer's concept was also taken up in 1900 by Hans Kuhn. He designed a flexible metal tube that could be introduced blindly over a stylet, and was long enough to project out of the mouth, an anesthetic agent being delivered through it.[29]

Though these individuals were able to pass tubes into the trachea, and to do so even in the absence of direct visualization by laryngoscopy, many anesthesia practitioners lacked the necessary skill. Laryngoscopy had yet to be perfected, so intubation had to be performed blind, and luck and the patient's cooperation were important to success. To be invariably successful in intubating the trachea, one had to actually see the larynx. That step was the next to be developed.

The Development of Laryngoscopy

For a long time, only laryngologists had any interest in visualizing the larynx. Levret, in France, attempted to do that in 1743. He looked through a speculum, using sunlight to help him see the image of a tumor in the throat on a metallic reflecting surface.[30] In 1807, Bozzini used a more elaborate piece of equipment, comprising a tin lantern and a wax candle, two mirrors, a metal speculum, and an eyepiece.[31] However, neither Levret nor Bozzini was successful. As Morell Mackenzie noted, quoting John Stuart Mill, in neither case were the tools suited to the art,[32] and their inventions did not take hold.

The earliest practical laryngoscope was that of Benjamin Guy Babington, of London. A medical student, he described his dual-mirror device in 1829.[33] He did not use artificial light but was able to see the epiglottis, which is why MacKenzie regarded Babington's as the first true laryngoscope.[34] A different approach was that of Manuel Garcia, a Franco-Spanish voice-teacher who lived in England. To understand the anatomy and physiology of the voice, he studied the movements of his own vocal cords with the aid of two mirrors, using indirect laryngoscopy. Garcia's account of 1855[35] was read by Ludwig Turck, a Viennese surgeon. In 1857, he obtained a set of mirrors, but the apparatus was clumsy, and he did not recognize the value of the laryngoscope.[36] He was followed by the Czech surgeon Johann Czermak, who used artificial light and improved mirrors. In Mackenzie's view, it was Czermak who finally created the art of laryngoscopy.[37] All these individuals used natural light and the technique of indirect laryngoscopy, but this, as Sykes has pointed out, has no application to the technique of tracheal intubation as used in anesthesia.[38]

The serendipitous development of direct, artificially illuminated laryngoscopy by Alfred Kirstein in Germany was another step forward. Kirstein heard that a colleague had accidentally passed an esophagoscope into the trachea and so obtained a fine view of the lower airway.[39] He fashioned the prototype of the modern laryngoscope by placing an electric light source within the handle of the instrument, attaching a blade so that he could lift the epiglottis and see the vocal cords. His "autoscope"[40] (fig. 6.4) was a forerunner of the first laryngoscopes to be used by anesthetists.

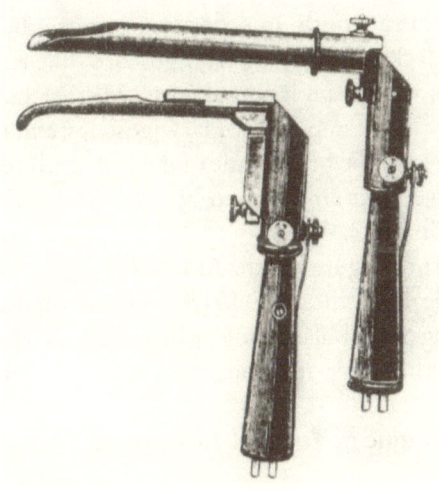

Fig. 6.4. Alfred Kirstein's 'Autoscope' (1895). (Source: N. Hirsch, G. Smith, p. Hirsch, Alfred Kirstein: Pioneer of direct laryngoscopy, *Anaesthesia* 1986; 41:42-45.)

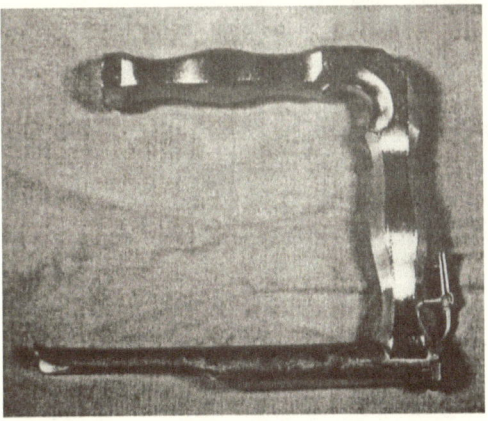

Fig. 6.5. Chevalier Jackson laryngoscope (1912). (Source: P. Koltai, R. Nixon, The story of the laryngoscope, *Ear, Nose and Throat J* 1989; 68:494-502.)

The ideas of two other individuals before World War I influenced progress in tracheal intubation. One was the leading endsocopist Chevalier Jackson. Influenced by Kirstein's work, he designed a direct-vision laryngoscope in 1903 (fig. 6.5).[41] It comprised arms that made three sides of a square, the fourth arm being nonexistent; the upper horizontal arm was the part that was gripped, while the parallel lower horizontal arm incorporated the laryngoscope itself. A key element was a distal illumination source; a second was insertion in the lateral part of the mouth, in order to minimize the distance from the lips to the larynx.[42] Jackson's work on laryngoscopy, like Kirstein's, influenced anesthesiologists, as well as otolaryngologists. His teaching emphasized the value of larngoscopy in anesthesia,[43] for laryngoscopy and tracheal intubation was an uncharted field in the first decade of the twentieth century. Anesthetists would therefore have been enlightened by an article on endotracheal tubes written by Jackson in 1913.[44]

The other influential figure was the American surgeon Henry Janeway, who wrote on intratracheal anesthesia in 1913.[45] His laryngoscope differed from Jackson's in consisting of a tubular handle, which contained two dry-cell batteries and a straight blade that projected from the handle at a right angle.

Perfecting the Technique of Tracheal Intubation

War expedites progress in surgery because new challenges face the surgeon in patient care; the anesthesia practitioner must adapt specialized knowledge and skill to fit the surgeon's. Accordingly, the next phase of development in tracheal intubation arose during and just after World War I.[46]

Among the types of trauma resulting from the war were severe facial injuries, which often compromised the natural airway and made direct visualization of the glottis difficult. A further challenge for an anesthetist looking after patients with maxillofacial injuries was to be sure of patency and integrity of the very part of the body that the surgeon was operating on. Figuring out a solution to this challenge was the task of two British anaesthetists, Ivan Magill (fig. 6.6) and Stanley Rowbotham. Their experience generated new concepts and techniques of tracheal intubation.

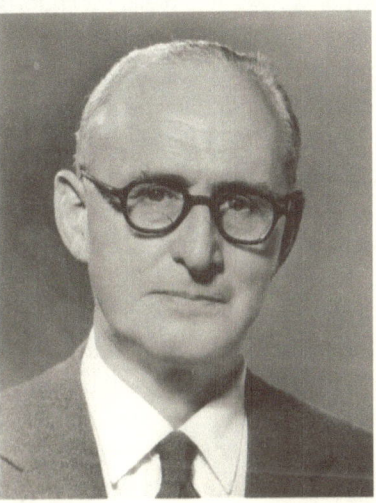

Fig. 6.6. Ivan Magill (1888-1986)
Ivan Whiteside Magill, born in Larne, Northern Ireland, graduated from Queen's University Belfast in 1913. After serving as a doctor in the military, Magill, with Stanley Rowbotham, gave anesthetics to patients with facial and maxillary injuries. Maintaining patency of the airway was always a challenge. He and Rowbotham used tracheal insufflation, then a single narrow tube, then two tubes, and finally a single wide-bore tube. Magill designed the forceps that bear his name to help pass the tubes, but he frequently passed a tube blindly through the nose. At London's Brompton Hospital, Magill designed an intubating bronchoscope, endobronchial tubes, and a tube to block off a bronchus, together with a suction catheter for use in one lung-anaesthesia. He favored the Magill (Mapleson A) attachment to the Boyle anesthesia machine and the rotameter in place of the dry gas flowmeter. In Great Britain, Magill influenced the development of anesthesia as a specialty by proposing an examination for a Diploma in Anaesthetics, which led to the founding of a body that could initiate this examination—the Association of Anaesthetists of Great Britain and Ireland. Like John Snow, Joseph Clover, and Frederic Hewitt before him, Magill anesthetized the highborn and well connected. He was knighted in 1960.

Initially, Magill and Rowbotham used the insufflation technique, which physiologists Samuel Meltzer and John Auer, of the Rockefeller Insitute in New York, had described in 1909.[47] They were able to maintain respiration in etherized animals if the lungs were continuously inflated through a tube in the trachea, even if the normal respiratory movements were stopped by an injection of curare. Magill and Rowbotham first modified this technique by passing two tubes into the trachea: one to introduce anesthetic gases and the other to allow vapor to escape. But since their surgeons frequently operated on the mouth, Magill and Rowbotham would instead pass a single wide-bore rubber tube, which seemed physiologically and economically to make greater sense. They also packed off the pharynx with gauze.

Thus did Magill and Rowbotham begin to prefer the endotracheal to the insufflation principle; thus too did they foster a new approach to general anesthesia.[48]

Despite the demonstrable efficiency and safety of endotracheal intubation, many anesthetists were slow to adopt it. However, several factors made practitioners more aware of its value. In 1924, Ralph Waters, of Madison, published an account of his carbon dioxide technique, using a canister of soda lime,[49] which mandated use of a leakproof circuit. Waters drew attention to the demonstration in 1915 by Dennis Jackson, of Cincinnati, that dogs could be safely anesthetized with nitrous oxide for long periods if they were intubated and if the expired carbon dioxide was absorbed with a sodium hydrate—calcium hydrate mixture.[50] Two years later, Guedel initiated studies of cuffs on endotracheal tubes,[51] which had been pioneered by Victor Eisenmenger in Prague in the 1890s[52] and which brought together the advantages of endotracheal intubation and the closed circuit. A circle form of closed circuit was introduced by Brian Sword in 1930[53] (see chapter 7), and in the same year, John Lundy learned more about tracheal intubation from Magill, when the latter visited the Mayo Clinic.[54] As noted in chapter 5, in 1934 Waters and his group began using cyclopropane,[55] which mandated use of a closed endotracheal technique.

Progress in chest surgery, which itself was facilitated by the use of cyclopropane and of ventilators, influenced progress in anesthesia also. Pioneer work on the use of ventilators had been conducted by P. Frenckner and thoracic surgeon Clarence Crafoord in Sweden in the 1930s.[56] A serendipitous incident also contributed. Waters learned that an endotracheal tube had been passed unintentionally into a bronchus, which induced one-lung anesthesia, and Guedel suggested that a double-cuffed but single-lumen tube might be used to facilitate chest surgery. This concept was put into practice by Emery Rovenstine.[57]

By 1940, therefore, a new approach to anesthesia was being developed, even though endotracheal intubation was by no means universal. This approach was furthered by curare beginning in 1942[58] (see chapter 5), which made it much easier for practitioners to directly see the glottis and pass a tracheal introduced in 1952.[59] It made intubation even easier and with even less delay after induction of anesthesia. Other factors that stimulated the use of laryngoscopes were the introduction of cyclopropane, the greater frequency of thoracic operations, and the recognition of the value of ventilators.

Variations in laryngoscopes, designed to overcome difficulties in visualization, also facilitated tracheal intubation. The straight-bladed instruments of Magill and Paluel Flagg, introduced in 1920 and 1928, respectively, heightened interest in the technique.[60] A straight-bladed laryngoscope was made and named after Lundy.[61] Like others, it was rigid, and Waters suggested that a folding one be made.[62] Various other laryngoscopes were designed as anesthesiologists, including Robert Miller in 1941, W. H. Cassels in 1942 and Robert Macintosh(fig. 6.7) in 1943. As with so many pieces of anesthesia apparatus, modification was the order of the day. Miller, of San Antonio, Texas, thought the available instruments were too thick and injured tissue besides not always facilitating visualization, and so designed a narrow blade that was curved near the tip[63]. Cassels decided that a curved blade would permit better visualization,[64] though it was Macintosh, of Oxford, England, whose curved blade[65] made the advantages of the curved blade better known in 1943.[66] Whereas the Miller blade was intended to pass posterior to the epiglottis, the Macintosh was meant to be placed immediately behind the epiglottis as the various structures near the glottis were lifted anteriorly.

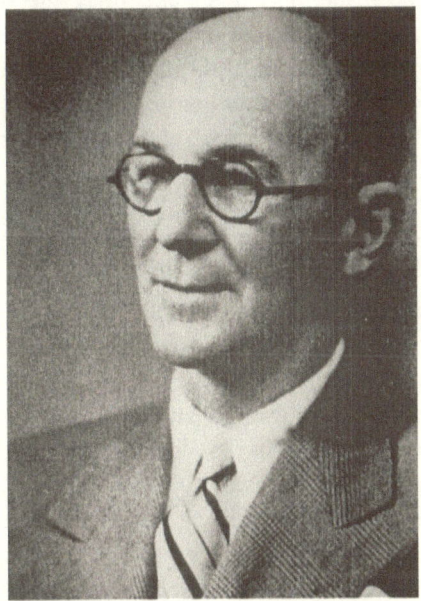

Fig. 6.7. Robert Macintosh (1897-1989)
Robert Macintosh was born in Timaru, New Zealand; served in the Royal Flying Corps in World War I; and, taken prisoner, attempted escape several times. He graduated in medicine at Guy's Hospital, London, in 1924. Macintosh practiced dental anesthesia in London, using entirely portable apparatus. This, plus use of a modified Flagg can during the Spanish civil war, gave him an interest in simplicity in techniques of anesthesia. In 1937, Macintosh was appointed Nuffield Professor of Anaesthetics in Oxford University, the first chair of anesthesia to be created in Europe. Macintosh was also interested in survival at high altitudes, self-righting life jackets, artificial ventilation, laryngoscope blades (he conceived the idea of a curved blade in 1943), curare, and complications in anesthesia. The department at Oxford, his research, the pieces of apparatus and the books on general anesthesia and regional anesthesia he was associated with, and his teaching in underdeveloped countries made him known round the world and a potent force in the development of anesthesia as a respected field of medicine. He was recognized by his peers by being awarded both the Hickman Medal and the John Snow Medal and by Queen Elizabeth by being knighted in 1955.

Despite the variety of blades, intubation was not always easy; the glottis could not always be seen. To help anesthesiologists overcome this problem, many ingenious laryngoscopes were invented. The Siker (1956), for example, incorporated a mirror,[67] and the Huffman[68] (1968) and the Belscope (1988)[69] a prism. Another problem was immobility or instability of the cervical spine, which limits any movement of the neck. The Bullard[70] and the Augustine Guide,[71] both introduced in the 1990s, were designed to overcome that problem.

Tracheal intubation made inhalational anesthesia safer and more efficacious, and to a large extent it overcame the problems of respiratory obstruction, the difficult airway, and, in thoracic surgery, pneumothorax. However, it was not free of complications. The action and effects of passing a tube into the trachea, its resting there sometimes for many hours, and the use of a metal instrument to aid intubation all were potentially traumatic to a part of the body that was designed to reject foreign bodies. To overcome those problems, two instruments were designed in the second half of the twentieth century: the fiberoptic laryngoscope and the laryngeal mask airway.

Fiberoscopy for Laryngoscopy

The fiberoptic laryngoscope, like the fiberoptic bronchoscope and gastroscope, is characterized by excellence of indirect visualization. Virtually abolishing the problem of difficult visualization of the glottis, it revolutionized the approach to the difficult airway.

The origin of the concept of light being guided down a tube goes back to the first half of the nineteenth century. The concept was popularized in 1854 by physicist John Tyndall, who showed that light could be guided down a jet of water.[72] The principle of fiberoscopy is analogous to this. Light enters one end of hair-thin glass fibers (diameter, 5-25 microns) and is continuously reflected off the fiber wall until it emerges at the distal end. Until the 1950s, such fine glass fibers were not available; and in 1954, Harold Hopkins, of Reading, England, and N. S. Karpany described a flexible fiberscope.[73] In February 1957, Basil Hirschowitz passed a prototype scope down his own throat and down the throat of a patient a few days later.[74] Ten years later, Peter Murphy, of London, reported using a choledochoscope for nasal intubation.[75]

Fiberoscopy then became a standard part of anesthetic practice, and the fiberoptic laryngoscope (fig. 6.8), a standard piece of anesthetic apparatus. It permits the anesthesiologist to see the glottis virtually perfectly—admittedly not with the naked eye but through a lens—in almost 100 percent of the patients. Andranik Ovassapian and his colleagues in San Diego, for example, in 1983 reported a failure rate in 413 cases of only 1.2 percent.[76] Fiberoscopy was then widely used for orotracheal intubation, as well as nasotracheal intubation. It greatly diminished the anxiety that was felt by anesthesiologists as they were about to anesthetize patients who were known to present difficulty in intubation and those in whom the difficulty occurred unexpectedly. Fiberoscopy was a boon to anesthesiologists and, though most of them were not aware of it, to patients also.

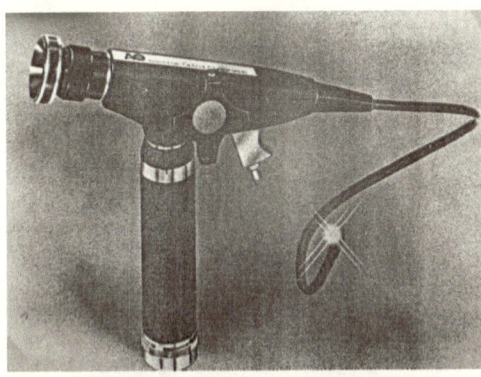

Fig. 6.8. Fiberoptic laryngoscope/bronchoscope. (Source: A. Conyers, D. Wallace, D. Mulder, Use of the fiber optic bronchoscope for nasotracheal intubation: Case report. *Can Anaesth Soc J* 1972; 44:654-66.)

The Laryngeal Mask Airway (LMA)

The development of fiberoscopy in anesthesia reflects the fact that in some patients, neither the face mask and the oropharyngeal airway nor tracheal intubation was invariably successful in controlling the airway. Though fiberoscopy met the problem of the difficult airway and difficult intubation head-on, as an effective solution to the age-old problem of respiratory obstruction, the technique had to be learned, and the instrument was complex and potentially fragile. A second development, late in the twentieth century, was simpler and more practical. It bypassed the problem not by ensuring insertion of a tube in the trachea but by optimizing control of that part of the airway immediately above the glottis. This was the invention of the laryngeal mask airway (fig. 6.9). Of the many devices that have been invented to make anesthesia safer and more effective, only a few are revolutionary in the sense of changing routine practice. This is what the laryngeal mask airway did after it was introduced in the 1990s.

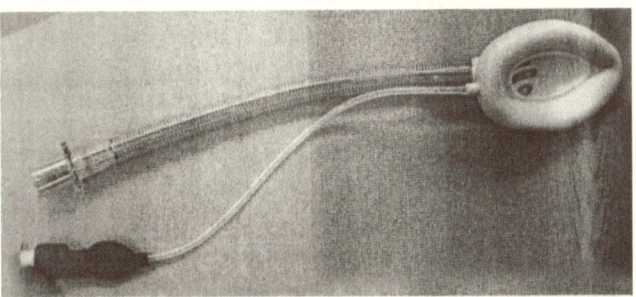

Fig.6.9. Laryngeal mask airway. (Photograph courtesy Dr. Francis Whalen.)

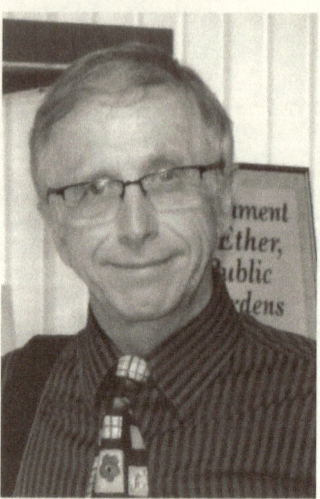

Fig. 6.10. Archie Brain (b.1942)

Archie Brain was born in Kobe, Japan, but left for England soon after he was born. With a scholarship to Oxford University, Brain studied modern languages and literature, but he switched to medicine, taking his basic-science education in Oxford and his clinical studies in London at St. Bartholomew's Hospital. Brain practiced anesthesia in England, Holland, and the Seychelles. In 1980, he worked at the London Hospital with James Payne. This stimulated his creative juices and his research talents, filing a dozen patent applications. One of Brain's brainy ideas was to overcome the deficiency of current airway devices by making an artificial airway join end-to-end at the glottis with the natural airway. That was the concept of the laryngeal mask airway, which surrounded the entrance to the larynx and trachea as the face mask does the entrance to the mouth and nose. The first model for the new airway became commercially available in 1988, and it soon changed the way anesthesia was administered, just as other innovations such as Snow's ether inhaler and Magill's endotracheal technique had done so earlier. Brain was recognized by his peers relatively early in his career, being awarded the Magill Gold Medal by the Association of Anaesthetists of Great Britain and Ireland, for example, in 1995.

The device was conceived by Archie Brain, an English anaesthetist (fig. 6.10). He reasoned that the traditional face mask and oropharyngeal airway did not always ensure a physiologically adequate and uninterrupted flow of air between the lips or nose proximally and the glottis distally. He also knew that tracheal intubation was sometimes traumatic. Research showed that a connection between an artificial and the natural airway was best made posterior to and around the glottis. He then designed a tube with an inflatable cuff that would encircle the entrance to the glottis; it was patented in 1982.[77]

Brain's new airway was indeed a mask around the larynx, and is thus a supraglottic device. However, it was not the first device to lie immediately proximal to the glottis. O'Dwyer's tube formed a seal as its conical tip lay in the glottis[78] and, in this sense, encroached on the physiologically sensitive trachea; and Beverly Leech, of Regina, Canada, designed an airway with a rubber excrescence that formed a seal in the pharynx,[79] though Leech had never proved that the seal was invariably effective and protective. In contrast, Brain showed that the laryngeal mask airway did make such a seal, with a pressure of some 20 cm H_2O.[80] The pilot study, conducted in 1982, showed that it had other clear advantages: it could be placed without the aid of muscle relaxants, and it protected the larynx from blood, saliva, and extraneous matter; and the throat was seldom sore after anesthesia. In large patients in whom intubation was unsuccessful, the laryngeal mask airway seemed to provide an airway that was patent and anesthesia that was safe.[81]

Much further research was necessary to validate the effectiveness and safety of the device that would ensure its acceptance by anesthesiologists. Various prototypes of the airway were tested over the next few years, and the number of patients in whom the LMA was used steadily increased. Commercial production of the LMA began in 1987.[82] Publications proliferated.

Clearly, a new era of anesthetic technique and technology was initiated, and the Brain airway generated production of a variety of other supraglottic devices. Whether time will unveil unexpected complications is not clear, but the device was rapidly accepted as a safe and effective means of airway control and lifesaving in the management of the difficult airway or failed intubation.[83] As Brimacombe has noted, "Probably no other airway device before, and certainly not since, has seen such a meteoric rise into the clinical firmament."[84]

*   *   *

Despite the complexity of some of the surgical operations of the twenty-first century, few could be performed without safe and adequate anesthesia; and that could not be achieved without patency of the airway and integrity of the respiration. This was recognized beginning in the earliest days of anesthesia, and anesthesia practitioners endeavored to find efficient and effective ways of securing control of the anesthetized patient's respiration so that it was not adversely affected by surgery or anesthesia.

When one considers the many problems that anesthesiologists have had to solve in relation to the airway, what might seem to be a simple matter of looking after a patient's breathing is actually a complex one. That is one more aspect of the complexity of anesthesia itself and of its evolution from craft through discipline to specialty.

Chapter 7

THE DEVELOPMENT OF ANESTHESIA
MACHINES, 1885-1935
THE EMERGENCE OF ANESTHESIA
AS DISCIPLINE ILLUSTRATED

One of the simplest ways of analyzing the evolution of anesthesia, especially as it emerged from craft to discipline, is to compare the anesthesia equipment of the nineteenth century with that of the first four decades of the twentieth century. In the former period, it was small, simple, and portable, and designed to be used in peoples' homes, where operations were often performed. Toward the end of the century, the apparatus became larger and complex and less portable, and the devices were no longer pieces of apparatus; they could be described as *machines* for hospital use. Their technological and innovative ingenuity then, and especially in the first decade and a half of the twentieth century, was in marked contrast to the stagnation that characterized anesthesia earlier. Machine design is in fact the clearest indication of the beginning of the transformation of anesthesia from a craft to a discipline.

There are several reasons for this transformation. One concerns changes in the practice of surgery. Antisepsis made longer surgical operations possible and their performance more appropriate in hospitals than in people's homes. Hence there was now no need for portability of anesthesia equipment and every need for more rugged equipment that was suitable for more "capital" operations and consonant with the growing concern about the safety of anesthesia. A second reason concerns the fact that from the latter part of the 1860s onward, it became possible to compress nitrous oxide and oxygen into metal tanks. That, added to the bulk and weight of the anesthetist's armamentarium, militated against minimalism of design.

Another reason relates less directly to anesthesia. That is the rapid progress that science and science and medicine made in the last years of the nineteenth century and the early part of the twentieth. In that period, an intellectual ferment revolutionized thinking among scientists.[1] For example, Wilhelm Rontgen discovered X-rays in 1895, Max Planck formulated the quantum theory in 1900, Willem Einthoven invented the string electrocardiograph in 1903, Albert Einstein announced the special relativity theory in 1905, and Charles Sherrington published his work on the integrative action of the nervous system in 1906. As Charles Singer pointed out, medicine in 1900 was based much more firmly in science than it had been in 1850, and medical thought was being redirected.[2] Such major discoveries opened many people's eyes to what could be done, and it is not unlikely that among those people were those medical scientists who designed the first generation of true anesthesia machines. The work of those scientists—who included surgeons, physiologists, and engineers as well as anesthetists—was of enormous importance not only because it focused a scientific approach on the design of anesthesia machines but also because it established some of the principles that would govern the design of anesthesia machines for long afterward.

As far as anesthesia machine design is concerned, the transition to a new era began in 1885. In that year, two notable events that were related occurred. One was Frederic Hewitt's article in the *Lancet* on nitrous oxide anesthesia.[3] Like many other anesthetists of his day, Hewitt was concerned about the mortality associated with anesthesia, especially with chloroform. Nitrous oxide was an alternative to ether and chloroform, and Hewitt's work made gas anesthesia safer, principally by showing how it could be mixed with oxygen. The second event was the manufacture of a two-cylinder anesthesia machine by the S. S. White Company, of Philadelphia,[4] which was the first of a new type of anesthesia equipment. Thus, our discussion of the development of the large freestanding machines will begin with the year 1885. Those two events, with others around this time, did much to lift anesthesia from the doldrums: consider Macewen's intubating the trachea in 1878 (chapter 6), Clover's efforts to improve ether administration (*vide infra*), and the advent of local anesthesia (chapter 4).

Hewitt is a significant figure for another reason. He was the first since the death of John Snow in 1858 to take a rigorous approach to research, as well as to the clinical practice of anesthesia. In this respect, he served as a link between the craft of the previous forty years and the discipline that would flourish in the next half century, before anesthesia was finally recognized as a specialty. With respect to the innovations in machine design, with which this chapter is mainly concerned, the impetus that Hewitt gave to anesthesia at the turn of the century certainly gives him a significant place in the history of anesthesia.

Brief Comments on Progress Between 1846 and 1935

Although the discussion in this chapter is mainly concerned with the period from 1885 (when the first freestanding anesthesia machine was designed) to 1935 (when the first anesthesia machine to have a modern look was manufactured), a brief return to 1846 will make even more obvious the contrast between equipment in the earliest period with that ninety years later. Few objects in anesthesia illustrate the contrast between *old* and *modern* better than two devices that were made in 1846 and in 1935. If figures 7.1 and 7.2 are compared, the simple ether inhaler used by William Morton in 1846 and the complex anesthesia machine designed by Karl Connell in 1935 show a world of differences. The Morton inhaler is simply a glass globe that had its functional origin in respiratory therapy. Handheld, it contained just a small ether-saturated sponge and a mouthpiece fitted with a crude leather valve through which the patient breathed the ether.[5] The Connell machine of 1935 was a stainless-steel wheeled cabinet suitable for administration of nitrous oxide, ethylene, cyclopropane, and carbon dioxide.[6] The differences reflect progress in anesthesia machine design and in anesthesia agents and, at the same time, the evolution of anesthesia from a new craft in 1846 to a discipline and a nascent specialty in 1935.

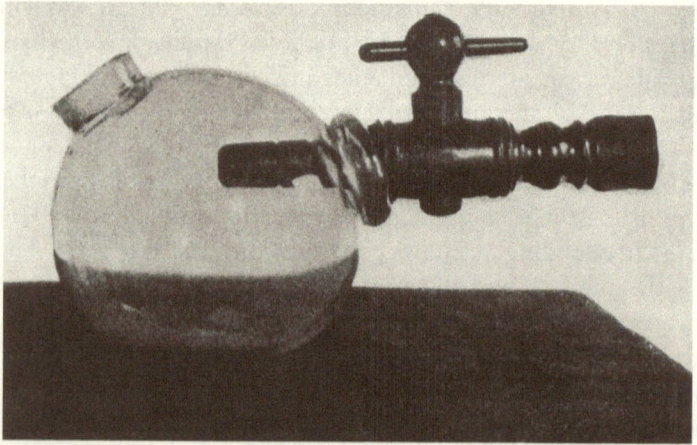

Fig. 7.1. Replica of Morton's inhaler, as used 16 October 1846. (Source: K. B. Thomas, *The Development of Anaesthetic Apparatus: A History Based on the Charles King Collection of the Association of Anaesthetists of Great Britain and Ireland* [Oxford: Blackwell Scientific Publications, 1975], p. 10.)

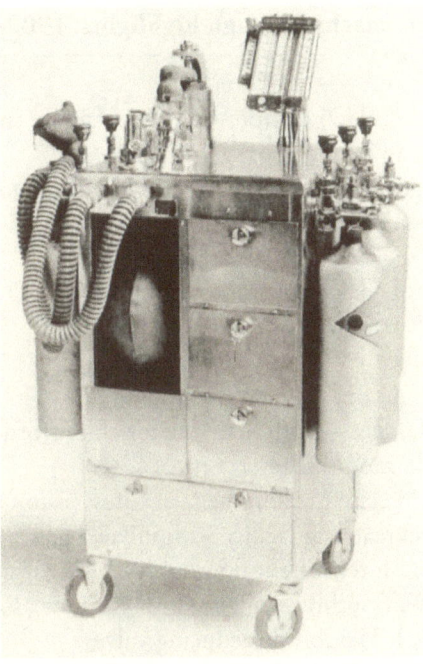

Fig. 7.2. Karl Connell's cabinet-type anesthesia machine (1935). (Photograph courtesy of Wood Library-Museum of Anesthesiology.)

Despite those differences, the objective inherent in the two pieces of apparatus was the same: to enable the practitioner induce and maintain anesthesia. What, then, are the significant differences? What was the evolutionary path that the many anesthetists, inventors, engineers, and entrepreneurs took between 1846 and 1935 in shaping the design of the anesthesia devices in that interval? More particularly, what specific principles governed the design of anesthesia machines in the period from 1885 (when the first two-cylinder White machine appeared) to 1935 (when the Connell was produced)? These questions form the background to the discussion in this chapter. Though some older devices are considered in this discussion, those of the first four decades of the twentieth century are emphasized, since many of the principles therein remained valid in the design of later, and technically more modern, anesthesia machines. For that reason, the development of anesthesia according to principles, rather than chronology, is what is emphasized in this chapter. Nor is it intended to go into the detail that the incomparable texts by Barbara Duncum[7] and Bryn Thomas[8] and the instructive chapter by David Wilkinson[9] provide. While the orientation is topical, a chronological guide to the highlights of development is, however, provided in table 7.1.

Table 7.1. Anesthesia machine design highlights, 1900-1930*

Preliminary Events

1868 Nitrous oxide (N_2O) compression, liquefaction in cylinders
      E. Andrews: advocacy of oxygen with N_2O
1873 W. Hele: regulatory device to control gas flow, temperature
1885 F. Hewitt: study of N_2O anesthesia
      S. S. White Company: N_2O machine
1893 F. Hewitt: stopcock for variation of O_2 with N_2O

Key Developments

c. 1900 C. Teter: N_2O machine production
1902 B. Dräger: Dräger—Roth machine for chloroform
1906 J. Heidbrink: modifies Teter; first of series
1908 K. Connell: precise measurement of gases; piston flowmeters
1910 W. Gatch: rebreathing facility with inhaled gases
      E. McKesson: intermittent flow, rebreathing; first of series
1911 F. Cotton, W. Boothby: sight-feed for gas flow assessment
1912 W. Boothby, J. Heidbrink: reducing valves
      C. Elsberg, R. Kelly, H. Boyle: insufflation apparatus
      K. Connell: rotary-vane gas flow, drop measurement of ether
      J. Gwathmey: with Woolsey, Foregger—anesthesia machine
1915 D. Jackson: machine with carbon dioxide (CO_2) absorption
1917 H. Boyle: machine, first of series
1924 R. Waters: to-and-from CO_2 absorption canister
1930 B. Sword: closed-circuit apparatus

*Sources: Duncum, 1947; Thomas, 1975; Wood-Library Museum of Anesthesiology

Nineteenth-Century Inhalers

In thinking about the design of an inhaler, Morton seems to have had his own ideas, though he did consult Joseph Wightman[10] and Nathan Chamberlain, instrument makers.[11] Most of the earliest inhalers, however, were adaptations of those that were relics of the eighteenth-century interest in gases and liquids as medicinal agents. One was the adaptation of Nooth's apparatus (see fig. 3.6) that William Squire used on December 21, 1846, in etherizing for Robert Liston in London's University College Hospital.[12] Often, however, instead of an inhaler,** a domestic item such as a handkerchief or a glove[13] might be used, with ether or

---

**An inhaler should strictly be regarded as a handheld device that enables a person to inhale vapor produced by a liquid. A vaporizer is a device that causes a liquid to be vaporized. (J. Robins, 2008, personal communication.)

chloroform simply poured drop by drop from a small bottle onto a rag or piece of cloth over the patient's face. Eventually, however, a more hygienic metal mask covered with lint or gauze was used. An early one was designed in 1862 by Thomas Skinner, of Liverpool[14] (fig. 7.3); later ones include those of Schimmelbusch, of 1890, and Yankauer, of 1910,[15] which were used well into the twentieth century.

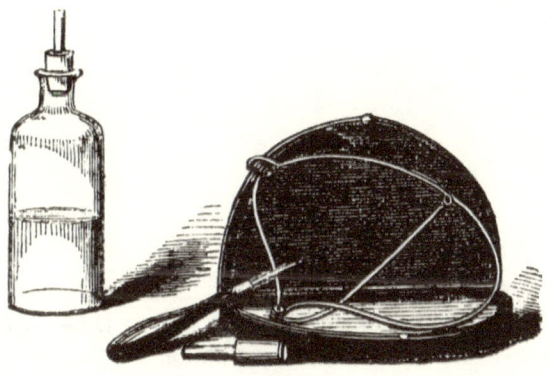

Fig. 7.3. Skinner face mask (1862). (Source: Thomas, 1975, p. 251.) (Photograph courtesy Wood Library-Museum of Anesthesiology.)

Even though Morton had taken some trouble with the design of his inhaler, he could not tell how much ether the patient actually inhaled. That problem was a deficiency of all early administration techniques. The nub of the problem was that some of the agent was lost by evaporation as it cooled. Therefore, the administrator could not be sure how deep anesthesia was at any one moment. That problem was one of many that Londoner John Snow recognized, and the one that he solved in 1847 by designing his temperature-compensated inhaler (strictly, though, it was a vaporizer; see fig. 3.4). In that way, he smoothed the way for others to follow—as did many of his successors.

Snow's Ether and Chloroform Inhalers

Snow realized, as others did not, that the efficiency of the earliest devices was hampered by their inability to keep the temperature of the ether or chloroform constant. Snow helped practitioners in two ways. One, as discussed in chapter 3, was to establish a clinical method of assessing anesthesia depth. The other way was to prevent the ether or chloroform from cooling, which is what Snow did in the definitive version of his ether inhaler of June 1847.[16] He placed the ether adjacent to a container of warm water so that the concentration of the vaporized and inhaled ether remained constant. Snow also designed a chloroform inhaler in 1848[17] (fig. 7.4).

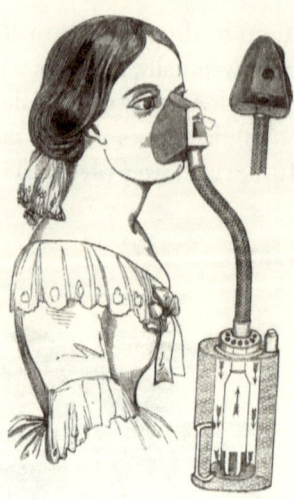

Fig. 7.4. Snow's chloroform inhaler (1848). (Source: J. Snow, *On Chloroform and Other Anaesthetics* . . . [London: John Churchill, p. 82.)

Snow's inhalers established the principle that it was only by controlling the concentration of ether or chloroform by mechanical means that one could hope to be precise—and safe—in administering an anesthetic. Even though ether and chloroform were given by the rag-and-bottle method for many years, Snow's principle eventually won out. Indeed, this principle governed the design of the larger and more complex anesthesia machines many years after Snow. It did so because of the paramount need for precise knowledge of the concentration of the anesthetic that was delivered at any one minute—knowledge that Snow's later experimental work[18] established.

The Duroy, Clover, and Junker Chloroform Inhalers

In the second half of the nineteenth century, ether and chloroform were administered by devices that combined a vaporizer with an inhaler that delivered the vapor to the patient's mouth. One was the chloroform "anaesthesimeter" that Paris pharmaceutical chemist Duroy designed in 1857,[19] but this was somewhat unwieldy. More practical was the reservoir bag, tubing, and face mask that London anaesthetist Joseph Clover designed in 1862. He put the agent in a reservoir bag of known volume, slung the bag and tubing over his shoulder, and had the patient breathe the agent in through the face mask (see fig. 3.2).[20] The apparatus was designed so that not more than 4% chloroform concentration could be delivered. Less unwieldy was the small chloroform inhaler designed by the German-origin surgeon Ferdinand Junker in 1867[21] (fig. 7.5). Junker's was easier to use, being suspended round the neck for all the world like a fashionable boa (fig. 7.5). Operating on the blow-over principle by means of a small hand bellows, the Junker inhaler, by including a graduated bottle that held a known amount of chloroform, was, like Clover's, designed to prevent an overdose of chloroform; a measure of safety was also provided by a feather valve in the face mask. However, incorrect assembly of the Junker inhaler led to at least one death.[22] Over the years, anesthetists modified it in various ways.

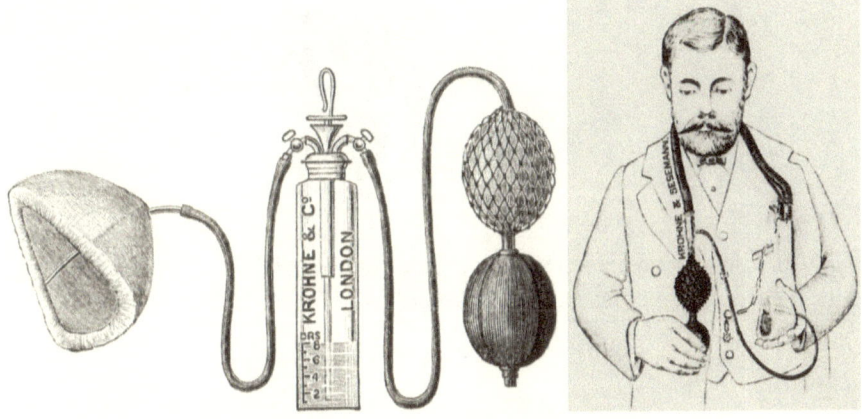

Fig.7.5. Junker's chloroform inhaler (1867). Note its suspension from anesthetist's neck, as shown in Duncum, 1947, p.270.

Clover and Hewitt and the Administration of Nitrous Oxide

Nitrous oxide presented different problems because it was a gas at room barometric pressure. Before 1868, when it was first liquefied and stored in pressurized cylinders,[23] nitrous oxide was manufactured from ammonium nitrate, stored in a bag, and given to the patient to breathe from a mask. The results were variable. In 1868, Clover modified his chloroform apparatus by adding a padded face mask and a supplemental breathing bag to a tube fitted with a stopcock.[24] He followed this up with two other pieces of apparatus. One, introduced in 1876, allowed nitrous oxide or ether to be given separately or combined.[25] The second, of 1877, was his portable regulating ether inhaler[26] (fig. 7.6). He could induce anesthesia with the non-irritating nitrous oxide and give the deeper-acting but pungent ether when the patient went to sleep. Ether could be breathed in, and its dose could be regulated more easily. Over the years, many modifications of the 1877 Clover were made by other anaesthetists, including Hewitt, who became interested in nitrous oxide when there was much concern about the safety of chloroform.

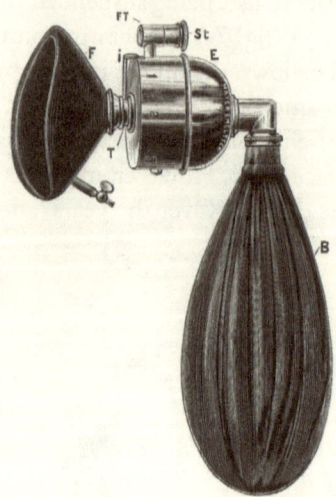

Fig. 7.6. Clover's portable regulating ether inhaler (1877). (Source: J.Clover, Portable regulating ether inhaler, *Brit Med J* 1877;1:69-70.)

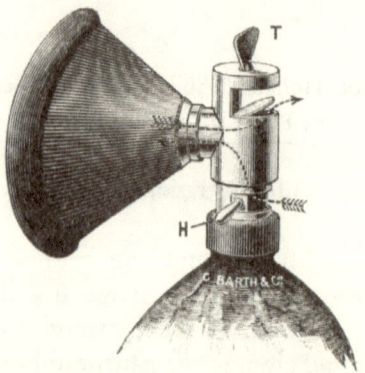

Fig. 7.7. Hewitt's stopcock for regulation of oxygen flow in nitrous oxide-oxygen anesthesia (1893). (Source: F.Hewitt [London: Griffin,1893], pp.95-101.)

Hewitt believed that the narrow caliber of the channel for air ingress in the Clover tended to cause hypoxia.[27] He enlarged the control tubes and ports and allowed the central tubes to rotate inside the ether chamber. This seemed to make respiratory difficulties less likely. Investigating nitrous oxide anesthesia, Hewitt also mixed oxygen rather than air with it, and his stopcock of 1893 allowed him to vary the amount of oxygen (fig. 7.7)[28] inspired.

Hewitt's original work was done when anesthesia was stagnant, and it spurred the development of anesthesia toward the end of the century. Wearing the mantle that Clover had worn after Snow (see chapter 3), his researches led him to stress the advantages of nitrous oxide and ether over chloroform.[29] He was inventive, and his stopcock was only one of several devices he produced, including a dental mouth-prop and the first oral airway (see fig. 6.2). Hewitt, wrote George Edwards, "fought an unceasing battle not only for the improvement of his own work but also for the good of sharing with others of such things as he had found and proved to be good."[30]

Hewitt, the doyen of anesthesia in his day, occupies an important place in the history of anesthesia. He was clearly more than a craftsman, and more obviously a medical scientist and physician. He showed others that anesthesia was a disciplined branch of medicine; indeed, he is one of the earliest representatives of anesthesia as a discipline. This is evident in the link he forged between the design of anesthesia machines in the nineteenth century with those in the twentieth. Like Snow and Clover, Hewitt understood and applied the principles of administration of anesthetic agents to anesthesia machine design, a quality that characterized those who designed anesthesia machines in the period before the First World War.

The understanding of the principles of anesthesia and of the design of anesthesia apparatus are, of course, linked: the degree of sophistication of apparatus design reflects the state of knowledge of anesthesia in any period. Thus from 1846 until early in the twentieth century, minimalism characterized the approach to anesthesia apparatus. The same could be said of use of knowledge in anesthesia; Hewitt's observation in 1896 about anesthesia that "the present state of our knowledge leaves much to be desired"[31] could be applied to anesthesia apparatus. Hewitt was one of few practitioners for whom the principles of anesthesia or of anesthesia apparatus were of deep concern, and he took the lead in explaining them so that the evolution of the specialty could move forward, as it soon did.

1900-1930: New Solutions to Old Problems

Anesthesia historians Peter Thompson and David Wilkinson remarked that "certain pieces of apparatus or innovative developments stand out as milestones in the continuing evolution of the specialty and are turning points in the development of apparatus."[32] Many of the milestones are marked by innovations in concept and principle, and those influencing the design of anesthesia machines in the first three decades or so of the twentieth century had a bearing on the design of later machines. They were, indeed, turning points that were related to advances in surgical and hospital practice.

Change was especially evident in the first decade of the twentieth century. The sudden growth of interest in anesthesia machine design was one example of change, but there were others, as practitioners began thinking more searchingly about the problems of anesthesia in general. The Society of Anaesthetists in London in 1893[33] and the Long Island Society of Anesthetists in 1905[34] were formed so that the members could discuss matters of mutual interest. Some physicians were by now giving much of their time to anesthesia in hospitals, and anesthesia departments were being established in hospitals. These developments marked not only the emergence of anesthesia from being a craft but also of professionalism in anesthesia.[35]

It was in this environment that some individuals formulated principles of lasting importance in the design of anesthesia machines. In England, Hewitt was one of those individuals, but two others, whose work highlights close attention to principles, were Vernon Harcourt and Augustus Waller. Before the larger American anesthesia machines are described, a detour to summarize the features of those two scientists' designs is worth taking because they introduce the roles that physics, as well as chemistry, would play in machine design.

The Vernon Harcourt Chloroform Inhaler

In 1903, the London chemist Vernon Harcourt designed an ingenious inhaler in an attempt to limit the amount of chloroform that could be given[36] (fig. 7.8). He wished to prevent chloroform being administered in a concentration of more than 2%. A double-necked pear-shaped bottle was filled with chloroform, which could be warmed by a naked candle. Two glass beads on the surface of the chloroform monitored its temperature: if it was below sixteen degrees Celsius, both beads would float; if it was greater, they would sink. A pointer and a scale were other parts of the device. The inhaler was efficient, but it did not remain in use; the structure was delicate, and as chloroform did, it lost popularity after the First World War.

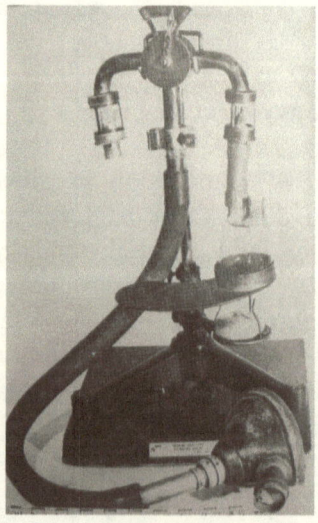

Fig. 7.8. Vernon Harcourt's chloroform inhaler (1903). (Source: Thomas, 1975, p. 86.) Characterized by portability; cf. fig. 7.5.

The Augustus Waller Chloroform Balance

The Waller Balance, also of 1903, was originally designed for use in the laboratory, where the percentage of chloroform in chloroform-air mixtures could be determined rapidly.[37] Its potential value in the operating room stemmed from the current interest in inhalers with chloroform percentage indicators. The balance, enclosed in a glass case that had inlet and outlet ports, consisted of a closed glass bulb of 250 ml capacity and a metal weight on each arm of the balance, together with a pointer. When the case contained only air, the weight was slightly lighter; when air and chloroform were pumped into the case, the bulb, which was larger than the metal weight, lost weight as the density of the mixed gases increased, a state that was reflected by movement of the pointer. Bulk and lack of portability, however, made the Waller impractical for clinical use. Waller, like Harcourt, knew a great deal about physiology and chemistry at a time when many anesthetists lacked an extensive knowledge of the scientific aspects of anesthesia. However, this changed when a brilliant group of anesthetists set to work in designing anesthesia machines in the first decade and a half of the twentieth century.

The Harcourt and Waller instruments originated in the increasing concern over safety in anesthesia, but other factors renewed interest in precision in the administration of anesthetic agents. Two were the longer and more complex surgical procedures that were being performed and the related increase in the numbers of patients being treated in hospitals. Larger and more rugged anesthesia machines, as opposed to devices, were needed.

Physically, the new generation of anesthesia machines, which initially appeared in the decade and a half before World War I, was characterized by their much larger size, which required their being supported by a base on legs, but more important were functional changes in design. They incorporated devices that made it possible, for example, to determine the dose of an inhalational agent being given and to visualize the flow of oxygen.

These larger machines were developed owing to the efforts of the generation of anesthetists and surgeons that followed Clover and Hewitt. The first members of that generation flourished in the decade before the First World War, particularly in the United States. They sought solutions that emphasized greater precision and control of gas flow and anesthesia agent concentration. They made a breakthrough, and their machines provided a template for the increasingly sophisticated machines of the second half of the twentieth century. Many of the basic principles of anesthesia machine design were, therefore, recognized early in the twentieth century, and it is on those principles that the discussion will now be focused.

Addition of Oxygen to Inhaled Nitrous Oxide

Although Edmund Andrews, the Chicago surgeon, stated in 1868 that giving oxygen with nitrous oxide improved the quality of nitrous oxide anesthesia,[38] his view was not widespread. Because nitrous oxide is not particularly potent, for many years, even well into the twentieth century, anesthesia was induced with 100 per cent nitrous oxide—that is, without oxygen. This is partly explained by the fact that until the 1870s, gases were not generally compressed into cylinders; hence nitrous oxide was supplemented with air in (often futile) attempts to avoid hypoxia. Even if the percentage of nitrous oxide was reduced to, say, 60, that of oxygen inspired would still only be 8, which was clearly less than normal. Therefore, French physiologist Paul Bert's recommendation of a mixture under increased atmospheric pressure[39] made sense. But the problem with this recommendation was that the high-pressure chamber required was cumbersome and impractical.

Hewitt's stopcock was one solution to the problem of hypoxia, but his methodical investigation into nitrous oxide—oxygen mixtures had a more far-reaching effect. It stimulated the development of machines for gas delivery, and the design of the earliest freestanding anesthesia machines, such as the White machine of 1885, already noted, was influenced by Hewitt's ideas.[40] The same is true of the White machine circa 1897, which appears to have been influenced by Hewitt's "non-asphyxial" method.[41] This had a metal framework that supported nitrous oxide and oxygen cylinders, the openings of which were controlled by disklike handles, a mixing chamber for the two gases. Though the White machine was one of the first to incorporate a yoke for the mixing and delivery of the gases, at these pressures, delivery of gases would be hazardous. One solution was the simple one of passing the gas into a reservoir bag first; the other was to incorporate reducing valves into anesthesia machines.

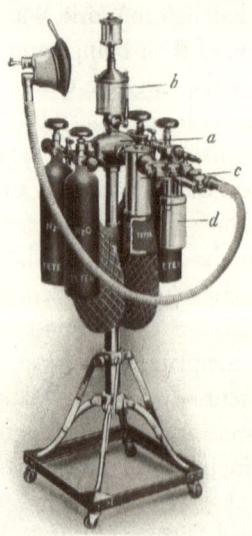

Fig. 7.9. Representative Teter anesthesia machine (c. 1912). (Source: M. von Brunn, *Die Allgemeinnarkose* [Stuttgart: Verlag von Ferdinand Enke, 1913], p. 313.)

Other machines that illustrate the freestanding concept and contained nitrous oxide, as well as oxygen cylinders, and that were supported on stands followed. Among them are the machines made soon after the turn of the century by Cleveland dentist Charles Teter (fig. 7.9).

The Need for Reducing Valves

In 1868, nitrous oxide was compressed in cylinders,[42] as a liquid, at seven hundred pounds per square inch (psi); oxygen was stored at 1500-1800 psi. These pressures were too high to be inhaled safely, a pressure of 20 psi being desirable. Until the first decade of the twentieth century, just hand valves and a bag were used to provide at least some control of the pressure of gas. But as Boston anesthetist Walter Boothby noted in 1912 in relation to his own machine, a smooth and constant flow of gas from a compressed liquid was not possible with a hand valve.[43] Automatic reducing valves were, therefore, essential. This was the opinion of an anesthetist who applied his original thinking to solve problems of anesthesia machine design—one in whom the very wellsprings of anesthesiology were said to have emerged.[44] Boothby's interest in reducing valves illustrates the concern with principles that characterized anesthesia as it passed from the stage of craft to discipline.

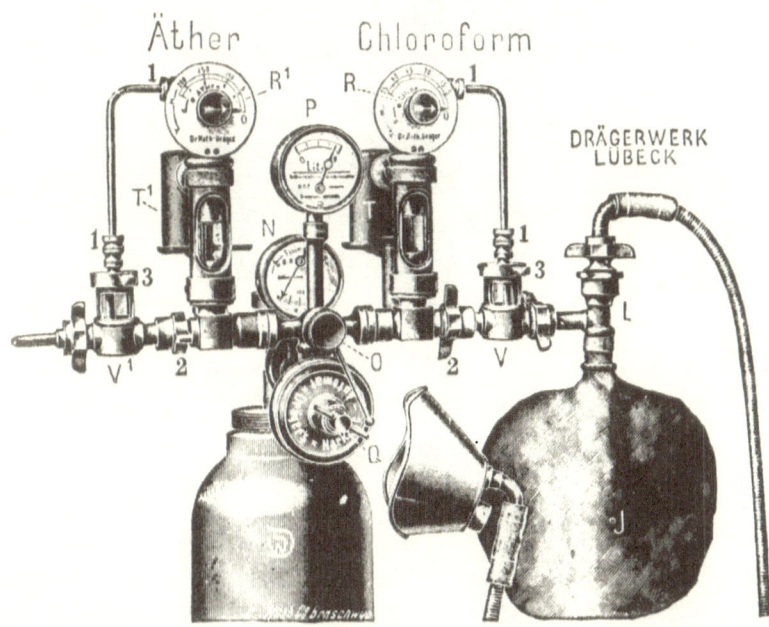

Fig. 7.10. Dräger—Roth anesthesia ether and chloroform machine (1903). (Source: Gwathmey, 1914, p. 318.) (Photograph courtesy Wood library-Museum of Anesthesiology.)

This topic concerned several other individuals besides Boothby and his surgical associate Frederick Cotton. One was Bernhard Dräger in Germany. The Dräger—Roth machine (fig. 7.10), which was based on machines attributable to Prochownick of 1895 and Wohlgemoth of 1901,[45] was manufactured in 1903, for use by Roth in Lubeck, Germany.[46] The Dräger—Roth was fitted with a main valve, as well as a hand valve, to allow the oxygen supply to be turned on and off quickly. It was supported by a metal base, four wheels, and four vertical metal rods. Oxygen was used to operate an injector that caused either ether or chloroform to be withdrawn from a bottle for evaporation. Though the amount of the anesthetic agent was measurable in terms of drops, its actual concentration was not measured; nor could the flow of oxygen be accurately measured. However, James Tayloe Gwathmey, of New York, thought that the Dräger—Roth was simple and satisfactory in operation, providing good muscle relaxation.[47] The consumption of chloroform made it economical.

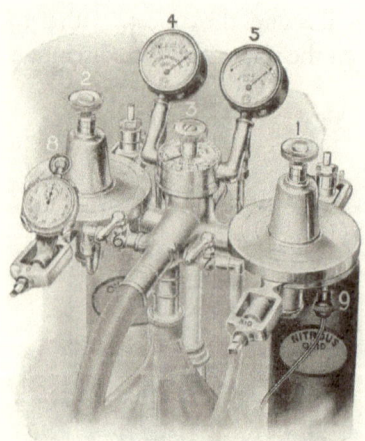

Fig. 7.11. Heidbrink anesthesia machine (1911). (Source: J.T.Gwathmey, [New York: Macmillan Company, 2nd ed., 1925], p.148.)

Reducing valves were included in several early twentieth century anesthesia machines in the United States. Both the S. S. White Company machine, circa 1910,[48] and the Heidbrink machine of 1912 (fig. 7.11)—designed by Jay Heidbrink, a Minneapolis anesthesiologist and dentist—had reducing valves. The valves on machines made early in the twentieth century by the White Company, which had been manufacturing anesthesia apparatus since 1871, were made of a tube turned in steel, a spring, and a brass diaphragm, together with a steel pin and wool packing.[49]

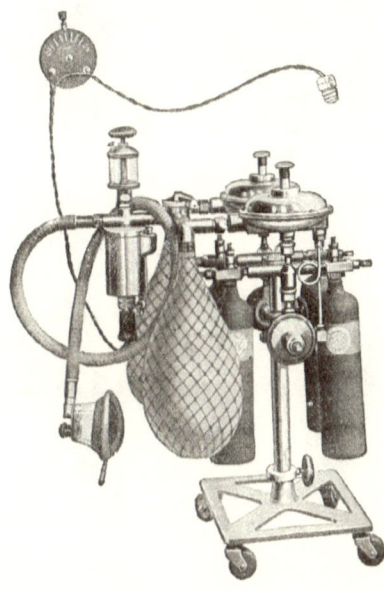

Fig. 7.12. Ohio Monovalve anesthesia machine (1912). (Source: Gwathmey, 1914, p. 158.)

Heidbrink was concerned by the lack of constant pressure in current machines. He was impressed by a machine that Teter showed him in 1903, and he acquired one, but he was mainly concerned about the inconstant gas pressure. He began to remodel the Teter and started production of anesthesia machines in 1906.[50] By 1912-1913, he had built his own model A. This incorporated a countervailing weight, reducing valves of a type that was commercially available, and bags for nitrous oxide and oxygen and for rebreathing.[51] From 1910 onward, his name was attached to many machines over the next few decades. Another machine of this era was the Ohio Monovalve, first made in 1910 (fig. 7.12). The gas passed through regulators to reduce the pressure and then through automatic valves, where the pressure was further reduced.[52]

Determining Ether Concentrations

Deficiencies in anesthesia machines also concerned Karl Connell, the Columbia University surgeon. Two were especially important to him: inaccurate knowledge of the amount of air in the flow of gases and of the percentage of ether vaporized.[53] He brought his interest in measurement of gases to bear on the design of anesthesia machines.

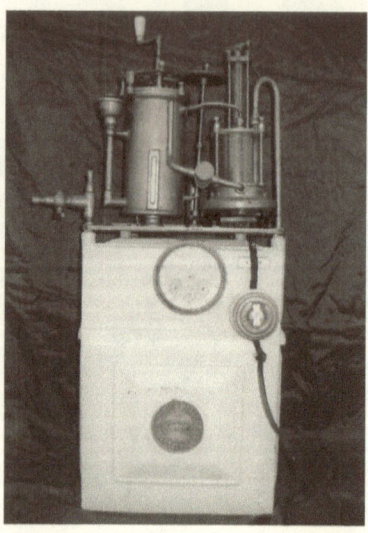

Fig. 7.13. Connell Anaesthetometer, modification of 1908 model (c.1912). (Source: P.Flagg, *The Art of Anesthesia* [Philadelphia:J.B.Lippincott Co., 1916], p.150.)

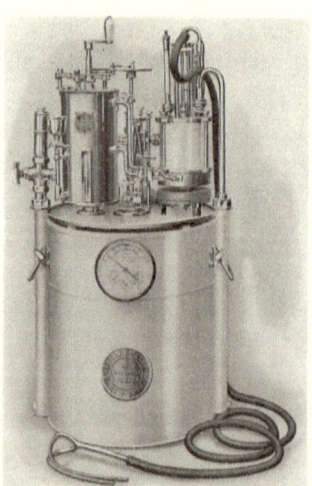

Fig. 7.14. Connell Anaesthetometer (1913). (Source: K.Connell, An apparatus – Anaesthetometer – for measuring and mixing anesthetic and other vapors and gases, *Surg Gynecol Obstet* 1913;16:245-55.)

Connell's contributions to machine design date from 1908. One, designed in 1908, was known as the Anaesthetometer.[54] Rectangular in shape (fig. 7.13), it delivered an air-ether mixture by insufflation. It was the first machine that measured the concentration of anesthetic gases precisely. It was fitted with kinetic piston-type flow meters. Connell described a second Anaesthetometer (fig. 7.14) in great detail in 1913.[55] Drum-shaped, air and ether, as well as nitrous oxide and carbon dioxide, could be administered. It comprised three main parts when used for the administration of ether and another when nitrous oxide was administered. Air or other gas under pressure actuated a recording mechanism (a gas meter in the "drum"), and simultaneously, the same mechanism automatically fed the "proper" amounts of ether from a reservoir into measured volumes of air into an ether vaporizer.

Connell described the ether vaporizer in a separate article in 1913.[56] He explained that the air delivered was indicated at all times in a glass tube containing a float and engraved so as to indicate liters of air passing each minute. Also engraved, opposite each airflow level, was the number of drops of ether required, from the number of drops of ether to be added per minute to make the air-ether mixture 14% by weight. Connell also indicated the number of drops of ether that would make a 1% mixture. In stating that "only by such knowledge can control and accuracy of dosage be secured and the effect of a given dose be foretold," Connell both followed the example set sixty years earlier by Snow and foreshadowed design requirements over the next sixty years.

Connell was a surgeon and an engineering sophisticate, but also a physician with vision. The 1913 Anaesthetometer could also be used in resuscitating persons poisoned by carbon dioxide or morphine, those with respiratory failure, or those in shock. He was evidently ahead of his time in suggesting that in cases of respiratory failure, "the nose and mouth are blocked for a few seconds at a time to expand the chest . . . or else the delivery pressure is increased and the flow interrupted four to eight times a minute for a few seconds."[57]

The validity of Connell's work was confirmed by others. Boothby found that surgical anesthesia was obtained by approximately 15% ether vapor in the alveolar air, and that induction might require approximately 30%.[58] Frank Mann found that in dogs, physiologic responses occurred consistently at various tensions of ether vapor.[59, 60] The Connell machine was state-of-the-art in its day. It was, however, large and more suitable for hospital than domestic use.

Estimating Gas Flows

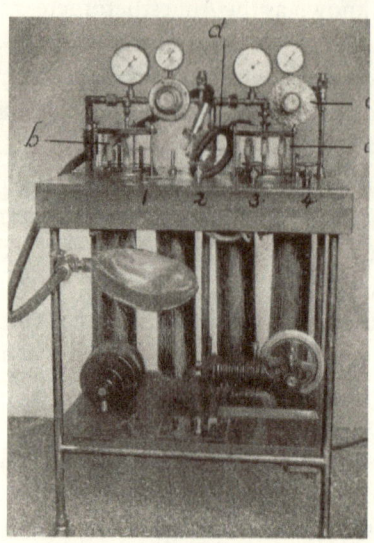

Fig.7.15. Cotton-Boothby nitrous oxide-oxygen anesthesia machine (1912). (Source: F.Cotton, W.Boothby, Nitrous oxide and oxygen anaesthesia and a new apparatus, *Surg Gynecol Obstet* 1912;14:195-201.).

Neither the handles on the top of cylinders nor reducing valves could, however, accurately control the flow of gases delivered to the patient's mouth or nose. Accurate control was obviously important in determining the concentration of anesthetic agent inhaled, and Connell and Boothby enhanced the understanding of that point. Contributing to progress in this aspect of anesthesia was the partnership of Boston surgeon Frederick Cotton and anesthetist Walter Boothby, also of Boston, before he moved to the Mayo Clinic. They designed the Cotton-Boothby machine in 1912[61, 62] (fig. 7.15). Boothby, like Connell, was a thinker who made original contributions to machine design. For example, in 1911, he listed certain essential points.[63] One was the ability to judge the flow of each gas being used—a point that Connell also worked on. Boothby bubbled gas through water, thus making its flow visible. Also important was the ability to regulate the flow so that nitrous oxide and oxygen could be administered in proportions as desired and to provide "smooth even flow." The third point was the importance of reducing the pressure of gases in cylinders by means of reducing valves; the volume of gas to be delivered to the patient, now reduced in pressure, was controlled by a valve that permitted fine adjustment.

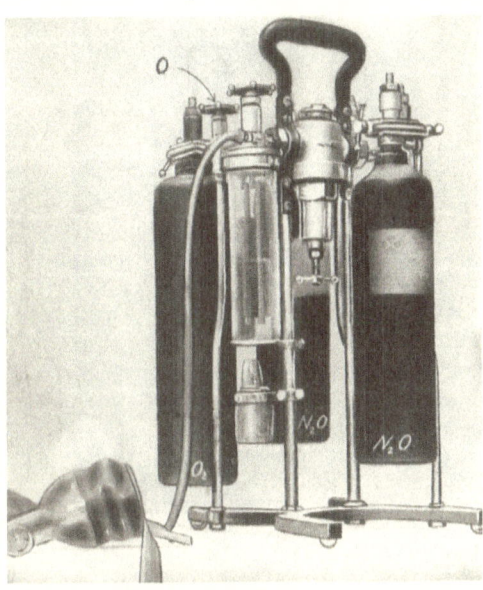

Fig. 7.16. Gwathmey-Woolsey nitrous oxide-oxygen anesthesia machine (1912). (Source: Gwathmey, 1914, p. 172.) (Collection of Wood Library-Museum of Anesthesiology.)

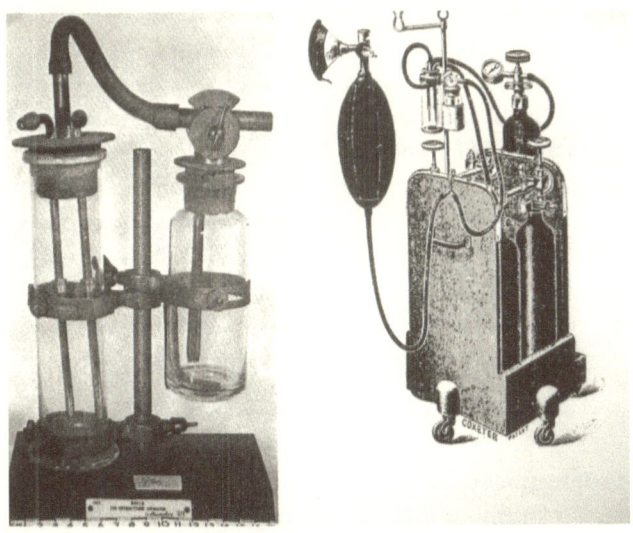

Fig. 7.17. Boyle nitrous oxide-oxygen-ether anesthesia machine (1917). (Source: Thomas, 1975, p. 148.)

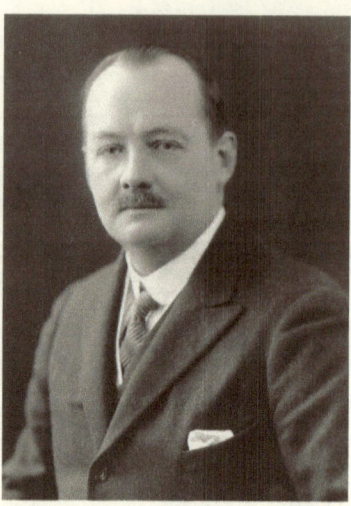

Fig. 7.18. Henry Boyle (1875-1941)

Henry "Cocky" Edmund Gaskin Boyle was born in Barbados. He studied medicine at St. Bartholomew's Hospital in London and graduated in 1901. His appointment there as junior resident anaesthetist taught him anesthesia, and he joined the anesthesia staff of St. Bartholomew's in 1903. The standby anesthesia techniques at that time included dropping ether onto some type of face mask and a nitrous oxide-ether sequence. For the latter, Boyle used a Gwathmey machine, but he sought to improve administration by modifying it and incorporating some ideas of Geoffrey Marshall. In the original Boyle machine, four cylinders were suspended from crossbars, and a bottle for ether was placed so that it could be warmed in a small basin of water and then passed through water so that bubbles would confirm the flow of ether, as a sight-feed. Like the McKesson and other machines designed by anesthetists, the Boyle machine was modified over the years. Boyle was one of the leaders of English anesthesia, authoring his own textbook in 1907 and introducing the mouth gag designed by American S. Griffith Davis into British practice as the Boyle-Davis gag. Boyle did much for anesthesia in Britain besides the foregoing, particularly with respect to the Section of Anaesthetics of the Royal Society of Medicine, the Association of Anaesthetists of Great Britain and Ireland, and the *British Journal of Anaesthesia*.

The fine-adjustment point was an important one. It was incorporated into two popular machines: the Gwathmey machine of 1912 (fig. 7.16),[64] in the United States, and the Boyle machine (fig. 7.17), designed by Henry Edmund Gaskin Boyle, of London (fig. 7.18), in 1917,[65] which spawned many descendants. A similar gas-ether Marshall machine that Geoffrey Marshall, also of London, designed at the same time was not described until 1920.[66]

The 1911 Cotton and Boothby machine was therefore a significant advance. Besides making for precision of administration, it was made of metal, was sturdy, and combined the portability of domestic anesthesia and the virtual stationary nature of machines for hospital use. Its dimensions could be halved as a central axis allowed the top half to be swung down and tucked in. It also provided for rebreathing, for this was an era when carbon dioxide was thought desirable in anesthesia,[67] since it stimulated the respiration. The machine also held ether in a separate chamber through which gases could either pass or not; air should be excluded from around the mask so that the inhaled mixture was not diluted. The machine was a milestone, incorporating technical innovations that shaped modern apparatus.[68]

In the United States, the Gwathmey machine was popular as it was small and portable. Gwathmey's ideas were influenced by those of other inventive individuals such as Dennis Jackson (a St. Louis, Missouri, physician and pharmacologist) and Cotton and Boothby in Boston. Gwathmey's thinking in turn influenced manufacturer Richard von Foregger, whom he met in 1907, and, in the United Kingdom, Boyle, whom he met in 1912.

Another way of making gas flow visible was the dry one achieved by using flow meters and rotameters. Connell incorporated a piston type of kinetic flow meter in his machine of 1908.[69] In Germany that year, rotameters were invented for use in industry,[70] and Maximilian Neu, of Heidelberg, made use of the principle in anesthesia in 1910.[71] In 1912, Connell used a rotary vane type of flow gauge,[72] and in his machine of 1930, a ball-bearing device.[73] Gas flow could also be measured by means of a pressure gauge.

Continuous or Intermittent Gas Flow?

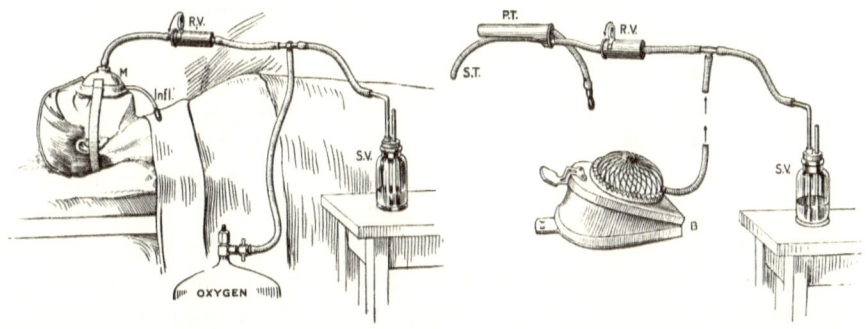

Fig. 7.19. Meltzer and Auer insufflation apparatus (1909). (Source: Gwathmey, 1914, p. 400.)

Continuous gas flow. All the nineteenth-century inhalers and early twentieth-century gas machines, such as the Teter, the Connell, the Cotton-Boothby, and the Gwathmey, delivered gas in a steady, or continuous, stream. So did the Meltzer and Auer Tracheal Insufflation apparatus (fig. 7.19) of 1909.[74] That apparatus, designed by Rockefeller Institute physiologists Samuel Meltzer and John Auer, had significance for anesthesia in a number of ways. The first was the finding that anesthesia, and life, could be maintained by continuously inflating the lungs of curarized animals with air and ether introduced through an oral O'Dwyer laryngeal tube (see chapter 6) or a tracheostomy. Meltzer and Auer believed that fresh gas reached the lower part of the trachea, that in distended lungs inspired and expired gas would be exchanged, and that the carbon dioxide would be returned to the atmosphere by a route that was different from the inspiratory route. The idea was not dissimilar to that of Robert Hooke, who in 1667 continuously inflated a dog's lungs,[75] and of Nagel, who in 1900 maintained respiration in curarized pigeons by continuously inflating their air sacs.[76]

The Meltzer and Auer technique influenced the development of anesthesia in four other ways. It affirmed the value of continuous gas flow, it had practical value in operations such as those on the thorax and the head and neck, it was a stimulus to later machine design, and it was one of the pathways that led to the practice of tracheal intubation (see also chapter 6).

The practical value of the Meltzer and Auer technique is apparent in two aspects of anesthesia. One was the occurrence of pneumothorax after the thorax was opened surgically. That had long been a serious problem for thoracic surgeons and for the practitioners giving anesthesia because it prevented the exposed lung from expanding, and, over time, in sick patients, which could be fatal unless it was managed appropriately. The Meltzer and Auer technique seemed to be an answer. In 1911, Charles Elsberg, of New York, adapted it to clinical use,[77] as did Liverpool surgeon Robert Kelly the following year.[78]

The Meltzer and Auer technique also influenced those who designed anesthesia machines. Henry Edmund Boyle, for example, in London, was interested in insufflation anesthesia,[79] and he designed the machine named after him with this clinical problem in mind. Air was pumped in a continuous stream by an electric motor, the flow being controlled by three cogwheels; in addition, the air and the ether were both warmed. This kept the lungs still during intrathoracic operations in the days before the routine use of endotracheal intubation and before muscle relaxants were introduced. The current of air could be interrupted when it was necessary to collapse a lung. The later techniques of *apneic oxygenation* and *passive gas flow* were derivatives of insufflation.

Rebreathing of gases. Continuous gas flow was expensive, and in order to economize, some anesthetists devised a method whereby some of the gases exhaled would be rebreathed. This was first developed with nitrous oxide anesthesia by Hewitt in 1886.[80] Willis Gatch, a Baltimore surgeon, wrote about rebreathing in 1910,[81] and it was a feature of the machine he designed (fig. 7.20). The practice caught on and was used extensively by Elmer McKesson, the Toledo anesthetist (fig. 7.21).

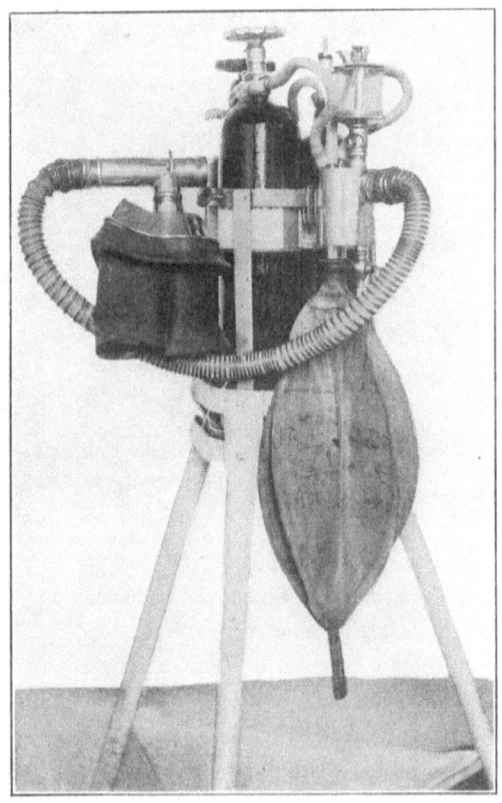

7.20. Gatch nitrous oxide-oxygen anesthesia machine (1910). (Source: J. T. Gwathmey, *Anesthesia* [New York: D. Appleton Company, 1914], p. 104.)

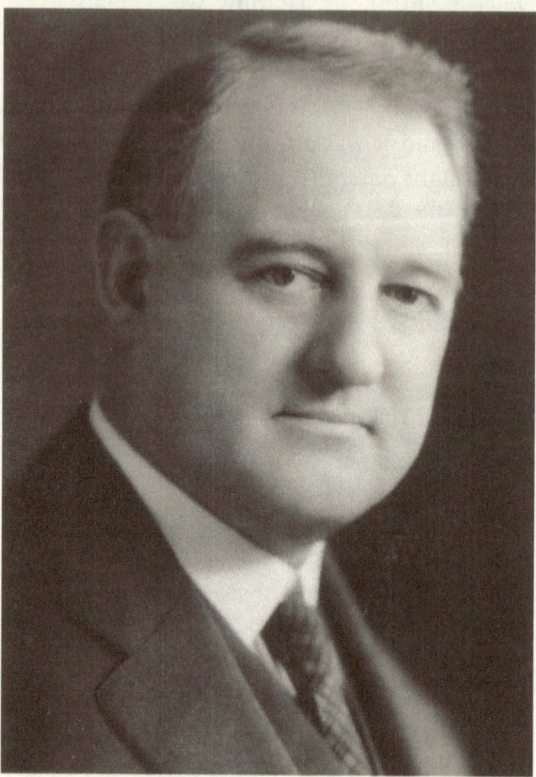

Fig. 7.21. Elmer McKesson (1881-1935)

Elmer Ira McKesson was a native of Walkerton, Indiana, where he later served as principal of a high school. He graduated from Rush Medical School in Chicago in 1906, interned at Toledo Hospital in Ohio, and spent his career in Toledo. His interest in anesthesia began while he was an intern, because little anesthesia equipment was available to provide safe and reliable pain relief for surgical patients, and because current anesthesia techniques with ether or ether and nitrous oxide frequently caused nausea and vomiting. McKesson's inventive genius led him to design anesthesia machines and pieces of apparatus. His first anesthesia machine appeared in 1910, while his inventions included mixing valves so that the proportions of nitrous oxide and oxygen could be changed rapidly and precisely, a rebreathing system based on a fractional and adjustable bellows arrangement, and valves that would facilitate on-demand gas flow. McKesson formed the Toledo Technical Appliance Company (later the McKesson Appliance Company), but McKesson remained a physician with academic interests and a talent for teaching, not only in anesthesia, but also in physiology. His contributions to anesthesia, though, were paramount, and his varied talents meant that the McKesson name was known the world over.

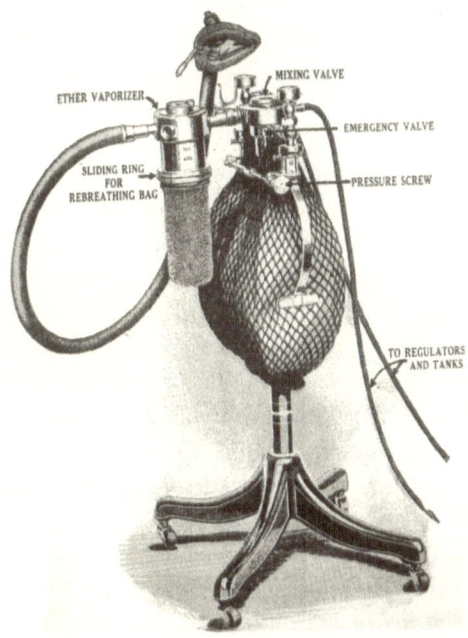

Fig. 7.22. McKesson nitrous oxide-oxygen anesthesia machine, Model F (*c*.1915). (Source: Toledo Technical Appliance Co., in *The American Year-Book of Anesthesia & Analgesia* [New York: Surgery Publishing Company, 1915], p. xii.)

Demand (intermittent) gas flow. McKesson, however, is particularly well known for the principle of intermittent gas flow, which ensures that gas is delivered only in the inspiratory phase of respiration. In 1910, he modified the principle of rebreathing by developing the technique of fractional rebreathing so that by means of valves and separate gasbags, some of the gases would be rebreathed and some fresh gases also, and he described the McKesson machine (fig. 7.22) that effected this in 1911.[82]

Like Connell and Cotton and Boothby, and also Heidbrink, McKesson had clear ideas of what an anesthetic machine should accomplish. He thought that it should have the right components, accurately control the gas mixture and its pressure, and regulate rebreathing.[83] A valve ensured that the bags for nitrous oxide and oxygen were kept filled and that the gas flow ceased when the patient stopped inhaling. Any difference in pressure in the two gases was minimized by pressure exerted by the walls of one bag pressing against the other. Like the Boyle machine, the McKesson spawned many succeeding generations. Such was its popularity. Bryn Thomas stated that it "represented a real advance in physiological and precision anesthesia,[84] and Zebulon Mennell, the London anesthesiologist, referred to it as "the Rolls Royce of nitrous oxide machines."[85] In the United Kingdom, the intermittent flow principle was the basis of the Walton series of machines (so-named, perhaps apocryphally, from a golf course of that name on which the individual was walking at the moment of enlightenment)[86] and the self-administration Minnitt machine,[87] described in 1934 for use by women during childbirth by Robert J. Minnitt, of Liverpool.

McKesson designed his machine with two objects in mind. One was to provide rebreathing of carbon dioxide in order to stimulate the respiration and thus expedite gaseous induction. This was considered quite acceptable to many anesthetists in his day. His other object was to accomplish primary and secondary saturation with nitrous oxide. McKesson would induce anesthesia by giving 100% nitrous oxide, to the point of cyanosis (primary saturation), after which some oxygen would be introduced, before reintroducing the nitrous oxide to flood the patient's lungs (secondary saturation). Only after this, when the patient was anesthetized, would oxygen be added again. Though the technique was condemned both in his day (by individuals like Gwathmey) and in the future by later generations of anesthesiologists, there is no doubt that the technique worked, and many practitioners made use of it. Almost as shocking, to anesthesiologists who did not practice in the pre-halothane era, was the deliberate addition of carbon dioxide, from cylinders placed equally deliberately on anesthesia machines, in order to speed up the anesthetized patient's breathing and uptake of nitrous oxide.

Carbon Dioxide Absorption

Rebreathing meant that some carbon dioxide accumulated in the patient's blood, and while this was favored by some anesthetists, including Gatch and McKesson, others took a different tack and sought to have carbon dioxide absorbed by the breathing circuit. In the nineteenth century, rebreathing had been studied by an anesthetist, a dentist, and a surgeon, each of whom used a chemical method to absorb the carbon dioxide. The first to do this was Snow in 1850. He realized, with respect to an anesthetic vapor, that "if its exhalation by the breath could in any way be stopped, its narcotic effects ought to be much prolonged."[88] He tested his supposition and confirmed its validity by breathing oxygen and chloroform in an experiment on himself. Next, in 1868, the London dentist Alfred Coleman used an apparatus for absorbing carbon dioxide in one hundred patients by adding caustic potash.[89] An estimated saving of two-thirds to three-fourths of the amount of nitrous oxide otherwise expected occurred. In 1868 also, Edmund Andrews laid limewater on the floor of a glass jar that housed animals he was experimenting on, evidently to absorb carbon dioxide.[90] Thus in 1915, when Dennis Jackson became interested in carbon dioxide absorption, he was following the experiments of notable predecessors, even though he pursued a different objective.

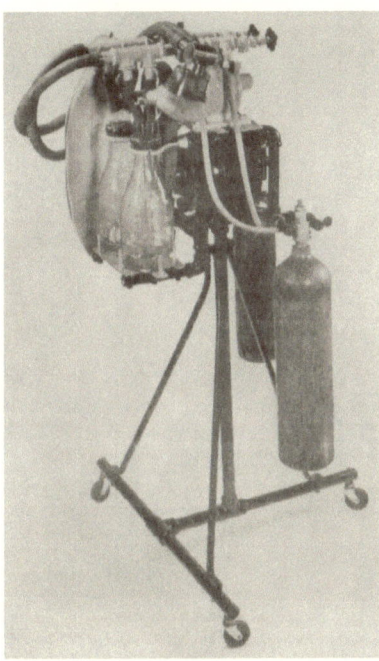

Fig. 7.23. Dennis Jackson's original nitrous oxide-oxygen anesthesia machine with apparatus for carbon dioxide absorption (1915). (Source: T. Keys, *The History of Surgical Anesthesia* [New York: Dover Publications, Inc., 1963], opposite p. 71.)

The paper that Jackson published in 1915[91] describes his own research and the names of a host of individuals besides Snow, Coleman, and Andrews who had been interested in the subject of carbon dioxide absorption. Jackson facilitated the production and maintenance of prolonged general analgesia or anesthesia by a variety of anesthetic agents with oxygen. Rebreathing would be made harmless by removing carbon dioxide with a solution of sodium hydrate and calcium hydrate. The very first Jackson machine—he was a great tinkerer and invented several machines, a Rube Goldberg of anesthesia—was built in 1914 (fig. 7.23). In a machine he built in 1915, he used a milk bottle as a safety trap and a cake pan to hold a solution of sodium hydroxide. Jackson tested his machines on dogs, but his colleagues did use them for clinical purposes. He hoped that his machines would be used clinically, if only because he wished to satisfy the need for some cheap, easy, and effective method for administering nitrous oxide. Jackson had social sensitivity and an empathetic understanding that many patients in Chicago's old West Side could only afford an anesthetic if he or she went without eating for the next day or two.[92]

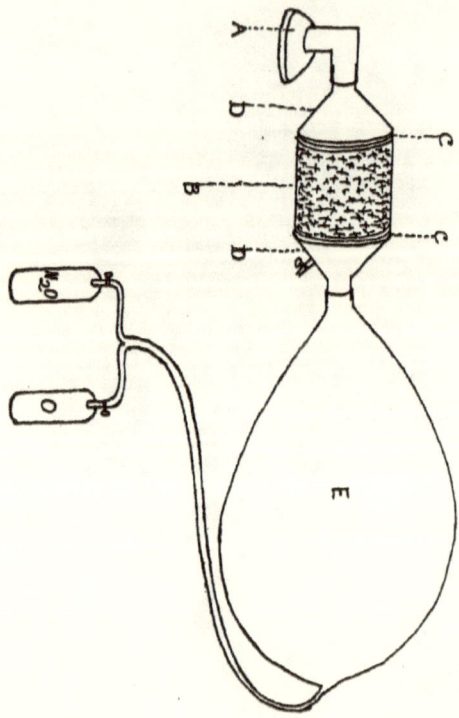

Fig. 7.24. Sketch of Waters "to-and-fro" carbon dioxide absorption apparatus (1924).A, face mask; B, soda lime in canister; C, D, metal canister; E, rebreathing bag. (Source: R. Waters, Clinical scope and utility of carbon dioxid filtration in inhalation anesthesia. *Anesth Analg* 1924; 3:20-22.)

The greatest impact that Jackson had, though, was on Ralph Waters, of Madison. The two of them carried on a correspondence beginning in 1920, and out of that connection emerged the Waters to-and-fro soda lime canister (fig. 7.24). After two and a half years of research, Waters described his device in October 1923 and wrote about it in February 1924.[93] Placed in the anesthetic circuit near the patient's face, breathing through it to and fro removed the carbon dioxide in the exhaled gases.

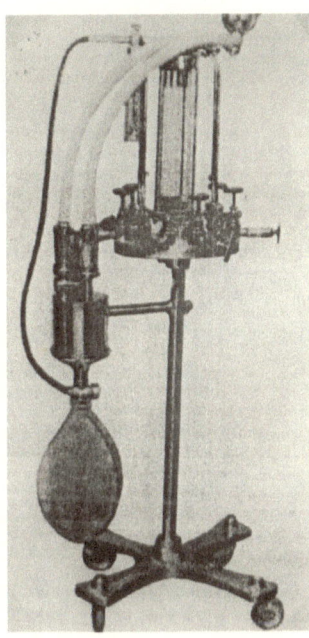

Fig.7.25. Sword's closed circle (carbon dioxide absorption) anesthesia machine (1930). (Source: B.Sword, The closed circle method of administration of gas anesthesia, *Curr Res in Anes Analg* 1930;9:198-202.)

The Jackson-and-Waters approach to carbon dioxide absorption was very successful in anesthetic practice. Brian Sword, of North Carolina and New Haven, Connecticut, thought that it did more than any other technique in the recent past to minimize difficulties with gas anesthesia. However, Sword did object to the placement of the Waters canister so close to the patient's face. To overcome this objection, he designed the closed circle absorption system. In the original closed circle, which Sword had been working on since 1926 and described in 1930,[94] inspired and expired gases flowed in the same direction but were separated by valves and two tubes, the one for inspiration and the one for expiration being attached to the face mask by a Y connection. The tubes were attached to a soda lime canister by means of flutter valves that operated in the two phases of respiration. The circuit also contained a rebreathing bag that equalized pressure (fig. 7.25). Sword acknowledged that carbon dioxide should be admitted to the rebreathing bag if the respiration became depressed, and positioned a valve to permit this. Sword listed several advantages of the circle system. These included simplicity of operation, flexibility of use, economy by reason of using 300 to 400 ml oxygen and 1000 to 1500 ml ethylene per minute. The circle system soon became a standard feature of anesthesia machines, being particularly valuable when cyclopropane replaced ethylene in the 1930.

Anesthesia in the Field: A Return to Portability

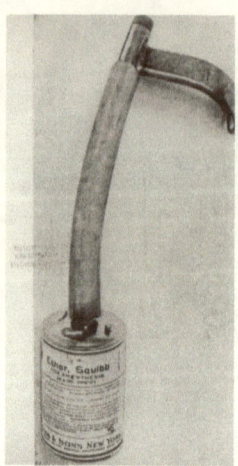

Fig. 7.26. Flagg can (1939). (Collection of Wood Library-Museum of Anesthesiology)

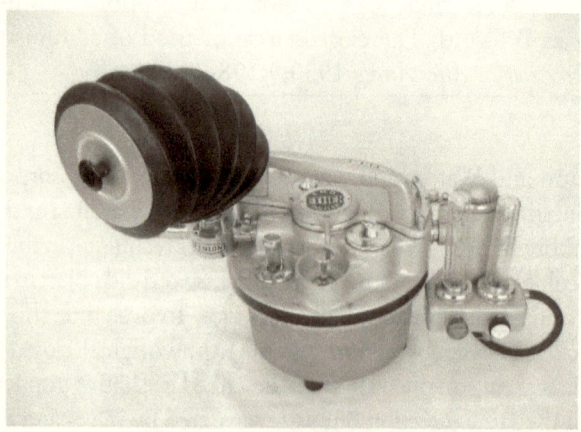

Fig. 7.27. Macintosh-Epstein Oxford Vaporizer (1941). (Collection of Wood Library-Museum of Anesthesiology.) (Source: Thomas, 1975, p. 9.)

In wartime, standard anesthesia equipment may be lacking, and innovative solutions to a variety of problems have to be found. One solution during the First World War was the Flagg (ether) can[95] (fig. 7.26). Consisting simply of a can of ether, a delivery tube, and an oral airway, it was used to provide ether anesthesia in the field. A similar response during World War II was the Macintosh Oxford Vaporizer[96] and the Epstein-Macintosh-Oxford (EMO) portable inhaler[97] (fig. 7.27). These two machines were draw-over vaporizers. The EMO inhaler was designed to deliver a certain concentration of ether vapor in air, the ether being kept warm by the presence in an adjoining chamber of calcium chloride crystals, which in turn had to be kept warm by warm water. Relatively high carrier gas volumes, exceeding 10 liters per minute, were required.[98] In later models, a bellows was attached.

*   *   *

Anesthetists working in the first few decades of the twentieth century recognized the need to solve certain problems of physical chemistry, and designed anesthesia machines that showed their understanding of the scientific principles involved. The machines of that period differed significantly from the smaller portable devices of earlier times that were used in homes as well as hospitals. The new designs took anesthesia from craft to discipline. In this way, anesthesia began to show evidence of greater maturity so that eventually it would justify being granted specialty status.

The development of the twentieth-century anesthesia machines reveals elements of the path that was followed by practitioners who came after Morton. The small portable devices of the nineteenth century might have been primitive, but they embodied important principles. Snow's vaporizers kept the concentration of ether and chloroform within safe limits, and Clover's controlled the concentration of chloroform and regulated that of ether. Hewitt, concerned with nitrous oxide, developed apparatus that allowed varying amounts of oxygen to be added and so made safety in administration potentially greater, a concern that Andrews had expressed earlier. Harcourt and Waller sought to attain even greater precision in the dose of chloroform administered. Early in the twentieth century, anesthesia machines became larger and freestanding, as more work was done in hospitals than in homes. Mechanisms to permit estimation of ether and chloroform used and visible control of amounts of gases were added, as were reducing valves to moderate the pressure of gas administered. Because of the dangers associated with chloroform, interest in nitrous oxide was renewed, as in the machines of McKesson, who also advocated rebreathing. In contrast, Dennis Jackson emphasized the value of carbon dioxide absorption, as did Waters a little later; and Sword designed a closed-circuit apparatus that made for economy, as well as carbon dioxide absorption.

While the anesthesia machines of the early twentieth century represented progress in anesthesia away from the less sophisticated devices of the nineteenth century, they also set a pattern for later progress in machine design. Marking that progress were in-machine devices that provided greater degrees of precision in the form of temperature compensation, so that volatilization was unaffected by ambient temperature. Also characteristic of later machines was the capacity to analyze the gases that were being breathed and to give warning if these were dangerously abnormal. In such ways, precision of dose was ensured, and safety was enhanced.

Chapter 8

THE EMERGENCE OF ANESTHESIA AS A SPECIALTY

While, as previous chapters have shown, steady progress was made in clinical anesthesia in the first half of the twentieth century, progress was also made in achieving the goal of recognition of anesthesia as a specialty. In both the United Kingdom and the United States, what was a long evolutionary process, which took the better part of a century, was finally completed in the latter part of the 1930s. Anesthesia, initially a craft and then a discipline, then took its place alongside other medical and surgical specialties as an autonomous specialty. Now both anesthesia practitioners themselves and their surgical and medical colleagues could view anesthesia from a more mature perspective than earlier.

This evolutionary process was complex as well as lengthy. Many requirements had to be satisfied. Three were paramount. One was evidence that anesthesia was based on a specific body of knowledge and techniques; another, that research was directed to create that knowledge and to disseminate it by means of a formal educational system; and the third, that an organization, or structure, was in place that could guide, support, and monitor anesthesia in providing patient care, including the training and certification of specialists, an appropriate academic environment, and specialty journals of anesthesia.

How this process was carried out is the subject of this chapter. The perspective is mainly American, but the evolution of specialization in the United Kingdom, Canada, France, and Germany highlights the way it developed in three other regions and points to the similarities to, and differences from, the process in the United States. Though there were differences, the regions shared one common factor: the desire of anesthetists to emerge from the often-well-meaning but still oppressive authority of surgeons and to gain professional autonomy.

The Need for Specialization in Anesthesia

When anesthesia was a craft, anesthesia was based primarily on experience, skill, and manual dexterity. Knowledge of anesthesia was empirical and not obtained from formal learning or research. It was a craft; in its simplest form, it consisted in pouring drops of ether or chloroform onto a face mask. To many people, this seemed the task of an artisan, not a physician. *It looked unchallenging*, and few physicians were drawn to it. That did not matter to surgeons, who wanted from anesthesia only a patient who was immobile, free of pain, and preferably soft-bellied. Anyone, surgeons thought, could give an anesthetic—and often, "anyone" did. That was the beginning of the poor image that so many physicians had of anesthesia.

Looks were deceiving, however. Safety in anesthesia became more and more of concern. As committees and commissions in the nineteenth century in the United Kingdom showed, many deaths were associated with anesthesia, especially with chloroform.[1] This would not change as long as anesthesia depended just on skill and empirical knowledge. Progress was possible only with understanding that was based on sound, scientific knowledge. That required training. When Frederic Hewitt, in London, asked in 1896 why the death rate had not seemed to diminish despite recent advances in anesthesia,[2] he said that physicians who gave anesthetics were often comparatively unskilled and did not understand the responsibilities of the task. So they should be trained. His colleagues agreed.

The same was true in the United States. Anesthetics were given by junior doctors, medical students, and nurses, who seldom were concerned with observing even simple physiological changes during anesthesia affecting the pulse and respiration. Anesthesia was "recklessly administered."[3] Postoperative complications—such as pneumonia, heart failure, and uremia—were not uncommon. Each hospital should therefore have a *special anaesthetizer*.

Training of would-be anesthetists was one answer, but to make anesthesia attractive as a medical occupation, the practice of anesthesia had to go beyond being a craft. As of 1896, the jubilee year of anesthesia, the answer for Hewitt was specialism.[4] However, by that, he meant the existence of physicians who gave most or all of their time to anesthesia. Nor did Hewitt say that it would take many years to achieve that goal, for the complexity of the process was not then apparent; much more was required than training and full-time physicians. What was needed was an entire structure that embraced education, research, and clinical practice and that, as well, would oversee the operation of full-time practitioners. This process actually required another forty years after Hewitt spoke. Anesthesia had first to emerge from being a craft that was based on experience and pass through the stage of being a discipline, when anesthesia was based on knowledge with a scientific base.

The Path from Craft to Discipline

Toward the end of the nineteenth century, then, on both sides of the Atlantic, the status and the standard and practice of anesthesia caused much dissatisfaction. Even before Hewitt mentioned specialism in 1896, other anesthetists realized that they had to correct the course of anesthesia. In the United Kingdom, the Society of Anaesthetists was founded in London in 1893[5] so that concerned physicians could discuss problems, like mortality, that were holding anesthesia back. In the United States, the Long Island Society of Anesthetists was founded in New York in 1905[6] for a similar reason. Such steps helped initiate the transition of anesthesia from craft to the next stage of discipline, when it would be based on scientific knowledge and on valid principles governing more precise administration of anesthesia.

The transition is evident in several ways. One was the desire to learn more about anesthesia from research. In England, John Snow did a great deal in the first decade of anesthesia,[7] and Hewitt, beginning in 1885, investigated variations in nitrous oxide and oxygen mixtures so he could make anesthesia safer.[8] In the early twentieth century, research included the design of anesthesia machines (see chapter 7) and studies of a number of inhalational and intravenous agents (see chapter 5). With the exception of Snow's, however, all this research was oriented to clinical practice, even if it yielded some basic knowledge. Basic scientific research was not yet under way.

Another indication of the transition from craft to discipline is the publication of textbooks on anesthesia. As Snow did so often, he led the way. As early as 1847, he wrote a text on ether in 1847[9] that was more authoritative than the short treatise by James Robinson earlier in the year,[10] and he wrote a comprehensive text just before he died in 1858.[11] Among others are J. Flagg's, of 1851,[12] and Henry Lyman's, of 1881,[13] both of which were published in the United States. Others by George Foy,[14] Laurence Turnbull,[15] Dudley Buxton,[16] Hewitt[17, 18, 19] and James Tayloe Gwathmey, in 1914,[20] and Paluel Flagg, in 1916[21] emphasize the awareness that practice had to be based on sound information. Those are just some of the many early texts, a complete listing of which has been compiled by A. G. McKenzie.[22]

The evolutionary nature of the process of transition is also apparent in that when anesthesia was a discipline, seeds were being sown that would germinate into the beginnings of anesthesia as a specialty. Hewitt's reference to specialism in 1896 was one of those seeds, though he emphasized "constant practice" and experience[23] rather than acquisition of knowledge through research and education. In the United States, at about the same time, S. Ormond Goldan publicized his ideas about the need for specialization in anesthesia.[24] He regretted the fact that anesthesia was still in its infancy, even after fifty years, and he deplored the view that anyone could give an anesthetic. Goldan thought it important that anesthetists establish independence from surgeons; like Hewitt, he stressed the special practice of anesthesia. While he knew that some physicians gave anesthetics willingly, he also knew that others did so reluctantly, or even fearfully. Skill in the absence of training and scientific knowledge was not enough to quieten the cry that, despite the growth of experience, people still died under anesthesia.

Even well into the twentieth century, death under anesthesia was an ever-present concern; in 1912, the mortality attributable to *chloroform anesthesia* was approximately 1 in 3,000,[25] though it is not possible to attribute any proportion to anesthesia and surgery. Today, however, it is estimated that *solely from anesthesia*, only one person in 185,000 will die, as opposed to a ratio of 1 to 2,860 totally attributable to surgery.[26] Statistics since the 1950s have been more precise, and they do suggest that there has been a trend toward a steady decrease in mortality associated with anesthesia over the years.[27]

Even so, it is not easy to find information that proves the hypothesis that evolving anesthesia—in this case, anesthesia as a discipline—is directly associated with a continuing decrease in mortality. Yet suggestive evidence is provided by an attempt to study the death rate due to, or associated with, anesthesia in England and Wales for the first one hundred years of anesthesia.[28] While it is impossible in that study to separate out disease, surgery, and anesthesia as independent causes of death, the fact is that after 1938, the absolute numbers of deaths due to or associated with anesthesia did begin to decline. It is not illogical to infer from that datum that over the years that preceded the point where the death rates began to decline, some factor or factors must have operated that were closely associated with the lowering of death rates. While such factors would include the introduction of the sulfonamides in the early 1930s and the greater use of blood transfusion, they might well include anesthesia-related factors. These include the availability of increasingly well-designed anesthesia machines in the period from 1900 to 1930 and of new anesthesia drugs and techniques in the 1920s and early 1930s, the greater degree of communication of knowledge that was initiated in journals and anesthesia societies in the first three decades of the twentieth century, and the overall and continuing concern with anesthesia-related mortality.

The changes in anesthesia that were occurring as it passed from craft into discipline from 1900 to 1938 coincided with a general view among anesthetists that they were becoming linked in a common and special endeavor and as a specific professional group. For as we trace the process, it becomes clear that in addition to the growth of knowledge of anesthesia and the research that creates it (and the ability of individuals to use it), a third aspect of the maturation of anesthesia was developing: the creation of an organizational structure that would shape anesthesia into a vehicle for optimum delivery of patient care.

These three aspects of the evolution of anesthesia, as well as some others, will now be considered in more detail.

I. Needs for a Specialty: A Knowledge Base

Though Hewitt was perceptive in stating in 1896 that the present state of knowledge left "much to be desired,"[29] it was not easy to create a necessary body of knowledge. However, at that time, a number of notable developments brightened the intellectual outlook and gave a sense of optimism to society. Of great import was the ferment in science and medicine in the last few years of the nineteenth century and the first few of the twentieth century, which helped to shape new perspectives. They might not have been apparent to all anesthetists, though the significance of advances in medicine—such as the existence of blood groups and of hormones, as demonstrated in 1902—would have. Progress was quite apparent. The First World War also expedited progress, even if only by showing that surgery demanded good anesthesia. After the war, which was thought to have put an end to all future wars, the general air of optimism served as a stimulus to advances in a number of fields, of which anesthesia was one. In fact, the 1920s and 1930s turned out to be a golden period for anesthesia, both in terms of creation of knowledge and for the quest for specialty recognition.

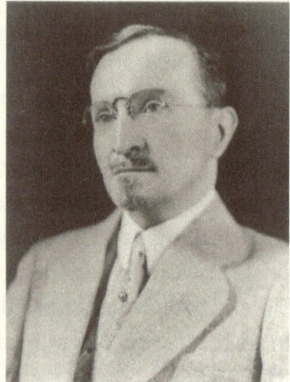

Fig. 8.1. Francis McMechan (1879-1939)

Francis Hoeffer McMechan was born in Cincinnati, Ohio. He came from a medical family, but he was a university teacher and a journalist before studying medicine. McMechan enrolled in Ohio Medical College in 1900 and graduated in 1903. He began his anesthesia career immediately, approaching it by close attention to its principles and its practice; but in 1911, arthritis made McMechan give up the clinical side of anesthesia. However, McMechan then gave his full attention to improving the organization of anesthesia. He facilitated the transition of the Long Island Society of Anesthetists into the New York Society; he was instrumental in founding the American Association of Anesthetists in 1912 and several regional organizations over the next decade; in 1914, he edited the *Quarterly Supplement of Anesthesia & Analgesia* in the *American Journal of Surgery*; and, in 1919, he founded the National Anesthesia Research Society in an attempt to foster a wider interest in anesthesia education. McMechan's influence began to spread further when the journal *Current Researches in Anesthesia & Analgesia* began publication in 1922. His name became known internationally as he traveled overseas, but arthritis progressively crippled him, and he was eventually forced to give up his unique activities in the service of organizational anesthesia.

For knowledge to grow, some individuals had to create it, and others use it. In that way, the type of situation that Goldan referred to in 1901 would be prevented: "as often as not the most available man gave the anesthetic,"[30] rather than the best trained individual. However, even after World War I, when more physicians had an interest in anesthesia, relatively few were actually in practice. In the United Kingdom, the slack was taken up by general practitioners; in the United States, by nurses. While each of these groups provided an important service, the ideal, as espoused by some individuals, was to have anesthesia administered by a specialist physician. This view was held firmly by some who were dedicated to such an ideal. One of them was anesthetist Francis McMechan (fig. 8.1), of Cincinnati. He argued that to ensure the safety of a patient, whoever administered an anesthetic had to be able to treat any complication that might arise—and that this lay in the purview of the physician rather than the nurse.[31] (That situation affected the United States more than the United Kingdom, where once the practice of anesthesia was established, it was only physicians who gave anesthetics.)

Though that view might be thought elitist, some surgeons shared McMechan's view. John B. Murphy, the Chicago surgeon, for example, stated in 1901 that "the present haphazard methods" of administering anesthesia were not acceptable.[32] His view was that only the hospital could lay the foundation for the skilled anesthetist, as it did for the surgeon, and even that the anesthetist would not be considered "a mere satellite" of the surgeon but would have an incentive to concentrate on administering quality anesthesia. Murphy understood that anesthesia should be taught by anesthetists, not by surgeons. The London surgeon Marmaduke Shield also thought there was "a strong and pressing case" for education of physicians in the theory and practice of anesthesia.[33]

If McMechan, Murphy, and Shield were justified in their view, then one must ask how knowledge specific to anesthesia was created for anesthetists in the early part of the twentieth century and how they applied it.

Although empirical knowledge is a feature of anesthesia as a craft, it is also an element of learning and of knowledge. Empirical knowledge can be learned by experience and stored in the memory, but it is more effective if recorded, in the form, for example, of physiological variables such as the pulse and respiratory rates and the skin color. Hence the significance of two Harvard medical students thinking in 1894 that they could put their observations on paper so that, over time, they might in that way become better anesthetists. The two were Ernest Amory Codman and Harvey Cushing, who recorded changes in pulse and respiration on a specially designed anesthesia record.[34]

That simple step was an early one on the path to objective—and verifiable—knowledge in anesthesia and, in a primitive form, of monitoring. (However, no warning alarm was built into anesthesia records; see also chapter 10). Objective knowledge could also be derived from a second contribution Cushing made to anesthesia: in 1903, he stressed the value of recording blood pressure readings in patients' records.[35] That heightened the awareness of the need to watch a patient and showed how knowledge of anesthesia could be built up. Moreover, only when anesthetists began to study the physiological effects of anesthesia could the craft of anesthesia evolve into a discipline, and later into a specialty.

Individual practitioners had a twofold relationship to knowledge. Some used knowledge to improve the clinical practice of anesthesia. Such individuals include Hewitt and his contemporary in London, Dudley Buxton. Hewitt's study of nitrous oxide and oxygen[36] and Buxton's analysis of mortality[37] are two examples of clinically oriented knowledge; another is Ralph Waters' study of chloroform.[38] The second type of knowledge was that derived from basic-science research. That type of knowledge, derived particularly from research by anesthetists, was, however, lacking until well into the twentieth century. And it is precisely that type of knowledge that would strengthen the hands of anesthetists when they were endeavoring to convince their peers that anesthesia could stand alone as a specialty and be recognized as such.

The relative lack of basic research in anesthesia, even up to the Second World War, is not surprising. Even in medicine, it was not until 1878 that researchers in physiology began using physical methods in the United States, and not until 1909 when it was recognized that clinical medicine had to branch into science and practice.[39] Nor is it surprising that much of the basic-science type of research applicable to anesthesia was carried out initially not by anesthetists but by basic scientists such as Samuel Meltzer and John Auer at the Rockefeller Institute in New York, Yandell Henderson and Howard Haggard at Yale University, and John Scott Haldane and Joseph Barcroft in Oxford and London in England. They created the basic knowledge of various aspects of respiration[40] that were so important to the understanding of anesthesia. Surgeons also contributed significant research, including William Halsted and his famous student Harvey Cushing, Rudolph Matas, Karl Connell, and Frederick Cotton.

However, while few anesthetists conducted basic-science research in the early decades of the twentieth century, some did carry out clinically oriented work. The work of two groups will be considered.

II. Needs for a Specialty: Research and Education

The First Wave of Research-Oriented Anesthetists

One of the first anesthetists to carry out significant anesthesia research was Walter Boothby in Boston. He is representative of the early-twentieth-century research-oriented pioneers and was the first real investigator in anesthesia[41] in this period. After working with J. S. Haldane in Oxford, Boothby became interested in the design of anesthesia machines. He confirmed Connell's dosimetric approach to ether administration (chapter 7), clarified the determination of ether tensions,[42] worked on the first water sight-feed apparatus and described a nitrous oxide—oxygen machine.[43]

As discussed in chapter 7, others were active in designing anesthesia machines, especially James Tayloe Gwathmey, Elmer McKesson, Dennis Jackson, and Jay Heidbrink. They helped fill the void in the knowledge base for that aspect of anesthesia to establish simple principles of the administration of anesthesia. In addition, they stressed education.

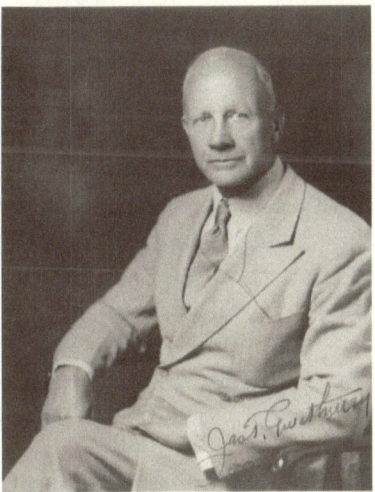

Fig. 8.2. James Gwathmey (1862-1944)
James Tayloe Gwathmey was born near Roanoke in Virginia. While at school, Gwathmey became fascinated by gymnastics and was adept in acrobatics, and when at Vanderbilt University, even while studying medicine, he was director of the gymnasium. He graduated in 1899. He interned in medicine in New York and trained in surgery and anesthesia. By 1904, Gwathmey was engaged in the practice of anesthesia full-time. He carried out some research, particularly on the use of oxygen in anesthesia and on anesthesia apparatus, and he began writing. In 1912, Gwathmey, with William Woolsey, published an article on the Gwathmey-Woolsey nitrous oxide—oxygen apparatus; and in 1913, he published his first article on oil-ether anesthesia. He became known for both of these contributions, but also as president of the New York Society of Anesthetists and as the author of his 1914 textbook *Anesthesia*. Gwathmey served in the U.S. Army in World War I, and did much to raise the status of young officers who were providing anesthesia. After the war, Gwathmey continued to practice, and articles continued to flow from his pen. He retired in 1939, but continued to write. By 1943, his publications totaled 113, on many aspects of the field in which he was for many years a leader.

Gwathmey (fig. 8.2), in New York, was a leading figure in anesthesia in the first two decades of the twentieth century. Like the other prominent anesthetists of his day, he was an authority on several aspects of anesthesia and, before World War I, was the doyen of American anesthesia. He was elected the first president of the New York Society of Anaesthetists in 1912,[44] he designed an anesthesia machine,[45] and he wrote many articles on clinical practice,[46] as well as his textbook.

McKesson, with an inventive mind that made him a natural in designing machines from 1910 to 1930[47] (see chapter 7), was another fine clinician, an inspired teacher, and a recognized authority on anesthesia. His interest in physiology made him one of the first anesthetists to stress the importance of measuring the blood pressure. An associate professor of physiology at Toledo Medical College until 1914, he enhanced the understanding of anesthesia when few anesthetists were concerned about principles of anesthesia that were based on physiology and physics. He stressed the changes in respiration as valuable physiological information. He was ahead of his time in advocating mouth-to-mouth insufflation for resuscitation of infants, and he incorporated a positive-pressure mechanism on his anesthesia machine as a means of ventilating a patient who might be apneic. Like Gwathmey, McKesson set an example of what an anesthetist might accomplish, so that surgeons, particularly, and other physicians could realize that anesthesia was based on science as well as art, worthy of full-time physician practice.

Jackson too was inventive, and his prototype anesthesia machines laid the basis for carbon dioxide absorption in anesthesia.[48] With H. Thomason, Jackson developed a circle system with nitrogen washout.[49] He influenced Waters in the 1920s when he was formulating his own ideas about carbon dioxide absorption, so his influence was taken forward by Waters and others. Heidbrink, the fifth member of this group of original minds, is remembered, like McKesson, for a long-lived series of anesthesia machines.[50]

These American physician-anesthetist investigators built up the knowledge base in anesthesia, based on sound, valid principles. This was important in the difficult environment of the First World War and then after it, when the importance of competence in anesthesia was more generally recognized.

The Second Wave of Research-Oriented Anesthetists

After the First World War, the practice of anesthesia was enhanced by research conducted by a second group of anesthetist-investigators. Teachers, as well as researchers, in the eyes of their peers, particularly the influential surgeons they worked with, they had high profiles as physician-anesthetists.

Surgeons valued their clinical work and thus that of anesthesia in general and so looked favorably on their colleagues' desire for anesthesia to become a specialty. Some, such as Edwin Schmidt in Madison and Charles and William Mayo in Rochester, were powerful in organized medicine and did much to convince their own peers of the need for specialty recognition of anesthesia.

An early member of this second group of anesthetists in the United States was Isabella Herb, of the Mayo Clinic and who later was entirely clinically oriented. More widely known, and with greater influence on the practice of anesthesia, were four who carried out fundamental clinical research in anesthesia: Ralph Waters in Madison, John Lundy at the Mayo Clinic in Rochester, Arthur Guedel in Indianopolis and Los Angeles, and Brian Sword in New Haven and North Carolina. All added to the knowledge of anesthesia, but Waters and Lundy are of special significance in their overall contributions, because those facilitated specialty recognition.

Waters, at the University of Wisconsin,[51] like Lundy at the Mayo Clinic,[52] was a pivotal figure in the evolution of anesthesia as a specialty. Indeed, Waters is the representative par excellence of this generation of anesthetists by virtue of his unique accomplishments in clinical practice, education, and research, and also by virtue of his vision. By demonstrating the potential of anesthesia as a force for good in health care, he perhaps did the most to justify recognition of anesthesia as a specialty. The significance of Waters' role is evident in his fourfold vision of his goals in anesthesia, which explains much of what he wished to achieve: enhancing care of patients undergoing surgery, teaching anesthesia, encouraging his junior in their own work in anesthesia, and cooperating in a research partnership with basic scientists.[53] Waters' contributions therefore merit consideration. They illustrate how a single individual had such an influence in the process leading up to specialty recognition.

Waters became interested in anesthesia in 1915, when he read the first issue of the quarterly supplement on anesthesia and analgesia that the *American Journal of Surgery* published. He soon started practicing anesthesia full-time and set up an anesthesia clinic in Kansas City. He showed what could be achieved by a full-time practitioner in anesthesia, and through his own results, he was able to influence others to become interested in the field. When he took charge of anesthesia in the new university hospital in Madison in 1927, nothing held him back. His desire to teach and to conduct research, to encourage others who showed any interest in anesthesia, and to engage in cooperative research knew no bounds. Waters did an enormous amount for anesthesia. With colleagues Arthur Guedel (fig. 8.3) and Lundy, he personified the desire for anesthesia as a specialty.

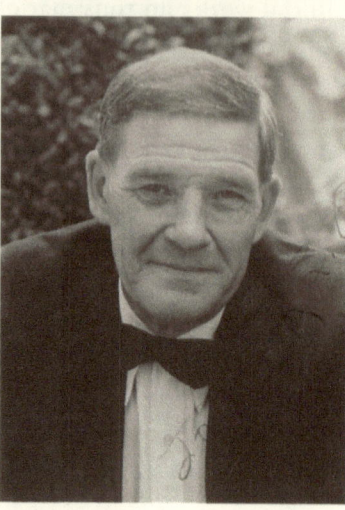

Fig. 8.3. Arthur Guedel (1883-1956)
Arthur Ernest Guedel's birthplace was Cambridge City, Indiana. He was a self-made
man, rising by his own efforts to overcome setbacks, and living by the philosophy that
one learns through mistakes. Guedel was too poor to attend high school, was apprenticed
to a machinist, lost three fingers in an accident, and studied at home after hours.
Nevertheless, he played the piano and organ and passed a special entrance examination
to enrol in the University of Indiana. He graduated from the university medical school
in 1908. Like his contemporary Ralph Waters, Guedel was a self-trained anesthetist
and practiced in several hospitals in Indianopolis. He served in the American military
in World War I, and was well known as the anesthetist who visited different hospitals
by means of a motor bicycle. In 1928, Guedel moved to Los Angeles. Guedel made
several important contributions to the practice and understanding of anesthesia: in the
technique of self-administration of nitrous oxide in labor, in the relation of physical
signs to depth of anesthesia, in the design of the cuffed endotracheal tube and of the
oral airway, in the introduction of divinyl oxide, and in education, by means of his own
textbook. His contributions to anesthesia were recognized in the United States in the
Guedel Lectureship and in England, in his being a recipient of the Hickman Medal.

Besides looking at the horizon when anesthesia might be a specialty, Waters
built up knowledge of anesthesia by conducting research in the operating room
and in the laboratory. In clinical anesthesia, besides introducing the to-and-fro
carbon dioxide absorption system,[54] he introduced cyclopropane[55] and sodium
thiopental[56] into anesthesia. In the laboratory, Waters worked with pharmacologist
Chauncey Leake in clarifying the effects of carbon dioxide on the body,[57] and
with scientists Meek, Hathaway, and Orth on the effect of anesthesia on cardiac
automaticity.[58] And he was close to the study conducted by pharmacologist Seevers
and physiologist Meek on the effects of cyclopropane in animals.[59] His initiative

in studying and introducing cyclopropane and thiopental illustrate his readiness to work with others and his awareness of the need to find and use better anesthetic agents. His work on carbon dioxide absorption did not require the same degree of laboratory cooperation, and Jackson's earlier work set him on the path to his own investigation and product. In turn, however, his to-and-fro device set an example for Sword to follow in designing his own circle, closed-circuit anesthesia system.[60] Waters also worked on an inflatable cuff for endotracheal tubes in 1928 with Guedel[61]. Guedel, who was widely respected for his knowledge of anesthesia, in 1920 had described eye signs in anesthesia as indicators of anesthesia depth,[62] amplifying his description in *Inhalation Anesthesia: A Fundamental Guide* in 1937[63]—another addition to the total body of knowledge of anesthesia.

Lundy, too, influenced fellow anesthetists and anesthesia and its development after World War I. An expert on local and regional anesthesia and head of anesthesia at the Mayo Clinic, his experience of barbiturates was even more extensive[64] than Waters'; and he first used thiopental sodium very soon after Waters, on June 18, 1934.[65] Lundy wrote prolifically, publishing a textbook on anesthesia[66] and articles on a variety of subjects besides anesthesia itself, such as the recovery room,[67] the blood bank,[68] and the plastic-styletted intravenous (Rochester) needle.[69] Having been taught the elements of regional anesthesia by Gaston Labat at the Mayo Clinic, Lundy was among those who, through education as well as research, expedited the development of regional anesthesia in the United States.[70]

The importance of anesthesia research, and of the knowledge that it creates and is spread, to the development of anesthesia as a specialty is profound. Yale University pharmacologist W. T. Salter observed that no professional group could maintain itself by service alone.[71] As do other specialists, anesthesiologists have to be able to look to the horizons of knowledge and to facilitate progress by exercising the vision that enables new knowledge to be applied clinically. In anesthesia, these requirements were within reach in the 1930s, and it is then that the process leading to specialty recognition picked up steam.

III. Needs for a Specialty: Organizations

Although the growth of knowledge precedes specialization in a particular field, knowledge must be used appropriately. This in itself is one rationale for specialization, but in medicine, it is essential that knowledge be used correctly, because patients' lives may be at stake. That is why clinical standards or guidelines are formulated. But they have to be enforced, and this is best done, in anesthesia as in other medical specialties, under the aegis of an organization of specialists who agree on how the standards should be applied and monitored.

As the number of would-be specialists increases, the need for, and later the existence of, an organization grows.[72] As anesthesia moved from craft to specialty, as it was increasingly characterized by use of knowledge, and as more physicians became interested in the work, anesthesia became increasingly professionalized.

The development of specialization, therefore, must also be seen in the context of professionalization.

A useful starting point is George Weisz' observation that underlying the rise of specialties, there is a fundamental transformation of intellectual perspective.[73] In medicine, specialization lagged behind that of the physical and chemical sciences, and it was necessary for physicians to catch up with scientists in this respect. In turn, anesthetists had to catch up with other specialists in medical fields with higher profiles. That could not begin until anesthetists discussed common problems among themselves, which was facilitated by professionally organized forums for discussion.

The Twin Roles of Individuals and Organizations

Individuals. In discussing the advent of anesthesia, Yale physiologist and historian John Fulton referred to the "vision and daring of youth,"[74] and he underlined the fact that the pioneers—Davy, Hickman, Long, Wells, and Morton—were all under the age of thirty. In contrast, the individuals who were instrumental in having anesthesia recognized as a specialty were mature physicians and so were much older than those we might paraphrase Fulton in calling them his "gang of five." In the vanguard in the twentieth century was the American "gang of six" that we have already met in their roles of creating the knowledge of anesthesia—Gwathmey, McKesson, MacMechan, Waters, Guedel, and Lundy—but their roles now were to build up the *image* of anesthesia so that other physicians in positions of influence would aid them in having anesthesia recognized as a specialty.

In the United States, the critical period for the evolution of anesthesia from a discipline to a specialty was from 1920 to 1938. It was then that the status of that gang of six physician-anesthetists, their dedication to the practice of anesthesia, their vision for its future, and the force of their personalities provided the momentum and the direction in the Sisyphean struggle to have anesthesia recognized as a specialty. While Gwathmey and McKesson before World War I had been especially influential as clinicians, after the war Waters, Guedel, and Lundy set examples as respected physician-anesthetists. Their presence around powerful surgeons of the day—Schmidt in Madison and the Mayos in Rochester, for example—and their ongoing efforts to have anesthesia recognized as a specialty eventually paid off. In Eckenhoff's opinion, Waters and Lundy were instrumental in accelerating the evolution of anesthesia into a specialty.[75]

The influence of the six physicians went beyond their being exemplars of physician-anesthetists in daily practice. They also envisioned a structure for anesthesia as a specialty. If that structure is a fabric, its warp was their vision for anesthesia and its woof was the composition of their ideas on how to manage anesthesia as a professional entity.

Organizations. Ideas for different elements in the organization of anesthesia had been forming ever since the founding of the Society of Anaesthetists and the Long Island Society of Anesthetists. In the United States, the process of building a structure was complex, because different people, in medicine as well as in anesthesia, had quite different ideas, and these people and ideas sometimes clashed. Also required was the cooperation of subsidiary organizations.

The fabric that was the development of the organizational structure for American anesthetists was woven from several different strands. There were two main strands and other minor ones. One of the main ones was derived from Adolph Erdmann's idea for the Long Island Society of Anesthetists of 1905. By 1912, the society had grown, and to reflect a broader membership, it became the New York Society of Anesthetists (NYSA), with Gwathmey as president. It steadily grew, and in 1936, it was renamed the American Society of Anesthetists, Incorporated. Then in 1945, it became the American Society of Anesthesiologists, Incorporated (ASA). This society became the main organization of American anesthesiology, representing anesthesiologists in professional and political matters, besides publishing the journal *Anesthesiology* and facilitating the continuing education of its members.

The other main strand was woven out of McMechan's original concept of societies providing regional representation. This too expanded and gained national, and even international, representation. Today, McMechan's web is still evident in the International Anesthesia Research Society and in the journal *Anesthesia & Analgesia*, first published in 1922. The society does not have the powers of the ASA, but it is highly influential in the educational sphere.

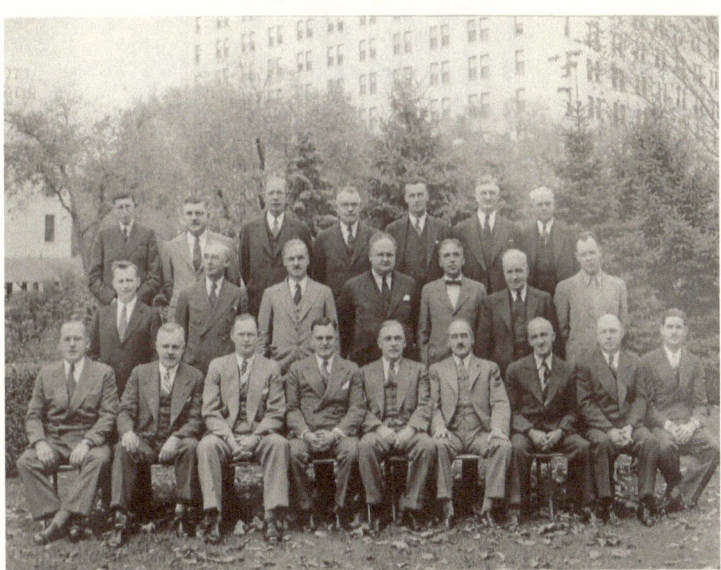

Fig. 8.4. Anesthetists' Travel Club, Annual Meeting, 1938. The Club included an Australian (G.Kaye, back row, extreme left) and Canadians (J.Blezard is seen front row, 3rd from right), while American Paul Wood (U.S.A) is seen in center of middle row. (Author's collection.)

In addition to these two strands, a third, thinner, one served as another socially cohesive force at a time when it was essential for American anesthetists to avoid feeling isolated and to develop a common front. This was the Anaesthetists' Travel Club, which was formed by Lundy and his colleagues at the Mayo Clinic in 1929. Its members were drawn from the United States and Canada (fig. 8.4). Although it was primarily an academic association—Henry Ruth wrote that it was "an ingenious arrangement whereby outstanding men in the field of anesthesiology could meet together annually to observe clinical work and discuss their problems"[76]—it did serve as a forum where the members, who included the protagonists of the movement for specialty recognition, could meet and exchange ideas about anesthesia as a whole. As Ron Stephen noted, the members were "bound by the concept of improving the status of anesthesia and forging it into a distinct and honorable specialty."[77]

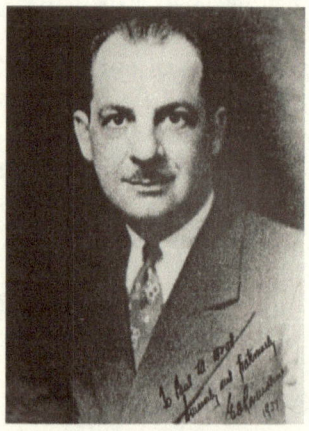

Fig. 8.5. Emery Rovenstine (1895-1960)

Emery Andrew Rovenstine was born in Atwood, Indiana. He graduated from college with a BA in 1917, served in the U.S. Army for three years, and, on returning from wartime duties, taught school for three years. He entered medical school in Indiana and got to know Arthur Guedel, who refereed basketball matches in which Rovenstine played. Rovenstine's interest in anesthesia was furthered by Guedel and by Elmer McKesson, who taught a course in anesthesia that Rovenstine attended. Guedel advised Rovenstine to study anesthesia under Ralph Waters in Madison, and he began his formal training in anesthesia in 1930. He joined Waters's staff in 1932, but in 1935, he joined the staff of Bellevue Hospital in New York, where a physician was required to develop an anesthesia program. Rovenstine, as assistant professor of surgery, organized the new department, added a residency program and a postgraduate course, and encouraged research. He himself was appointed Professor of Anesthesia in 1937. Rovenstine did a great deal for the growing specialty of anesthesiology, helping to launch the journal *Anesthesiology* and involving himself in the American Board of Anesthesiology. He also did a great deal by training the many residents who went on in their turn to train others.

Over the years, many of the leaders of North American anesthesiology, including many who expedited specialty recognition, attended the meetings of the Anesthetists' Travel Club. Some were among that postwar generation that worked hard in the 1920s to demonstrate the achievements of anesthesia, such as Lundy, Waters, and Guedel. Others were of the next generation, such as Emery Rovenstine (fig. 8.5), of New York, who trained under Waters and carried on his ideas to the next generation still. The Anesthetists' Travel Club enabled Waters and his peers to create a matrix in which the ideas of anesthetists in the 1930s could germinate.

Genesis of the Specialty of Anesthesia

Initial initiatives. How the fabric was woven out of the two principal strands, even though at times they became tangled as anesthetists strove to have anesthesia recognized as a specialty, may be understood by examining certain events that began in 1912. During Gwathmey's presidency of the NYSA, the society asked the American Medical Association (AMA) at its annual meeting to approve the creation of a Section on Anesthesia.[78] However, approval was not granted, mainly because the society was not national. But at the same time, some physician-anesthetists who had been at the AMA meeting formed another society with the national name of the American Association of Anesthetists (AAA). This group met next time the AMA met, the following year, which is when McMechan's name first became prominent. Seen by those who would come to admire him as a human dynamo and by others as the "little corporal,"[79] he had a vision of a national structure for physicians practising anesthesia.[80] Corporal or not, he was highly successful. Under his aegis, the Interstate Association of Ohio and Kentucky was formed in 1915; he helped found the Canadian Society of Anaesthetists in 1920; the Southern Association of Anesthetists and the Pacific Coast Association of Anesthetists were established in 1922; the Eastern Association of Anesthetists, in 1923; and in 1926, the AAA morphed into the Associated Anesthetists of the United States and Canada (AAUSC). The McMechan web was a national one. Now there were two organizations of anesthetists in the United States: those derived from the original Long Island Society and the NYSA, and those deriving from the AAA.

McMechan also envisioned a society that would seemingly be focused on research. He named this the National Anesthesia Research Society. One of those who encouraged the existence of this society was McKesson, who wanted manufacturers of anesthesia drugs and equipment to be members of an anesthesia society. The society grew, and in 1925, it became not only wholly professional but also international, changing its name to the International Anesthesia Research Society (IARS). Thus was initiated McMechan's grand international plan, whereby the IARS would attract members from all over the world.

McMechan, though progressively disabled by rheumatoid arthritis, traveled widely, and he added the conception of an International College of Anesthetists to his vision of a worldwide specialty. He even hoped that certification might be granted by 1936. McMechan's plan had earlier included a literature for physician anesthetists, including the supplement to the *American Journal of Surgery* on anesthesia and analgesia. Literature was important; Waters, for example, then beginning to take a "special interest" in anesthesia, discovered the anesthesia supplement with "considerable joy."[81] The success of the supplement was such that its offspring, *Current Researches in Anesthesia and Analgesia*, could contain material that was of specific interest to physician anesthetists; it preceded the *British Journal of Anaesthesia* by one year and, like its British cousin, is still thriving.

Meanwhile, the New York Society was growing.[82] By 1915, it had fifty members, including physicians from New Jersey, Pennsylvania, Connecticut, Massachusetts, and Maryland. This suggested that the society was national, and in 1921, it sought again to have the AMA approve an anesthesia section. However, the efforts failed. By this time, the idea of certification of specialists was growing, not only in the United States but also in Canada and in England, and the members of the New York Society, just as McMechan had, decided to plan for the certification of anesthetists. This was well under way by 1934.

All this time, the New York Society continued to grow, with physicians from Ohio, Texas, Georgia, Minnesota, Oklahoma, and Nevada applying. Much of the credit for the increase in membership goes to the secretary-treasurer, Paul Wood, who in this respect was analogous to McMechan. When the NYSA granted the first certificates to Fellows in Anesthesiology, one of the certificands was Waters.

Final initiatives. The New York Society was clearly thriving despite its unsuccessful efforts to have a section in the AMA recognized. Wood stressed the advantages of a national identity; as anesthesia-historian Douglas Bacon has observed, the name *New York* was "parochial."[83] That is why the society's name was changed in 1936 to the *American Society of Anesthetists Incorporated*.[84] That name, however, would be on the books for less than a decade. Toward the end of World War II, and as American anesthesia showed more signs of separating into two types of practitioners—physicians and nurses—Wood proposed renaming the society the American Society of Anesthesiologists, Incorporated. This was done in April 1945.[85] It was a logical development, for many physicians who had become interested in anesthesia during the war were turning their thoughts to formal training. Moreover, it was generally recognized that the underlying objective of American physician-anesthetists was to encourage the science as well as the art of anesthesia—which had been the objective of the original Long Island Society.

Despite the rebuffs from the AMA in the 1930s, some physicians persisted in seeking the cooperation of the AMA with respect to specialty recognition.

Two pathways seemed possible. One was via an AMA Section of Anesthesia. The other was by way of a body to oversee specialty development in medicine as a whole: the Advisory Board for Medical Specialties (ABMS). Plans for the latter were drawn up in 1933 and 1934, and, when the ABMS was founded in 1936, prospects for specialty recognition for anesthesia brightened.

The founding of the ABMS was significant; some have traced the beginning of the era of medical specialization in the United States to it.[86] For anesthesia itself, it is perhaps more accurate to state that the founding of the ABMS served as a stimulus that encouraged those anesthetists who were interested in specialty recognition to continue their efforts, even though in 1936, the time was still not ripe. But in that year, the American Society of Anesthetists appointed Lundy to represent it at a meeting of the AMA and ABMS, though, again, negotiations stalled. Neither organization appeared to be enthusiastic, and nothing came of that step. While one part of the problem had always been a lack of validated national representation, another was the separation of the two pathways that were being forged to gain specialty recognition. On the one hand, the efforts of the NYSA group were negated by the failure of McMechan's organizations to support a request for specialty recognition and their wish not to be subordinated to any other medical organization; on the other, the AMA did not see eye to eye with McMechan, who insisted on physicians being anesthesia providers.[87]

At that point, two other strands in the fabric became apparent. One developed from the support of one of those surgeons who favored recognition of anesthesia as a specialty. This was E. R. Schmidt, head of surgery at Wisconsin, who recognized the value of Waters' vision and his concept of residency training. Schmidt's solution was simple: certify anesthetists through affiliation with the American Board of Surgery.[88] But another wrinkle had to be ironed out, which is where the second strand becomes evident. The American Board of Surgery required that a request for specialty recognition be accompanied by representation of some of the national societies of the specialty. Because the IARS and the AAUSC—under McMechan, who had spent much effort on his own plans for certification—did not wish to join in, the others solicited the support of a society with a respectably national name: the American Society of Regional Anesthesia, which had been founded in 1923.[89] Now two "national" anesthesia societies could proceed to devise a stratagem whereby an American Board of Anesthesiology could legitimately be taken under the wing of the surgery board. In 1937, the ABMS approved the affiliate board's statement that anesthesiology was a specialty and that an American examining and certifying board for anesthesia was being formed with representatives from two national organizations.

In 1939, McMechan died. It became clear that the AMA's opposition an anesthesia section was no more. The chairman of the AMA Council on Scientific Assembly went so far on November 24, 1939, to announce that "the establishment of a Section on Anesthesiology would be for the good of the

American Medical Association and . . . would help your specialty very much."[90] The AMA's approval was formalized in June 1940,[91] and anesthesiology was now, finally, recognized as a specialty.

IV. Needs for a Specialty: Training and Certification

Implicit in anesthesia's being recognized as a specialty was a fourth need: for training programs, examination of would-be specialists, and their certification. In a sense, these were in place before anesthesia was formally recognized as a specialty. Waters had initiated a residency program soon after he joined the faculty in Madison in 1927, and many of his trainees took the Waters system to the university departments that they later headed all over the nation. In 1937, only four hospitals were approved for residency programs, but by 1945, forty-nine were approved. Similarly, examinations modeled after the ABMS requirements had been developed earlier in the 1930s by the NYSA, though modeled after the much less rigorous requirements of the International College of Anesthetists.[92]

V. Needs for a Specialty: Communication Media

Communication of knowledge also influenced the evolution of anesthesia. While books provided an established knowledge base, newer knowledge could only be communicated by journals. In the United States, the publication in 1915 of a quarterly supplement to the *American Journal of Surgery* and of *Current Researches in Anesthesia and Analgesia* in 1922 showed that anesthesia was maturing and worthy of the request for specialty recognition. *Current Researches*, the first journal on anesthesia published anywhere, showed that the nascent specialty was founded on knowledge that was unique to anesthesia.

As the number of anesthetists nation-wide grew in the 1930s, it seemed logical to explore the prospects for a second American anesthesia journal.[93] However, discussions with the AMA provided no firm basis on which to proceed. The AMA was testy too, for McMechan was charged in 1935 with poaching contributions for his journal that should have gone to the AMA.[94] Once again, the incipient specialty of anesthesia was riven by squabbles. Though the NYSA had agreed not to proceed with a "publication" while *Current Researches* and McMechan were active, the NYSA-derived strand continued to ponder the question of another journal. By 1937, a special editorial committee was set up, evidently to start "definite proceedings toward the securing of a journal for The American Society of Anesthetists,"[95] and there did seem to be a place for a journal with a higher content of scientific material as opposed to the clinical content of *Current Researches*. As Bacon has pointed out, when McMechan died on June 29, 1939, "the world of anesthesiology changed, and during the next several years McMechan's organizations would fade into oblivion and the other main organizations would become the voice of anesthesiology in the United States."[96] Matters were organized apace, and *Anesthesiology*, the new journal, was first published in July 1940, with Henry Ruth, of Philadelphia, as editor. Its success in publishing basic science material, clinical topics, and reviews provided one more piece of evidence that affording anesthesia specialty recognition was justified.

The Academic Component of Specialization: Universities

If development of an intellectual perspective is a requisite of specialization, such is most likely to be found within universities. In anesthesia, this was a late development. Until Waters was appointed professor of anesthesia in Madison in 1933, there was no university department of anesthesia in the United States. The integrated approach to anesthesia of clinical practice, education, and research—so essential to the potential of anesthesia as a specialty—did not exist before then. Clinical practice was service-oriented; education in anesthesia was most commonly an apprenticeship, and anesthesia research was carried out in physiology and pharmacology departments. This situation began to change with Waters in the 1930s, and it was followed up by Henry Beecher at Harvard in the 1940s.

The background and the visions of the two men were somewhat different, and it is appropriate to consider some of the differences that bear further on the topic of specialization.

Waters at Wisconsin

Some aspects of Waters' contributions have already been noted, but here his fourfold vision should be considered purely in the university setting. While his emphasis on clinical practice and research were significant in this context, the most long-lasting was the residency program in anesthesia that he started at the University of Wisconsin. His residents were able to see Waters in action, whether providing excellent anesthesia, engaging in unique research such as his study on chloroform,[97] or, especially, teaching. His program became a model for other universities. In a sense, since Waters was self-educated without having had a university appointment or any academic training before going to Madison, Waters' ideas were homegrown.

Waters' residency training program was the first of its kind anywhere, and its development in a university setting was evidently appropriate. It gave a clinical purpose to the university, and this had other benefits with respect to the quest for specialty recognition. Besides other anesthetists, surgeons and internists who were high in the medical hierarchy were enabled to see what anesthetists were doing, not only as versatile practitioners, but also as anesthetists who were fully justified in wanting anesthesia to be recognized as a specialty. In this sense,

Waters was himself a model for anyone who wondered what kinds of attributes a specialist in anesthesia might have. Like Snow much earlier, Waters married the art and science of anesthesia. Waters was evidence enough that anesthesia was, indeed, worthy of being regarded as a specialty.

Beecher at Harvard

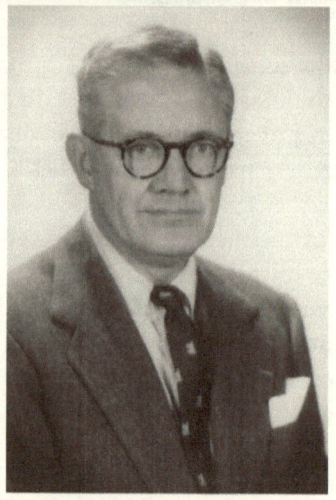

Fig. 8.6. Henry Beecher (1904-1976)

Henry Knowles Beecher was born in Wichita, Kansas. A graduate of Harvard Medical School, which he entered in 1928, Beecher took three years of training in surgery and for one year worked with Nobel laureate and physiologist August Krogh in Copenhagen. With this background, and without having formal training in anesthesia, he established an anesthesia program in Boston, based at Massachusetts General Hospital (MGH). He started this new career in 1936. A carrot of uncertain size was the existence of an endowment fund, which had been inaugurated in 1917, to be applied to the Henry Isaiah Dorr chair in research and teaching in anesthesia at Harvard, where anesthesia was in need of attention. Beecher was appointed to the chair—the first chair anywhere to be endowed—in 1941. He served with the MGH unit in North Africa, and as a military doctor, he made important observations on pain, resuscitation, and therapy in the wounded. Beecher became well known for his work in clinical pharmacology and, later, for his views on medical ethics, especially in relation to brain death. He also became known as the coauthor of the 1954 study of deaths associated with anesthesia, in which use of curare was unjustly faulted. Beecher's contributions to anesthesia were principally academic, but in anesthesia in the 1940s and 1950s, such contributions were sorely needed.

A second university chair was that at Harvard University. This differed from the Madison chair, for it was a research chair: the Henry Isaiah Dorr Professor of Research and Teaching of Anesthesia, and the first such chair in the United States. It was endowed in 1917, but remained unoccupied until Henry Knowles Beecher (fig. 8.6) was appointed in 1941. This appointment was made after anesthesia was recognized as a specialty, but at a time when it was important to consolidate, by providing evidence that specialty recognition was, indeed, justified.

Beecher, like Rovenstine, was a member of the generation that followed Waters and Lundy. His background was unlike that of Waters. He trained as a surgeon at the Massachusetts General Hospital, not as an anesthetist; he was primarily an academic, having studied physiology with Nobel laureate August Krogh in Denmark toward the end of his surgical residency. Beecher brought the standards of the university to anesthesia.[98] That is how Beecher influenced the growth of the new specialty, in contrast to the influence of Waters, who came to anesthesia from general practice. After being trained in surgery and physiology, and after returning from Denmark in 1935, Beecher was drafted into anesthesia. With an academic perspective on anesthesia, Beecher thus contributed to the intellectual matrix that anesthesia needed as a young specialty. He established the first laboratory purely for the study of anesthetic agents and anesthesia, he developed methodological approaches for the resuscitation of wounded soldiers and for the measurement of pain, and he provided leadership on ethical issues such as the study of drug effects and the definition of death.[99]

Ralph Waters and Henry Beecher thus illustrate the two sides of the coin that is the art and science of anesthesia, both of which had to be developed in order to justify the recognition of anesthesia as a specialty in the United States.

Specialization in Great Britain and Ireland, Canada, and Germany

The way anesthesia evolved in England, Canada, and Germany is considered to compare and contrast the process of specialty recognition there with it in the United States. In all three countries, the evolution of anesthesia from craft to specialty took many years, as it did in the United States. Even in England, where the process had begun, critical efforts to recognize anesthesia as a specialty did not bear fruit until the 1930s. At the other extreme, in Germany, specialty recognition was delayed until the 1950s.

Great Britain and Ireland

In England, physicians who specialized were associated with the Royal College of Physicians if they practiced a medical specialty or with the Royal College of Surgeons of England if a surgical specialty. Anesthesia lay within the domain of, and as an adjunct to, surgery. As more medical practitioners in Great Britain became interested in special work, they raised concerns in the forums of the parent Royal College, though not always with success. Anesthesia was not highly regarded, and for much of the first century of anesthesia, the cry from anesthetists in England was similar to that in the United States. Though trained as physicians, they were regarded as technicians; at the beginning of the twentieth century, anesthesia had no place in the medical curriculum,[100] and it was not thought to require high-powered knowledge or skills for its practice. Anesthesia was commonly entrusted to general practitioners and hospital interns rather than to physicians with particular knowledge and understanding of anesthesia. Even so, the special knowledge and competence of men like Snow (anaesthetist to a queen), Clover, Buxton, and Hewitt (anaesthetist to a king) did serve, in contrast to the situation in the United States, to remind surgeons and others that anesthetists were indeed physicians.

With the advances in medicine and surgery—and anesthesia—in the 1920s, the time seemed ripe to formalize efforts to improve the standard of anesthesia that Hewitt had urged in 1896.[101] Anesthesia had obviously matured—the *British Journal of Anaesthesia* was launched as early as 1923—but it was not clear where the efforts should be directed. The Section of Anaesthetics of the Royal Society of Medicine, the descendant of the original Society of Anaesthetists, was inappropriate because the Royal Society of Medicine was a forum just for scientific debate. Therefore, in 1932, members of the section founded the Association of Anaesthetists of Great Britain and Ireland (AAGBI).* Its objects were comprehensive: to promote the development and study of anesthesia and the recognition of anesthesia as a specialized branch of medicine, to coordinate the efforts and activities of anesthetists and promote their various mutual interests among them, and to promote the establishment of diplomas and degrees in anesthesia.[102]

Emphasis on education was still necessary, for many general practitioner-anesthetists regarded themselves as having special skills in

---

*Though events in Australia are not discussed in this history, it may be noted that the Australian Society of Anaesthetists was founded at about this time, in 1934.[103]

anesthesia, despite their never having been formally trained in anesthesia. Because of the concern that general-practitioner anesthesia was not always of a high standard, and in response to a request made by the AAGBI, the Conjoint Board of the two Royal Colleges in 1935 introduced the Diploma in Anaesthetics (DA) as a means of assessing anesthesia competence of general practitioners. The DA was the first such examination and certificate in anesthesia anywhere. In 1946, it was proposed that fellowship be inaugurated, and examinations for a higher diploma recognizing a full-time specialist qualification in the form of Fellow of the Faculty of Anaesthetists of the Royal College of Surgeons (FFARCS) was held for the first time in 1953.[104] However, not until 1989 did the faculty become an autonomous college with its royal charter.[105]

Though the manner in which British anaesthetists prepared for specialty recognition differed from that of their American counterparts, the timing of the formation of the AAGBI and the introduction of the DA suggest that the broad outlines and the timing of the movement were similar. The evolution of anesthesia, its recognition as a specialty, and also its later development, proceeded at much the same pace in the United Kingdom and the United States, even though the organizational structure was different.

As in the United States, a university chair was lacking in England for many years; similarly, the first university chair was created at about the time the movement for specialty recognition was picking up pace. That chair was established in 1937, for the Nuffield Professor of Anaesthetics. The first person to be appointed to the chair was Robert Macintosh.

Canada

As in the United States, specialization in Canada was discussed in the latter part of the nineteenth century. Interest was furthered by the experience of military medicine in World War I, when the potential of anesthesia was self-evident. However, even in 1920, the idea of specialization in medicine and surgery in Canada met with little enthusiasm.[106] At that time, the formation of a Canadian Royal College was mooted, though the idea of "advanced study of, and postgraduate work in Medicine and Surgery"[107] was not taken any farther. Just as the question of forming a Canadian College in 1920 had come from physicians in Saskatchewan,[108] so the question of standards for the qualification of specialists, first asked in 1922, was raised not in Quebec or Ontario but in far-off Alberta.[109] The Royal College of Physicians and Surgeon of Canada was finally founded in 1929, and its one object related to specialists. It was stated that "it is considered necessary and advisable that a practising physician essaying to do 'special work' should have the opportunity of obtaining a distinguishing designation . . . whereby it may be known that he is properly qualified."[110] However, as the 1920s gave way to the 1930s, no one gave any thought to anesthesia as a specialty, for the Royal College was primarily thought of as a means to encourage further training for academic internists and surgeons.

Initially, the Royal College was not regarded as a certifying body. But in 1933, it was estimated that 35 percent of the medical profession restricted their practice to a particular field, and though the irregularities of training for specialists was deplored, the need was stressed to identify the well-trained specialist.[111] Most people thought that a central body, such as the Medical Council of Canada, an examining and licensing organization, should formulate standards for specialist practice. Deliberations proceeded slowly, and because of this, radiologists threatened to set up their own college, as in England, while others, including anesthetists, considered a specialist board, as in the United States.

Eventually, however, the Canadian Medical Association (CMA) invited the Royal College to look after specialty matters; and in 1937, plans for certification of practitioners from several specialties were underway. Typically, though, in view of the barriers that anesthetists had always had to overcome, anesthesia was not among the specialties first approved for certification; not until 1942 did the College Council approve anesthesia for certification. In that year, forty-two certificates were issued,[112] without examination, to anesthetists; but in 1946, specialist certificates were granted only by examination.[113] Certificates in anesthesia were grandfathered at first and issued after examination, as from 1947. A separate fellowship for anesthesia, in addition to certification, was established in 1951.

Following specialty recognition, other developments strengthened the position of specialization in anesthesia. The Canadian Anaesthetists' Society was founded in 1943[114] (the earlier Canadian Society of Anaesthesia, founded in 1920, had folded into the CMA in 1928), with Harold Griffith, of later curare fame, as president. The *Canadian Anaesthetists' Society Journal* (later the *Canadian Journal of Anesthesia*) began publication in 1954,[115] with Roderick Gordon as editor.

The two qualifications that had come about in 1951 now created a problem: there was, in essence, a dual standard of specialty qualification. The fellowship as an elitist designation and Certification, one that marked run-of-the-mill specialist competence. This proved unacceptable, and in 1972, the single certification examination replaced the two previous examinations.[116] Requirements were changed so that a physician who passed the single examination could, on payment of a fee, be entitled to be referred to as a Fellow of the Royal College of Physicians of Canada, and thus a recognized specialist. Careful examination of the last sentence reinforces the minor difference from the English anesthesia fellowship: in Canada, fellows in anesthesia are members of the physicians' division of the college rather than the surgeons'.

Research did not play the same part in the evolution of anesthesia in Canada as it did in the United States, perhaps because it had more of a separate, ivory-tower aspect. However, some notable research work was done by Canadian anesthetists. In Montreal, Wesley Bourne carried out many biochemical and pharmacological studies, such as one on Avertin.[117] And Griffith, as well as advocating endotracheal intubation,[118] subarachnoid anesthesia,[119] and cyclopropane,[120] later introduced curare into anesthesia.[121] As well, Easson Brown carried out research in Toronto. He investigated the effects of ethylene[122] at the same time as it had been investigated in the United States.[123] The development of cyclopropane originated in Toronto, where the first studies on this versatile agent by pharmacologists George Lucas and Velyien Henderson[124] were conducted before being aborted. Farther west, in Alberta, Irving Bell and Samuel Gelfan, though not practicing anesthetists, introduced vinyl oxide in 1933.[125]

Despite that research, a university chair was not endowed in Canadian anesthesia until 1945. Then one was established at Montreal's McGill University, with Wesley Bourne as professor.

Germany

Though some of the progress in anesthesia at the end of the nineteenth century and early in the twentieth originated in Germany, anesthesia was recognized as a specialty much later there than in the United States, England, and Canada.[126] Anesthetists were held back quite firmly by their surgical colleagues, just as they were in France, where physiologists as well as surgeons ruled the roost. Not until 1922 did E. von der Porten, who is regarded as the first professional anesthetist in Germany, call for instruction of medical students in anesthesia.[127] In 1928, surgeons Hans Killian and H. Schmidt visited the United States and were impressed by the professionalism of anesthesia there. However, Killian concluded that economic and cultural conditions in Germany would prevent German anesthetists from creating a system that was similar to that of the Americans.[128] Schmidt, impressed by his American experience, practiced anesthesia for two years, but economic conditions were such that he returned to surgery.[129]

Other interesting developments occurred in 1928. That year a German congress on anaesthesia was held in Hamburg. McMechan then expressed the hope that specialism in German anesthesia might develop. His hope would not be realized because the prevailing medical (i.e., surgical) opinion was that the specialty of anesthesia was not necessary. Even so, two German anesthesia journals appeared in 1928.[130] *Der Schmerz* was founded to promote scientific interest in narcosis as a first step toward the establishment of the anesthetists "profession" in German medicine, and *Narkose und Anaesthesie* also began publication. These journals, however, were edited by different groups, neither of which included an anesthetist; their independence of each other illustrates the lack of unity in German anesthesia in the 1920s.

Finally, however, several significant developments occurred in 1952 and 1953. One was the publication in 1952 of the journal *Der Anaesthetist*. In the same year, a German Study Group for Anaesthesiology was founded. In 1953, the Council of German Physicians endorsed a policy that recognized training requirements leading to autonomy of anesthetists,[131] and the German Society of Anaesthesia was founded. The hopes of a specialty of anesthesia in Germany were now realized.

There are several reasons why specialty recognition in Germany was delayed. These highlight the greater influence of social and economic factors in Germany than in English-speaking nations. One factor was the hierarchical structure of medicine in Germany. Another was economic: it was considered economically risky to specialize in anesthesia in comparison with surgery, for example. A third factor was the isolation of German medicine in the interwar years; German anesthetists were thus out of touch with North American and English anesthesia. Yet, as Schmidt noted, another factor was the fear on the part of older German surgeons of "a second, jointly responsible person placed at their side."[132]

*   *   *

The evolution of anesthesia from a craft, via a discipline, to a specialty, was a lengthy and complex process. The process began at the end of the nineteenth century when the need for "special anesthetizers" was recognized and when practitioners with a particular interest in anesthesia began to meet to discuss common problems. It was not enough, however, for anesthetists to practice anesthesia full-time for anesthesia to develop as a specialty. While full-time practice and communication among anesthetists did lead to the development of a unique ethos of anesthesia, more was required before anesthesia could be recognized as an autonomous specialty. Three factors were especially important. One was a vision of what was required among practitioners for the development of anesthesia—a vision that was formulated by men like Ralph Waters in the United States and Robert Macintosh in England. The second was the creation of a unique body of knowledge by means of research and the daily practice of anesthesia and its integration into clinical practice and education. The third was the need for an organizational structure. Though this process took the better part of ninety years, when it is considered against the fact that anesthesia developed de novo in 1846, and that it was not highly valued for many years, the fact that a specialty was in fact created is in itself notable.

Chapter 9

Continuing Progress in the Practice of Anesthesia

Just as anesthesia in the first half of the twentieth century differed in many ways from anesthesia in the preceding half century, so anesthesia was different in the second half of the twentieth century from that in the earlier fifty years. Differences resulted from innovations in drugs and techniques and equipment, and also from change outside anesthesia itself. The most extensive cause of change was the Second World War; anesthesiologists Keith Sykes and John Bunker noted that it "changed everything."[1] In the United Kingdom, the armed forces' surgical teams gained new knowledge about resuscitation and trauma; in civilian practice, the greater incidence of trauma led to the formation of the emergency medical service (EMS). Though in England the greater need for anaesthetists was met partly by older general practitioners, the continuing shortage in the face of the increase in trauma surgery and the lack of anesthesia equipment generated new problems and solutions. An example of one solution was the development of new types of anesthesia machines and ventilators, the Oxford Vaporizer[2] and the Blease ventilator[3] being two examples.

The war had other effects. In both the United Kingdom and the United States, knowledge of anesthesia grew—new drugs such as curare and lidocaine, for example, were both introduced during the war—and physicians acquired a greater understanding of anesthesia. In the United States and in Canada, short training courses for physicians bound for military service were in some ways akin to the residency training that Ralph Waters had set in the 1930s, and they confirmed its value after the war. In the United Kingdom, the creation of the National Health Service, which was modeled on the Emergency Medical Service, established the British system of consultants and trainees.

Change continued after the war. Anesthesia continued to evolve. Innovations in drugs and techniques and advances in surgery made clinical practice vastly more exciting than anesthesia had been when it consisted of dripping ether or chloroform on a mask over a patient's face. The new intravenous drugs and inhalational agents are discussed in this chapter, and other innovations are discussed in succeeding chapters: the development of monitoring (chapter 10); the involvement of anesthesiologists in critical care (chapter 11); the expansion of local anesthesia into regional and neuraxial forms of block, and its application to pain management (chapter 13); and the widening of the scope of anesthesia as cardiac surgery and neurosurgery and other surgical fields stimulated the emergence of anesthesia subspecialties (chapter 14). Anesthesia also evolved outside hospital walls, as anesthesiologists became involved in resuscitation medicine (chapter 13).

Intravenous Anesthesia

A great variety of intravenous drugs were developed after the war. Some, such as the benzodiazepines, synthetic opioids like fentanyl and sufentanil, muscle relaxants such as pancuronium, and induction agents like propofol found a permanent place as anesthetic drugs. Others, like phencyclidine,[4] were used until side effects caused them to be withdrawn, while propanidid, which was used in Europe[5] and Canada,[6] was never used in the United States because of cardiovascular depression and hypersensitivity. But whether the drugs turned out to have a place or not, their development reflects well on those who researched them, tested them, and marketed them. Eight of the classes of drugs that were found useful are considered here. None was regarded as an ideal intravenous drug, and each is compared in table 9.1 with that ideal. Though each had some drawbacks, progress in developing intravenous drugs in this period was such that the quest for the ideal anesthetic seemed less and less of a mirage.

Table 9.1. Comparison of intravenous agents,* 1950-2000, with theoretically ideal intravenous agent**

Variable	Phen	Benz	Ket	Steroid	Etom	Propofol	Opioid	MR
Potentcy	+	+	++	++	++	+++	+++	+++
Stability	+++	+++	++	++	+++	+++	++++	+++
Safety	++	+++	++++	++++	+++	++++	++	++
Ease of use	++	+++	+++	+++ +++	+++	++++	+++	++
Fast action &recovery	+	++	++++	+	+++	++++	+++	+++
Nontoxic: body,postop; little biotransformn.	++	++	++	++	+++	+++	++	++
Nonallergic	++++	+++	+++	0	+++	0	+++	++
Drug compatibility	+++	+++	++	++	++	+++	+++	+++
Action***	S	S	H, A	H	H	H, S	A	R

*Abbreviations: Phen=phenothiazine; Benz=benzodiazepine; Ket=ketamine; Etom=etomidate; MR=muscle relaxant

**Given ranking of +++++

***S=sedation; H-hypnosis; A=analgesia; MR=muscle relaxation.

The guiding principle in the synthesis of these new drugs was that of achieving great specificity of action. The objective was to have each drug produce a different and specific physiological and pharmacological result on the nervous system. Use of just intravenous drugs, for example, made it possible to induce and maintain anesthesia, including muscle relaxation and analgesia. In contrast to the blunderbuss nature of the inhalational agents of the nineteenth century, anesthesia with twentieth-century drugs had a laser-like quality; drug use could be "tailored" to the precise anesthesia need. This principle was consistent with the concept that the several aspects of anesthesia are mediated by different drugs acting specifically at different sites in the nervous system, so that different aspects of the anesthetic state are achieved.[7]

Precision of drug effect was made possible in part by utilizing the relationship between chemical structure and pharmacological activity. Some drugs were used to tranquillize or sedate a patient before operation; others, to induce hypnosis; others, to achieve analgesia; and yet others, for muscle relaxation. The anesthesiologist's armamentarium in the second half of the twentieth century was varied and extensive as never before.

Use of these intravenous drugs modernized the concept of George Washington Crile's much earlier "anoci-association"[8] and John Lundy's succeeding concept of balanced anesthesia.[9] The principle was sound: relatively small doses of drugs with specific actions induced anesthesia that was both light and adequate; it was no longer necessary to induce deep anesthesia to obtain muscle relaxation, for example, as it had with ether or chloroform. Long-term effects were avoided as drugs, which had undergone rigorous testing before being used clinically, were given in smaller and less toxic doses.

In practice, the intravenous drugs were usually given in combination with inhalational agents, though, as noted, they were sometimes used as the sole anesthetic agents, along with oxygen as the sole inhaled substance. In addition, intravenous drugs were given to sedate a patient who received a local anesthetic agent for regional anesthesia or for infiltration at the site of surgery. In general, the intravenous drugs greatly expanded the scope of anesthesia.

Phenothiazines: The "Lytic Cocktail" and Neuroleptanalgesia

Phenothiazine derivatives were studied in France soon after World War II. Some found use as antihistamines or would combat Parkinsonism,[10] but because promethazine potentiated barbiturate action in experimental animals, French naval surgeon Henri Laborit used it to supplement nitrous oxide and meperidine anesthesia. The addition of chlorpromazine (L'Argactil, Thorazine), which was synthesized in 1950,[11] curiously induced greater detachment in the patient from the surgical environment. This effect of the drug cocktail introduced another new concept into anesthesia: depression of the central nervous system and the sympathetic nervous system, but not of consciousness. Diminished initiative, emotional response, and interest in the immediate surroundings seemed to result. Chlorpromazine was a "neuroleptic" (literally, one that "takes the neuron").

Laborit thought that surgical stimulation sometimes made the sympathetic nervous system overly active and that the neuroleptic state might benefit surgical patients. This concept was established with chlorpromazine as a tranquilizer and meperidine as an analgesic, with the objective of preventing shock in wounded French soldiers in the Indochina conflict. Hypothermia added to the regimen produced artificial hibernation.[12] And when haloperidol (and later droperidol) and a potent opioid phenoperidine were administered, a dissociative state known as neuroleptanalgesia[13] resulted. Though, in the first ten years of their use, these potent drugs to some extent depressed both the nervous and the cardiovascular systems, no deaths were associated with their administration.[14]

The concepts of artificial hibernation and neuroleptanalgesia, however, went beyond the aims of anesthesia of relieving pain and maintaining homeostasis, and certainly beyond that of attaining balanced anesthesia. The latter was still a reasonable objective, for the combination of hypnosis and light anesthesia, analgesia, depression of reflex activity, and muscle relaxation was effective. Originally, this combination of effects was achieved with a single agent like ether or chloroform, though relatively deep anesthesia was needed for surgery. That was why Crile and Lundy had argued that it was physiologically preferable to take a two-pronged approach: to combine relatively light general anesthesia with a volatile agent to protect the brain against harmful psychic stimuli, and local anesthesia to block noxious stimuli from being transmitted from the operative site to the brain. As anesthesia evolved, especially after curare was introduced in 1942, their concept was modified to achieve anesthesia with light general anesthesia with induction by a barbiturate, maintenance with nitrous oxide, analgesia with a drug like meperidine, and muscle relaxation with curare or one of its analogs.[15, 16, 17] Though seemingly designed to protect a patient by reducing body temperature and cellular metabolism, artificial hibernation and neuroleptanalgesia were better for the surgeon and the anesthesiologist than the patient. Patients often remained semicomatose for hours, and their anesthetized bodies had to withstand the insults of an imposed vegetative state and cardiovascular and respiratory depression, despite the theoretical benefit of hypometabolism.

Other phenothiazines also were synthesized by German researchers.[18] These provided premedication and countered postoperative nausea and vomiting. They include the following: promazine (Sparine) and promethazine (Phenergan), with a dimethyl amino propyl side chain; prochlorperazine (Stemetil), trifluoperazine (Stelazine), and perphenazine (Trilafon) with a piperazine side chain; and pecazine (Pacatal) with a piperidine side chain.

Benzodiazepines

A second group of drugs comprised the benzodiazepines. The benzodiazepine story is another that illustrates the dependence of anesthesia on many other professionals other than anesthesiologists and on industry. Behind the development of the benzodiazepines lay a world in which the pharmaceutical industry was aided by numerous chemists, pharmacologists, psychiatrists, and industrialists. Though the drugs were marketed originally for psychiatrists, anesthesiologists used two in particular, diazepam and midazolam. There was an obvious place for these drugs in anesthesia, since general anesthesia is based on deliberately modifying consciousness. In addition, their effect on the nervous system was relatively gentle.

The benzodiazepine story[19] began when the head of pharmacology at Roche Laboratories, Lowell Randall, asked his chemist colleagues to produce new compounds for use as tranquilizers. Randall originally wished to find a substitute for myanesin. The chemists, under Leo Sternbach, a Pole with knowledge of dyestuff chemistry, began working on compounds that were known as benzheptoxdiazines. Of the forty compounds that were then submitted for pharmacological testing, one was a sedative that was ten times as strong as meprobamate in blocking strychnine-reversible cat spinal reflexes. It was actually not a benzheptoxide but a benzodiazepine.

Randall asked Sternbach to produce this compound in quantity. Intensive pharmacological scrutiny showed that the compound (chlordiazepoxide [CPZ, Librium]) had properties that warranted production of its analogs. For a while, it was used in anesthesia for premedication.[20] Among the analogs, one had potent properties as a muscle relaxant and anticonvulsant, and became known as diazepam (Valium). Psychiatrists and family practitioners used this as an anxiolytic and a sedative, while anesthesiologists, understanding its dose-related effect on the brain, started using it as a premedicant[21, 22] and as an induction agent.[23] Diazepam was not soluble in water, but midazolam (Versed), which was produced specifically for use in anesthesia and which affected neuronal transmission, was, and so was of more practical value as an injectable agent.[24]

Ketamine

The cyclohexylamine compounds provided another approach to intravenous anesthesia. Patients were unaware of pain even though conscious and detached emotionally and intellectually from the surroundings; they even lapsed into a cataleptic state. This dissociative state was more like the neuroleptic state, though cardiovascular and respiratory depression was absent and loss of consciousness was less profound.

The most important representative of this class of drug was ketamine (2-[o-chlorophenyl]-2methylamino cyclohexanone). It was was synthesized in 1962, and laboratory studies[25] and testing on state prisoners[26] followed. As Ketalar and Ketaject, it was released for clinical use in 1970.

Yet another concept in the practice of anesthesia was formulated. Small doses of a drug, not large enough to induce unconsciousness, produced sedation and analgesia, as well as detachment from the environment and protection of the upper respiratory reflexes; larger doses induced unconsciousness, yet without cardiovascular or respiratory depression. Clinically, ketamine given by intramuscular or intravenous injection facilitated surgical care in several different conditions: as the sole anesthetic for minor operations, including changing burn dressings; to produce immobility, especially in children, in diagnostic procedures;

for induction of anesthesia in patients in shock; for the management of mass casualties; and for sedation or induction of anesthesia.

Steroids

Research into various steroids showed that the effects and the applications of intravenous anesthesia are more diverse than those of inhalational anesthesia. Intravenous drugs may affect components of anesthesia that are different from those of inhalational agents. Steroid anesthetics intrigued because they induce anesthesia in a unique manner.

Interest in anesthesia-inducing steroids originated in the discovery by Hans Selye in Montreal in 1941 that injections of progesterone made rodents sleep.[27] Selye attributed this to an oxygen atom at either end of the steroid molecule. The most efficacious compound was pregnanedione.[28] By 1955, the drug hydroxydione was shown to be capable of inducing general anesthesia,[29] and it was introduced into anesthesia the same year.[30] Hydroxydione fascinated because hypnosis was delayed for several minutes following intravenous injection. This unique feature made people wonder further about the still-unclear mechanism of anesthesia. However, because the duration of action of hydroxydione was prolonged and thrombophlebitis sometimes occurred, its use was discontinued.

Interest in steroid anesthesia did not fade, however, and a two-steroid combination—alphaxolone and alphadolone, known together as Althesin—generated interest at a conference in London in 1972.[31] Alphaxolone was the primary hypnotic component; alphadolone facilitated the solubility of its fellow steroid, which was increased further by putting up Althesin in Cremophor EL. The advantages of Althesin were its short action, its administration by continuous infusion, and its use to induce sedation or anesthesia. However, because of hypersensitivity reactions, in 1984, Althesin too was taken off the market. A further, and unsuccessful, attempt to "resuscitate" steroid anesthesia came with the introduction of minaxolone in 1979, but excitatory reactions and prolonged recovery led to its being banned from use as well.[32]

Propanidid and Etomidate

Another drug of this period also had a brief clinical life. This was propanidid, a eugenol derivative. Eugenol, obtained from cloves and cinnamon, has anesthetic properties. Following work by M. J. Thuillier and his associates in 1957,[33] propanidid was introduced as an intravenous anesthetic in the 1960s, and it was used in Europe and Canada.[34] Because its effects were of short duration, it was popular for ambulatory procedures. Two problems led to its downfall:

hemodynamic depression when large doses were given, and hypersensitivity to the drug, which was solubilized in Cremophor EL.

Etomidate, an imidazole derivative, did remain in use, though, as with Althesin, it was the solvent that caused problems. Synthesized in 1964,[35] the first clinical report was not published until 1974.[36] Experience was needed before it could be given safely. A benzodiazepine and fentanyl given first facilitated induction with etomidate. The drug could be given as a single dose or in an infusion, and instability of the cardiovascular system and respiratory depression did not occur. The European experience was favorable. However, as has occurred not infrequently with intravenous anesthetics, favorable initial opinions as to its use were later offset by unfavorable developments. These included temporary inhibition of pain on injection, occasional thrombophlebitis, myoclonus, nausea and vomiting, and, as reported in 1983, temporary inhibition of steroid synthesis by the adrenal glands.[37] Its use was restricted to management of patients at risk for hemodynamic instability and polyallergic reactions.

Propofol

The use of propofol (Diprivan) too was at first limited by adverse reactions, but it turned out to be one of the great innovations in intravenous anesthesia. From the 1980s onward, propofol was widely used as a hypnotic in the operating room and as a sedative in the intensive care unit.

Propofol is a substituted derivative of phenol, formally named 2, 6-di-isoprofol. Studies on phenols were initiated in the 1970s, and propofol in its original form was investigated clinically and reported on in 1977.[38] Because of low solubility, it was originally put up in Cremophor EL. Concerns about anaphylaxis initially caused it to be discontinued, but reformulation in an egg-containing lipid emulsion resuscitated propofol, and it was reintroduced in 1983.[39]

Propofol usurped the throne that had been occupied by thiopental in its reign of half a century. A highly satisfactory anesthetic, propofol is used outside the operating room also, particularly for deep sedation. Yet like thiopental, propofol is not the ideal intravenous agent so many had searched for over the years. The search for the holy grail of an ideal intravenous anesthetic therefore continued.

Opioid Analgesics

Morphine has advantages besides analgesia, such as euphoria and anxiolysis, but also side effects such as nausea and vomiting, pruritus, addiction, and respiratory depression. The analgesic meperidine also may upsets people. The side effects can be countered by an antagonist like nalorphine,[40] but it seemed preferable to seek drugs with greater analgesic specificity and fewer side effects. Beginning in the 1960s, it became possible to synthesize clinically superior opioids.

When Paul Janssen, in Belgium in 1960, synthesized fentanyl, anesthesia took a quantum leap forward. A highly productive physician, chemist, and entrepreneur, Janssen realized that the analgesic effect of the traditional opioids was due to the presence of the piperidine ring.[41] This clue led him to synthesize an analgesic with greater potency, specificity, and efficacy of action than morphine, and without affecting body homeostasis and producing fewer side effects.[42] Chemical manipulation of the piperidine moiety provided greater analgesia; fentanyl was one hundred to three hundred times as potent as morphine, with a higher therapeutic index than with morphine or meperidine. Sufentanil and alfentanil followed,[43] though sufentanil was not approved for use in the United States until 1984.[44] The ultra-short-acting remifentanil appeared later.[45, 46]

These new opioids, which provide further evidence of the relationship between chemical structure of drugs and anesthetic activity, enhanced the administration of both general and regional anesthesia. Methods of pain relief became more versatile, not only as part of the anesthetic in the operating room but also in the surgical ward after surgery and in the obstetric suite. Opioids could be injected intravenously, intrathecally, or epidurally by health care professionals or by patients themselves by means of a patient-controlled analgesia (PCA) pump in relieving their pain (see chapter 12). They refined balanced anesthesia when combined with a local anesthetic agent, and they allowed anesthesiologists to tailor analgesic needs to individual patients. Fentanyl was also used as a component of the technique of conscious sedation, which facilitated care of the patient who was undergoing surgical or dental procedures that required a combination of analgesia and sedation rather than general anesthesia.

Because the opioids brought a new dimension to the practice of anesthesia and the anesthesiologist's understanding of the action of analgesic drugs, their intriguing story of science and scientific discovery merits telling here.

Advances in pharmacology: opioid receptors and endorphins. In 1964, W. R. Martin posited the existence of spinal opioids,[47] and Tsou and Zhang, in China, conceived of delivering opiates directly to the neuraxis.[48] Since nalorphine,[49] pentazocine, butorphanol, and buphrenorphine had mixed agonist-antagonist (i.e., action-opposition) activity, Martin concluded that analgesics acted on more than one site in the nervous system, and in 1967 he concluded that there was more than one type of receptor for opioids.[50] Such receptors uncover another facet of the relationship between chemical structure and action of a drug.

Progress was also made in the early 1970s in John Liebeskind's laboratory in Los Angeles.[51] Stimulation of the periaqueductal gray in the brain led to a pain-free state known as stimulation-produced analgesia (SPA). In view of the work by Tsou and Zhang on the analgesia effect of morphine in the core gray regions,[52] SPA was thought to be related to the anatomical basis for opioid analgesia. Graduate student David Mayer then proposed that stimulation attenuated pain "by activating a neural substrate that functions normally in the blockage of pain."[53] This idea was formulated before the next steps—the demonstration of opioid receptors or endorphins—were made.[54] Huda Akil then found that naloxone blocked the effects of SPA. In 1972, it was concluded that the analgesia of SPA and of morphine resulted from the effect of a mechanism at the same site (the periaqueductal gray) and by the same mechanism.[55]

The definite existence of opioid receptors was demonstrated next. The story of the pertinent research from 1971 to 1973 has been told by Marcia Meldrum[56] and notably by one of the participants, Solomon Snyder.[57] The main points are the following. In 1971, Avril Goldstein suggested that stereospecific opioid receptors do exist in the brain,[58] and the next year, Lars Terenius identified the hypothesized receptors,[59] though his report was not published in 1973 in a journal that was not read by many scientists in English-speaking countries.[60] Also published in 1973 was the corroborative paper in the journal *Science* by Solomon Snyder and Candace Pert,[61] which generated the greatest attention, as well as a third paper, by Eric Simon and his group.[62]

The final steps in this story concern the endorphins, or the body's own opiates. Their existence was described at a meeting in 1974 at which many of the principal researchers were present.[63] One was John Hughes, who worked with Hans Kosterlitz, of the University of Aberdeen. Hughes announced, first, that an extract of SPA-active regions of guinea pig brain would inhibit contractions of the guinea pig ileum as though the extract were morphine, and, second, that this effect was blocked by naloxone. The conclusion: the extract was an opiate-like substance that interacted with the opiate receptor—or a morphine-like substance that was produced in the body of the guinea pigs who had "donated" their brains to science.[64]

How was this work to be interpreted by anesthesiologists? The new knowledge clarified understanding of how the brain and the spinal cord mediate the effects of opioids[65] and how compounds with one set of actions (as "agonists") interacted with those with opposing actions (as "antagonists"). Four points can be made. First, both agonists and antagonists exist, each with specific actions and natures. Second, agonist analgesic drugs such as fentanyl, like hormones and neurotransmitters, are efficacious at very low concentrations. Third, their structure is similar to that of the antagonists, and agonists may be transformed into antagonists as the molecular configuration is altered. And fourth, antagonists act rapidly, so that morphine poisoning, for example, can be counteracted without delay if an antagonist such as naloxone is given. This suggested that agonists and antagonists have common sites of action—in the opioid receptors—and these were shown to exist, as stereospecific sites binding opioids.[66] Two years later, the first endogenous opioid receptor ligands were shown to be the pentapeptides met—and leu-enkephalin.[67] Later work revealed three families of endogenous peptides and three distinct types of receptors.[68] Of these, the endorphins are the significant peptides as far as pain is concerned; as far as opioid activity is concerned, the *mu* receptor is significant.

In anesthesia, this new understanding expanded the horizons of anesthesiologists by updating the background to the use of the opioids. They were found efficacious in quite small doses, in surgical patients or women in labor, for example; and they could be administered intravenously, intrathecally, or epidurally. The fact that analgesia and respiratory depression are mediated through separate subgroups of the *mu* type of receptor suggests that research will lead to the synthesis of drugs with even greater specificity for pain control, with consequently less concern about respiratory depression.

Synthetic Replacements for Curare

Continuing research into neuromuscular transmission. The introduction of curare in 1942 (see chapter 5) stimulated continuing basic and clinical research into the neuromuscular junction. At first, it was not clear whether impulses were transmitted there by electrical or chemical means (i.e., by sparks or soup). As curare was replaced by more effective muscle relaxants, this research intensified, with anesthesia being partly responsible for illuminating this aspect of physiology. The key points of this research are the following.[69]

The 1950s began with the work of Bernard Katz and his colleagues in London on transmission across the junction between the nerve and muscle. With Paul Fatt, Katz found first that an "end plate potential" at the junction is generated by an inward current at the end plate and that it spreads passively from there along muscle fibers. Acetylcholine was then released at the end plate, which caused a rise in the end plate potential, which in turn could be prolonged by applying cholinesterase. After that, the release of acetylcholine was followed by essentially short-circuiting of the membrane at the end plate so that it was momentarily permeable to sodium and potassium ions, but not to the chlorine ion. Muscle fibers then contract.

Part of this remarkable research story, which earned Katz a share in the Nobel Prize for Medicine or Physiology in 1970, concerned the way acetylcholine was released. In 1951, Fatt and Katz detected continuous discharges of end plate potential at very low amplitude in the end plate region, even when the presynaptic region was not stimulated. However, these "miniature" end plate

potentials could be abolished by a drug like curare, which competitively blocks
the site of an acetylcholine receptor. Three years later, Jose del Castillo and
Katz found that when the regular type of end plate potential was stimulated
to rise, it did so stepwise in such a way that each end plate potential was an
integral multiple (0, 1, 2, 3 or more) of the miniature end plate potential. Two
conclusions followed: the normal end plate potential consisted of an integral
number of miniature *units*; and with a decrease in the calcium concentration
at the end plate the end plate potential was reduced in *definite quanta*. These
conclusions led to a third: acetylcholine is released in discrete multimolecular
packets, from vesicles, which are termed *quanta* also.

All those findings clarified the actions of the various muscle relaxants, or
neuromuscular blocking agents, that replaced curare. In essence, they interfere
with the ability of acetylcholine to occupy receptors in the end plate region of
the neuromuscular junction. This was the background of the work that led to
replacements for curare.

Research into replacements for curare. The value of curare was limited by several
side effects, including histamine release, bronchospasm, and hypotension. Part
of the problem was that because curare was a plant product, its composition and
potency might vary. The answer was to develop synthetic curariform drugs.

The chemistry and pharmacology of curare-like compounds goes back
to 1869. In that year, A. Crum and T. R. Fraser reported on quarternary
derivatives of the alkaloids methylstrychnine and methylbrucine.[70] Some of
their properties seemed to be analogous to those of South American curares,
but the relationship of the quarternary ammonium molecular structure and
the neuromuscular blocking was not clear; indeed, it was not clarified until
after World War II.

In 1948, two teams discovered that decamethonium bromide blocked
neuromuscular transmission,[71, 72] and this was used widely for a while as a
muscle relaxant in anesthesia. During the research into other compounds
that followed, one compound was found to contain 10 atoms (8 of carbon
and 2 of oxygen) positioned between two quarternary nitrogen atoms. It
was similar in this respect to decamethonium, and its molecular structure
was not unlike that of acetylcholine. That was succinylcholine, also known
as suxamethonium.

Succinylcholine is historically interesting because it was first used in 1906,
though not as a muscle relaxant. It was among compounds that Reid Hunt and
Rene de Taveau, of Washington, investigated when analyzing effects of choline
derivatives in blood pressure studies.[73] They missed its paralyzing action because
the experimental animals were immobilized by being curarized. Nor were the
neuromuscular effects recognized by J. Le Heux in 1921[74] and David Glick in
1941.[75] The initial lack of recognition of a property of a drug that is later found

to be valuable is, of course, not uncommon, and in anesthesia, one only has to think of ether, nitrous oxide, and chloroform, as well as curare.

In contrast to the nondepolarizing end plate action of curare, the action of succinylcholine at the motor end plate was to depolarize it. This made it impossible to reverse its action by giving an antagonizing drug. This mode of action was recognized in 1949, when Daniel Bovet, in Rome,[76] and G. Buttle and Eleanor Zaimis,[77] in London, described the depolarizing action. At the same time, Arthur Phillips[78] and he and J. Castillo and E. de Beer[79] published the results of similar work.

Beginning in 1951, many papers on the clinical effects and use of this potent muscle relaxant were published, first in Continental Europe[80, 81, 82] and England[83] then in the United States.[84] It was given by single injection or by continuous intravenous infusion. The onset of action was speedy, and its action was of a few minutes' duration, both features making it quite different from curare. Soon, however, troublesome side effects were reported. One was prolonged respiratory depression after its administration.[85, 86, 87, 88] Some cases were related to the genetic absence of pseudocholinesterase in the blood, and this opened up the new field of pharmacogenetics[89] as another fascinating aspect of the use of muscle relaxants.

Meanwhile, research into other replacements for curare had continued, and this yielded the first synthetic nondepolarizing substitute for curare in the form of gallamine triethiodide (Flaxedil). Its pharmacological nature was clarified by Bovet and his group in 1947.[90] One disadvantage of gallamine was its effect on the heart in causing tachycardia. In the next half century, some fifty nondepolarizing agents were added to gallamine.[91]

One muscle relaxant was a semisynthetic compound that was developed out of the knowledge that had been gained from the study of curare. This was metocurarine a trimethylated derivative of *d*-tubocurarine, described in 1948.[92] Like gallamine, the clinical use of which was reported in 1948,[93] metocurarine was used for many years.

Superior to both gallamine and metocurarine was the next relaxant to be used clinically: pancuronium. The pancuronium story underlines the way drugs are developed long before they reach the operating room. Like that of curare, the story concerns a South American plant. In 1862, Don Ramon Paez told of a poison known as guachamaca that was used during hunting in Venezuala.[94] This may have been derived from a plant known as *Malouetia nitida* or *M. schomburgki*. A century later, from another *Malouetia* species, *M. bequaertiana*, a bisquarternary steroidal alkaloid named malouetine was isolated. This had neuromuscular blocking activity that was similar to that of d-Tubocurarine,[95] and so stimulated a search for an aminosteroid drug that could be used as a neuromuscular blocking agent. Two teams worked on this.[96] At the University of Glasgow and the University of Strathclyde, M. Alauddin and his colleagues eventually reported on the nondepolarizing activity of a group of androstanes,[97] and working for Organon, C. L. Hewett, W. R. Buckett, and D. S. Savage, who benefited from the advice of Alauddin's team, reported the synthesis of pancuronium in 1964.[98]

The development of pancuronium was made possible by the existence of several factors. One was the cooperation of chemists and pharmacologists in clarifying the advantages and disadvantages of the several investigational paths that should be followed. Another was business decisions that pharmaceutical companies had to make, which enabled Organon to succeed over at least two other pharmaceutical companies. A third factor was the cost, of both time and money, that was spent in efforts to synthesize a drug that might or might not be efficacious. One consequence of this work on pancuronium, however, was that it led to the development of an even more widely used relaxant, vecuronium.[99]

Research into muscle relaxants was highly productive. Two main classes of muscle relaxants were synthesized: a group of steroidal compounds (pancuronium, vecuronium, and also rocuronium), and a group of compounds (atracurium, doxacurium, mivacurium, and cisatracurium). In developing the synthetic relaxants, as with other anesthetic agents, many different individuals were involved besides anesthesiologists. Chemists, pharmacologists, botanists, and scientists in pharmaceutical companies—all contributed their expertise, to say nothing of the patients and the countless animals that took part in the numerous studies.

The development of the many neuromuscular blocking agents is another clear example of the relationship between chemical structure and pharmacological activity. This relationship was elegantly demonstrated in the work that led very recently to production of a compound known as sugammadex, chemically a cyclodextrin.[100] The compound was devised specifically to encapsulate the molecule of the neuromuscular blocker, the active form of which can thus be removed from the circulation. Side effects are minimal or none. This work on structure-activity relationships is of a high level and may be applied to other classes of agents.

Inhalation Anesthesia

Among the advances in anesthesia that originated in the Second World War was the introduction of compounds containing fluorine, which in turn was an outcome of intensive research into fluorine chemistry. This led to the synthesis of an entirely new group of volatile inhalational agents, the fluorinated hydrocarbons, which was one of the characteristic features of anesthesia after World War II. Though the inhalational agents were not as numerous as the intravenous agents of this period, they changed anesthesia so that it was more precise and predictable for anesthesiologists and safer and pleasanter for patients. Together with new forms of respiratory management (see chapter 6) and monitoring, including real-time measurement of concentrations of anesthetic agents and rapid measurement of concentrations of electrolytes and gases in the blood (chapter 10), these various advances did much to change anesthetic practice in the latter half of the twentieth century. In addition, with desflurane, anesthesiologists could say that they were close to finding an agent that was almost ideal. In this connection, aspects of the inhalational agents are summarized in table 9.2.

The nature of anesthesia also changed with invasive operative procedures on the heart and lungs, and the new inhalational agents served anesthesiologists well as they fashioned appropriate anesthesia regimens in trying to solve problems presented by explorations of new body frontiers.

In solving those problems, anesthesiologists also made use of advances in other fields that were developing apace at the same time, such as those in electronics, computers, and the plastics industry. Some of those advances facilitated the administration of the new volatile inhalational agents, which were delivered from temperature-compensated and agent-specific vaporizers and the analysis of inspired and expired concentrations. In such ways, practitioners were greatly aided in the causes of precise dosage and safety.

Table 9.2. Comparison of fluorinated inhalational agents,* 1950-2000, with theoretically ideal agent**

Variable	Fluroxane	Halo	Methoxy	Enflur	Iso	Sevo	Des
Potentcy	++	+++	++	++	++++	++++	++++
Stability	++	++	++	+++	+++	+++	+++
Safety	++	++	++	++	+++	+++	++++
Fast action, recovery***	++	+++	++	++	+++	++++	++
CNS action-specific	++	+++	++	+++	+++	+++	+++
Nonflammable Nonexplosive	++++	++++	++++	++++	++++	++++	++++
Odorlessness	+	+	+	++	++	++	++
Muscle relaxation	++	+++	++	+++	+++	+++	+++
Nontoxic: body,postop; little biotransformn.	+	++	+	++	+++	+++	+++

*Abbreviations: Halo=halothane; Methoxy=methoxyflurane; Enflur=enflurane; Iso=isoflurane; Sevo=sevoflurane; Des=desflurane

**Given ranking of +++++

Fluroxene

Beginning in the 1950s, the fluorinated hydrocarbons changed anesthesia practice in a number of ways. In general, they were less pungent and irritating than ether and less toxic than chloroform; and they had fewer unpleasant side effects than either of the two older agents. Their synthesis was an outcome of the continuing search for the "ideal" inhalational anesthetic, which, in the 1930s, had begun to emphasize the value of the fluorine atom. Research actually began as early as 1930, when chemists investigated the properties of hydrocarbons that produced fluorocarbon as the refrigerant Freon.[101] They found that incorporating fluorine made a compound stable and less toxic and less flammable. Anesthesia-related research was reported first in 1932,[102] and though a suitable anesthetic was not synthesized in the 1930s, the research did suggest that incorporating an organic fluoride might yield an efficacious anesthetic.

Wartime did not interrupt research on anesthetic agents; instead, two factors, indirectly, expedited it. One was the enhancement by hydrogen fluoride of the catalytic alkylation of isoparaffins, which were needed in the production of high-octane fuel. The second was the use of uranium hexafluoride in separating isotopes of uranium from uranium oxide. Some of the work on this was done by Earl McBee, a chemist at Purdue University, who was interested in fluorinated hydrocarbons. With a grant to develop anesthetic agents from Mallinckrodt Chemical Works, which manufactured ether and cyclopropane, McBee did develop anesthetic agents.[103] Fluorinated compounds then became available for testing.

Another link in the chain of events was Mallinckrodt's support of the work of Benjamin Robbins at Vanderbilt University. Head of anesthesia there, Robbins was a pharmacologist, and he tested some of McBee's compounds in mice and dogs. Though Robbins did not produce an anesthetically suitable compound, his work led the way toward success by others.[104] One was John Krantz at the University of Maryland, who identified ethyl-vinyl ether, which had potential anesthetic value, as being worth fluorinating.[105] This was done by Julius Shukys.[106] That is how trifluorethyl vinyl ether, or Fluroxene, came to be introduced in 1954, as the first of a new class of volatile inhalational agents.

Fluroxene was used until 1974. It was supplanted by halothane, partly because of the discovery of a toxic metabolite, and partly because halothane was more potent. Though never used widely, fluroxene initiated the use of a long line of fluorinated inhalational agents that were much less flammable than ether. Fluroxene also illustrates the impact on anesthesia of the knowledge of fluorine chemistry that originated in the needs of industry in the 1930s and of the military in World War II. It also reminds us of the general point that anesthesia has never developed in a vacuum.

Halothane

The fluorinated compound halothane (Fluothane) was developed after
Charles Suckling, a chemist at Imperial Chemical Industries (ICI), in
Manchester, England, asked practitioners what properties of an inhalational
agent they considered ideal. They said it should be volatile, nonflammable,
stable, and potent; Suckling also considered factors such as partial pressure
and vapor pressure. Use of newer techniques such as gas chromatography
eventually led to the synthesis of halothane, which, with single chlorine and
bromine atoms and three fluorine atoms, seemed to be an ideal anesthetic
agent.[107]

After conducting initial research himself, and discovering that halothane
anesthetized houseflies, Suckling passed halothane over to James Raventos, also
of ICI.[108] Finally, halothane was studied clinically by Manchester anaesthetist
Michael Johnstone, who described halothane as an anesthetic in 1956.[109] A report
by R. Bryce-Smith and H. D. O'Brien[110] followed. Halothane immediately
became an anesthetic best seller.

Halothane revolutionized anesthetic practice. It had significant advantages
over ether and chloroform. It was potent and noncombustible, induction was
rapid, partly because it was not pungent, and it was seemingly nontoxic. It was
favored for induction of anesthesia in children, even replacing the earlier favorite
of cyclopropane. Yet halothane was not the elusive ideal, the holy grail, among
anesthesiologists. Light-sensitive, it had to be stored in amber-colored bottles;
and for developing countries, it was costly. Two more serious disadvantages were
its tendency to sensitize the myocardium to catecholamines and the occasional
development of jaundice.

The occurrence in 1962 of jaundice in a sixteen-year-old girl was a
setback. Her liver was severely poisoned, and this, with other cases of post-
halothane liver damage, set off a hue and cry for the causative factor in cases
of jaundice.[111] The National Halothane Study, organized by the National
Academy of Sciences / National Research Council and its Committee on
Anesthesia, was launched to sift through data of anesthetized patients.
Data from some 865, 000 patients[112] were analyzed. The main finding was
of halothane-associated massive hepatic necrosis in eighty-two patients.
The precise cause of liver damage was not established, though genetic
predisposition and sensitivity were suspected. Many anesthesiologists
switched to other fluorinated hydrocarbons that were coming on the market.
Even so, halothane continued to be used for many years, and it was only
the availability of isoflurane, beginning in 1971, that led to its disuse. Until
then, halothane had its place in the sun as the search for an ideal inhalational
anesthetic continued.

The National Halothane Study was the second large study of an anesthetic in the United States. Would halothane suffer the same fate as curare? Opinions about halothane and its hepatotoxic potential were divided, and the study was designed to answer the question, did halothane damage the liver? The study had two benefits. First, it showed that computers could facilitate large-scale studies in anesthesia; second, it generated a large body of data on overall postoperative mortality. As John Bunker, chair of anesthesia at Stanford University noted in 1972, the halothane study unearthed "the most comprehensive data on surgical deaths ever collected."[113] If nothing else, it was an epidemiological triumph.

Methoxyflurane

Regarded initially as an alternative to halothane, methoxyflurane (Penthrane) was introduced in 1960. It was used for self-administration for analgesia in labor and for general anesthesia. Its use, however, was limited by disadvantages. One was high solubility, hence slow induction and recovery.[114] Another was kidney damage by the inorganic fluorine atom on the caused its downfall and exile into veterinary medicine.

Enflurane and Isoflurane

Between 1959 and 1966, Ross Terrell and his colleagues at Ohio Medical Products worked systematically to synthesize a fluorinated anesthetic agent.[115] Their goal was to develop a compound that would approach the anesthetic ideal. Of more than seven hundred compounds, only compounds 347 and 469 had anesthetic potential. They were the methyl ethers containing fluorine and chlorine, the isomers known as enflurane and isoflurane.

Enflurane was discovered in 1963. Its chemical stability made it superior to halothane, but it caused cardiovascular depression and, occasionally, convulsions. More suitable was isoflurane, which was synthesized in 1965. Concern that it might be carcinogenic delayed its introduction. This was the era of the 1960s, so different from that of the 1920s and 1930s, when ethylene, cyclopropane, and divinyl ether were introduced in quick succession without any requirement of government approval—to say nothing of James Young Simpson's using chloroform in 1847, where almost immediately, he had observed its effects on himself. However, animal studies of isoflurane[116] gave the signal for clinical studies, and it was introduced as an inhalational agent in 1971.[117] Isoflurane became one of the most frequently used agents. Some concern was expressed about side effects such as maldistribution of coronary blood flow[118] and about a degree of biotransformation. The holy grail remained a mirage.

Sevoflurane and Desflurane

Another page in the chapter of inhalation anesthesia was turned with the advent of sevoflurane. A halogenated methyl isopropyl ether, it was synthesized by Bernard Regan and described for anesthesiologists in 1975.[119] It is potent, lacks pungency, and acts rapidly. It is excellent for the induction of anesthesia in children. It is administered from a standard type of vaporizer.

Among the many compounds that Terrell investigated, the 653rd was desflurane, a fluorinated methyl ethyl ether. Its chemical structure indicated low blood solubility, and hence rapid uptake.[120] Its vapor pressure (88.53 kPa at 20 C) makes desflurane different from other inhalational agents and necessitates a special vaporizer. Desflurane is potent, though its irritability when inspired makes it necessary for it to be administered for maintenance rather than induction. Other features are its stability and the lack of degradation in the body. These various factors mean that patients recover from anesthesia very rapidly.

In the opinion of R. M. Jones, of London, desflurane comes closest of all the inhalational anesthetic agents to the ideal inhalational agent; as of 1990, its properties were thought to be "a distinct improvement on those of existing anesthetic agents."[121] Yet as the twentieth century closed, it appeared that the ideal had actually not been reached. Nor would it be reached as long as it remained uncertain where general anesthetic agents act to produce their effects.

*   *   *

With the introduction of new intravenous and inhalational drugs in the second half of the twentieth century, anesthesia continued to progress. Innovations that were generated and applied reflect both the improvements in anesthetic practice and the justification of the recognition of anesthesia as a specialty that was making many contributions to health care delivery. However, as is apparent throughout modern anesthesia, progress was only made possible by other contributions by individuals and organizations in other fields besides anesthesia. This merits discussion in concluding this chapter's account of intravenous and inhalational agents.

Closely associated with the introduction and use of intravenous and inhalational agents was a technical support system underlying the production and use of those agents. It it is, therefore, appropriate to explain how that support system functions and has developed. Otherwise, it may be thought that anesthetic drugs appear de novo without research or by chance, which—except in rare circumstances such as those surrounding the development of ethyl chloride and ethylene—is far from the case.

Consider how drugs are discovered or synthesized, and manufactured and prepared. This occurs long before they reach the operating room. Years—sometimes decades—of activity, unrelated to anesthesia, is necessary first as chemists work in the laboratories of pharmaceutical companies. Just that reflects an entirely separate dimension of historical events and of smart, even inspired, thinking. No new drug ever reaches the operating room today in the absence of a great deal of research guided by that thinking. Then the chemists' discoveries or manipulations are followed by drug testing by pharmacologists. And lying behind their work are the knowledge and the techniques, the equipment and the materials that they work with, none of which remained static, any more than anesthesia did. Thus progress in anesthesia has very largely depended on progress in chemistry and pharmacology, whether this concerns the relationship between the structure of a chemical compound and its activity in the body, for example, or the effects of potentially useful drugs on the heart and nervous system. Nor is this progress made by these tests in vivo, both in animals and in patients and sometimes healthy volunteers.

The point here is a simple one: many factors have influenced the evolution of anesthesia, besides the work of anesthesiologists themselves. Surgical advances, of course, have made a large impact, but so has engineering—whether it concerns the production of anesthesia machines, electronic equipment, or computers—and the plastics industry. Thus has the history of anesthesia been shaped in many ways by the history of other facets of society.

Chapter 10

MONITORING IN ANESTHESIA

After the Second World War, many of the surgical procedures were complex and were performed on parts of the body that surgeons had not broached before. In some of these operations, particularly on the heart and lung,   n o r m a l functions of the body were taken over by machines, which added a complicating technical factor. Moreover, many of the patients who underwent these new procedures were extremely sick and liable to respond poorly to the stresses of surgery and anesthesia. Anesthesiologists, therefore, faced enormously complex challenges in keeping up with innovative surgical procedures and in devising anesthesia regimens that would be appropriate to complex surgery and be safe for very sick patients.

Part of the challenge that anesthesiologists faced was the fact that in caring for the sick and endeavoring to deal appropriately with the often-rapid physiological changes that occur in them, the ability of the human senses to detect critical responses of the body to surgical or anesthetic encroachment is limited. The need to detect such physiological changes *promptly* is frequently urgent, for otherwise, especially in sick patients, a cascade of potentially lethal events may be set in motion. The situation might well be dire if, under such circumstances, anesthesiologists rely only on their "normal" senses, such as sight and hearing, in trying to keep abreast of such critical events, for they may lack the acuity that is likely to be essential.

That the sensitivity of the senses in detecting physiological change is indeed limited was shown in 1947. The test question was this: can the human eye accurately detect the blue color in the skin that develops when the blood is oxygenated inadequately? The answer: human eyesight is definitely *unreliable* in accurately detecting cyanosis of the skin and mucous membranes.[1] This observation must be linked to a second, more recent, one that is pertinent to anesthesia: the human organism is also unreliable in detecting serious mishaps that occur during an anesthetic, termed critical incidents,[2] and that may lead to grave disability, or even death.

As more invasive surgical procedures were developed beginning in the 1950s, it was therefore vital to find ways of improving the ability of the human organism to detect and correct abnormal trends and critical incidents during anesthesia. Two such ways were found. One was to heighten the awareness in anesthesiologists of the importance of increased vigilance so that potentially serious abnormalities might be detected early. The second was to use instruments that are designed to measure or detect changes in physiological parameters with great sensitivity and accuracy. This latter modality, known as monitoring, became a vital part of the administration of an anesthetic because its use aids anesthesiologists in the detecting changes in physiological values. Since monitors are fitted with alarms, they are also capable of bringing a warning to the attention of the anesthesiologist.

The increasing use of monitors was a notable feature of anesthesia in the second half of the twentieth century and is the topic of this chapter.

The Relationship between Monitoring and Anesthesia

Monitoring has been part of anesthesia care since the beginning, as is shown by a case report of 1846. One month after William Morton demonstrated ether anesthesia in October 1846, Boston surgeon Henry Jacob Bigelow noted the changes in pulse rate, respiratory rate, and pupil size in a patient during anesthesia and the corrective action that was taken.[3] The last point emphasizes the fact that corrective action is important, even vital, because, otherwise, monitoring—whether by the human senses or by artificial means—is valueless. In the Bigelow case, slowing of the pulse and respiration and coldness of the hands led him to suggest "the propriety of desisting." To return the circulation and respiration to normal, "affusions" were applied to the head, the ears were syringed, and ammonia was given. This did the trick; consciousness was soon restored.

Bigelow was describing monitoring by the human senses, and his report foreshadowed two aspects of later monitoring by artificial means. One is that monitoring aids are intended to *complement* the human senses, not to replace them. The second is that monitoring should serve as an early warning system (the term *monitor* is derived from the Latin verb *monitare*, meaning "to warn"), providing information that can be acted on before an incident becomes critical. The 1846 report shows that monitoring is not really a recent development, and indeed, there is a close temporal relationship between monitoring and anesthesia. Monitoring evolved as anesthesia evolved, and as anesthesia evolved, so did monitoring. To follow the development of monitoring is to follow the development of anesthesia.[4] The state of anesthesia at any one time is reflected by the state of monitoring, and vice versa.

Initially, when anesthesia was an empirical craft, the only monitors that were available were indeed the human senses—as is apparent in figure 3.2, which shows Joseph Clover relying on his finger palpating his patient's pulse. As anesthesia developed, monitoring was refined; and as the twentieth century progressed, anesthesia machines were fitted with increasingly sophisticated means of monitoring gas flow and anesthesia agent consumption, as well as means of displaying many other valuable data (see also chapter 7). As the twentieth century progressed, the practice of anesthesia and the availability of information-rich monitors advanced together. Therefore, as the evolution of monitoring is discussed, the state of anesthesia at any particular time should be borne in mind.

Phases in the Development of Monitoring

The history of monitoring may be divided into three phases:1846-1901, 1902-1955, and 1956-2006.

Monitoring in the Nineteenth Century

In the nineteenth century, most practitioners gave anesthesia only from time to time, and so their knowledge and experience were limited. Yet the challenges were often overwhelming, and tragedies occurred all too often. In the absence of artificial monitors in this period when anesthesia was a craft, human inadequacies became all the more noticeable. Consider the case of Hannah Greener, for example. She died suddenly on January 28, 1848, as anesthesia was being induced with chloroform.[5] Would the presence of a monitor have stimulated corrective action and prevented her death? No one can say, but it is likely that Hannah died because her heart stopped suddenly, probably from the lethal combination of fear, light chloroform anesthesia, and the rhythm disturbance known as ventricular fibrillation. Today, that arrhythmia can be diagnosed electrically, but no such means was available in 1848, so no corrective action could be taken. (Compounding the problem was the fact that regardless of the lack of electrocardiography, ventricular fibrillation was unknown in 1848.) With only their senses to aid them, practitioners were at a serious disadvantage.

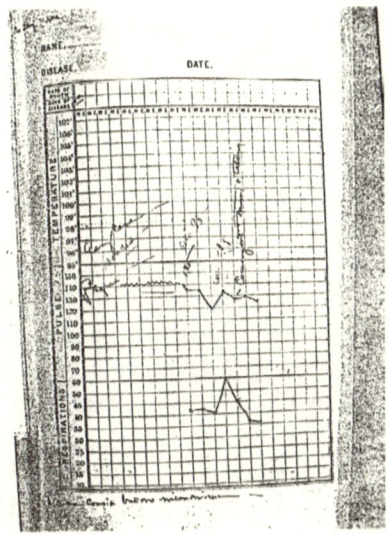

Fig. 10.1. Early anesthesia record completed by Harvey Cushing, 5 April, 1895. (Source: Treadwell Library, Boston.)

One of those who felt disadvantaged was neurosurgeon-to-be Harvey Cushing. In 1894, as a medical student, he anesthetized a patient who, to his dismay, died under anesthesia.[6] This made him and fellow student Amory Codman think that they might be better anesthetists if they had a picture of how an anesthetic was progressing all the time. So they designed a record on which clinical data could be entered *during* an anesthetic. That is how the anesthesia record (fig. 10.1) originated.[7] Though the anesthesia record was only indirectly a monitor—it did not have a built-in alarm, for example—it did serve to indicate potential warning signs. It may be regarded as a precursor of an alarm, and thus of an anesthesia monitor. For Cushing, the anesthesia record also monitored his own progress and competence. He stated that "the careful recording of the pulse rate throughout the operation"[8] was indeed beneficial.

The anesthesia record was used to collate data regarding physiological variables. That and a practitioner's five senses, constituted monitoring in the nineteenth century.

Monitoring from 1902 to 1955

In the second phase of monitoring, the advances expanded the practitioner's awareness of changes in the body's physiological systems. The principal variables monitored included the blood pressure, the heart rate and rhythm, and brain activity, as well as the breathing.

Monitoring of blood pressure. During his study year in Europe in 1900 and 1901,[9] Cushing saw Scipione Riva-Rocci, of Turin, use an instrument to measure blood pressure. Known as the sphygmanometer, Riva-Rocci had reported its use in 1896.[10] Cushing himself first noted the use of sphygmomanometry in 1902[11] and recommended its use in the operating room in 1903.[12] (In doing so, Cushing made the second of his contributions to monitoring, and the second of his four contributions to anesthesia.[13])

As this history shows, many aspects of anesthesia have an often long prehistory. Blood pressure measurement, like other monitoring modalities, is no exception. It was first determined in the eighteenth century, though not clinically then: in England, Stephen Hales described his experiments on the blood pressure of animals in 1733.[14] Basic physiological work was continued in the human in the nineteenth century. In France, J. L. M. Poiseuille used a column of mercury for this purpose in 1828; and in 1856, J. Faivre attached a Poiseuille manometer to the artery of amputated limbs.[15] Thus, when Riva-Rocci attached a mercury column to a rubber cuff and estimated the blood pressure by palpating the radial artery,[16] he was following a path that had been opened up by earlier physiologists. Cushing's surgical foresight enabled him to follow the path further, and his recommendation of sphygmomanometry inaugurated the era of monitoring in anesthesia with instruments.

Blood pressure measurement was furthered by Nicolai Korotkoff, of St. Petersburg, Russia, in 1905. He inflated a cuff on the arm until the circulation was occluded and then *listened* for the sounds in the brachial artery as the cuff was deflated. He wrote that "the manometric figure at which the first tone appears corresponds to the maximal pressure. The time of cessation of all sounds indicates . . . that the manometric figures at this time correspond to the minimal blood pressure."[17] The stethoscope was thus essential to sphygmomanometry, but Cushing also showed later that it could be used to monitor the breath sounds during anesthesia.[18]

Use of the stethoscope to measure blood pressure and as an intraoperative monitor was encouraged by anesthesiologist Elmer McKesson, of Toledo, Ohio. He made an important point: blood pressure recordings might indicate "the gradual development of shock so far in advance of its serious consequences that treatment may be instituted, or the causes modified in such a way as to avoid its complete development."[19] This echoed what Bigelow had said seventy years earlier, just as McKesson's remarks were echoed in 1995 by Casey Blitt: "Appropriate monitoring facilitates timely therapeutic intervention to prevent undesirable outcomes."[20]

Monitoring of cardiac rate and rhythm. The second monitor that came into use in anesthesia practice was the electrocardiogram (ECG). Einthoven described this in 1903,[21] but it was not used routinely as an anesthetic monitor until the 1960s. Instead, cardiac rate and rhythm were monitored mainly by palpation (feeling the pulse) and by auscultation (listening with the stethoscope).

At first, the ECG machine was cumbersome and not portable. Even in the early 1950s, when practitioners began to realize that the ECG might help them evaluate the cardiac condition of an unusually sick patient, the cathode-ray device was not a fixture in the operating room; it would have to be trundled in on its wheeled stand and set beside the anesthesia machine. Not until the era of cardiac surgery dawned later in the 1950s did changes in the electrical activity of the heart appear to have everyday, and even vital, relevance to anesthesia. That is apparent also from the fact that a textbook on the ECG for anesthesiologists and written by an anesthesiologist was not published until 1964.[22] In due course, ECG tracings would be found on every anesthesia machine.

The ECG, like the sphygmomanometer, was noninvasive. That reflects two facts of the first half of the twentieth century. First, before the era of cardiac surgery, anesthesiologists did not use invasive forms of monitoring; second, technological development had as yet not made a notable impact on monitoring. Again, progress in monitoring reflects progress in anesthesia. Though anesthetists in the 1920s and 1930s were concerned about mortality associated with anesthesia, especially when chloroform was used, they had no overt concern with patient safety, and monitors were not designed with that in mind. Rather, it was still the signs of anesthesia that were emphasized. That is evident from Arthur Guedel's emphasis of eye signs in assessing depth of anesthesia in 1920,

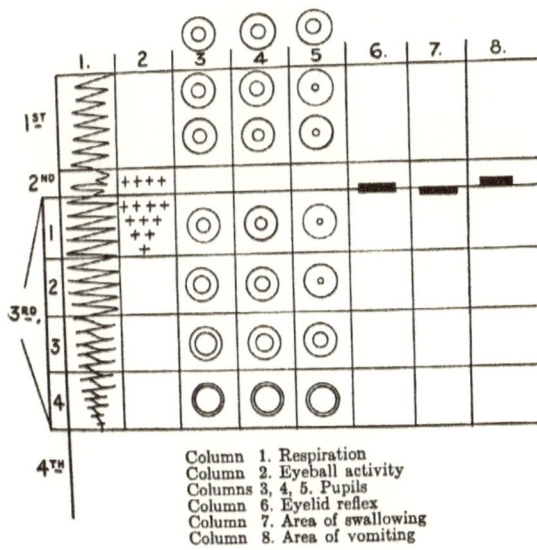

Fig. 10.2. Guedel chart of signs and stages of anesthesia. (Source: A. Guedel, *Inhalation Anesthesia: A Fundamental Guide* [New York: The Macmillan Company, 1937, p. 25].)

when he published a modification of Snow's original signs and stages of anesthesia[23] (fig. 10.2). But like the anesthesia record, Guedel's signs were not so much a monitor as an indication of the anesthesia status in a patient. Noel Gillespie did much the same in 1943, when he argued that one could best determine the depth of anesthesia by observing the way in which reflexes were modified.[24]

Monitoring of brain activity. The electroencephalograph (EEG) was another noninvasive monitor of this period. It was thought to have possible *practical* value in assessing the depth of anesthesia in 1937,[25] but not until 1950 did Albert Faulconer, at the Mayo Clinic, confirm its value in the operating room.[26] Yet the EEG, unlike the ECG, is still not routinely used as a monitor of anesthesia. Compared to the ECG, the EEG is costly, more difficult to set up, and less obviously applicable.

Faulconer's ideas and his research illustrate the lack of development in monitoring soon after the Second World War. In the 1940s, advances in the clinical aspects of anesthesia were beginning to be overshadowed by advances in the scientific aspects of anesthesia. Faulconer conducted his research into monitoring with the technological equipment that was then available, and as he did so, he was the first to continuously measure anesthetic gas and vapor concentrations and to make use of the EEG as an index of depth of anesthesia with ether and thiopental.[27] He also applied the knowledge gained in research to develop, with Bickford, the technology of servo-anesthesia.[28] Faulconer was ahead of his time, even a "forgotten pioneer."[29] He carried out this work in the 1940s, when there was relatively little interest in instrument monitoring as a valuable aid to anesthesia. This may be confirmed by looking at the first edition of J. Alfred Lee's *A Synopsis of Anaesthesia*,[30] published in 1947, in which there is no reference to monitoring as such.

Monitoring Beginning in 1956

Beginning in the 1950s, progress in monitoring picked up speed. It progressed in two ways. First, it became possible to monitor many more physiological variables. Devices became available for measurement of oxygen, carbon dioxide, and anesthetic gas concentrations in the blood. Second, some monitoring became invasive: instruments were inserted into parts of the body such as arteries and veins.

Why was such rapid progress made in monitoring from the 1950s on? One reason is that technological development was expedited by the impact of such devices as the computer (built first as recently as 1946), the diode valve, and the transistor. Microprocessing in particular influenced the ability of physicians to process information. Along with these advances, progress in the plastics industry facilitated the use of invasive monitoring.

The inauguration of cardiac surgery and the associated need for real-time, in-body measurements also moved monitoring along. Heart surgery itself came about partly after surgeons in World War II realized that the heart was actually quite robust and that it could be handled with impunity, as for example when they manipulated it while removing bullets that had lodged in the heart.[31] The need to know how anesthesia affected the brain during neurosurgery similarly spurred progress in monitoring.

A fourth explanation for the advances in monitoring is more general. It takes time for new technology to modify and expand the scope of what can be done in an operating room, and it was only sometime after peace returned in the mid-1940s that surgeons used monitoring devices more extensively. And only after the mid-1950s and the affluent 1960s did expenditure of further energy, and money, generate more monitors.

The beginning of the third phase in monitoring is marked by two events that occurred in 1956. One was a landmark in monitoring: the invention of Leland Clark's oxygen electrode.[32] The other was a landmark event in anesthesia: the introduction of halothane as a versatile fluorinated inhalational agent.[33]

The principal monitors of the second half of the twentieth century are listed in table 10.1. Some were essential in that they gave warning of dangerously low tensions of oxygen (hypoxia) or high tensions of carbon dioxide (hypercapnia, or hypercarbia) in the blood. Mandatory monitors included the pulse oximeter, the sphygmomanometer, the electrocardiograph, the capnograph, and those that measure oxygen and gas pressures and anesthetic agent partial pressures in the anesthesia machine; the availability of thermometry is another essential feature of monitoring. Some monitoring techniques were not as basic and essential because they were invasive, intra-arterial, central venous, and pulmonary pressures being recorded. Other monitors provided information about vital functions relating especially to the heart, the respiration, the nerve-muscle junction.

Table 10.1. Monitoring devices, 2006.

SYSTEM	MONITOR
Standard*	
General	Automated anesthesia record**
Cardiovascular	Pulse oximeter, automated noninvasive sphygomamometer, stethoscope, oscilloscopic electrocardiograph
Respiratory	Pulse oximeter, capnograph, exhaled gas flowmeter, spirometer, gas analyzers, circuit low-pressue alarm
Temperature	Thermometer
Neuromuscular	Peripheral nerve stimulator
Advanced	
Cardiovascular	Direct vascular pressure wave regulators, transesop hagealechocardiograph
Central Nervous	Electroencephalograph, BIS/PSA, evoked potentials analyzer
Additional	
	Blood-gas, electrolyte analyzers
	Pulse plethysmograph
	Transcutaneous O_2, CO_2 analyzers
	Noninvasive cardiac output analyzer

*Qualified administrator of anesthesia a sine qua non.
**Unaccompanied by an alarm, hence not a true monitor.

Of these monitoring techniques, pulse oximetry, capnography, and intravascular pressure measurement are historically interesting in illustrating the complexity of development. They are therefore discussed in detail, as are issues and questions concerning use of the monitors.

Blood Oxygen (pO_2) and Carbon Dioxide (pCO_2) Tensions and
Acidity/Alkalinity (pH)

Attempts to measure the blood oxygen and carbon dioxide concentrations and
pH go back many years. Much research preceded the capacity for measuring
these parameters at the bedside. Over the years, such efforts consumed an
enormous amount of time and effort[34] and provided many examples of how
chemistry and physics contributed to monitoring techniques that became part
of routine anesthesia care.

Oxygen Tension. The story of how devices that were used to measure oxygen
tensions in the blood extends over more than half a century. It includes
research by chemists in the nineteenth century and the early twentieth century,
research in the Second World War that included studies of aviation and visual
physiology, and analyses of oxygen tensions.

The concentration and the saturation of oxygen in the blood were of interest
to H. L. Daneel, in Germany, in 1897. He found that dissolved oxygen reacted
with negatively charged metals, including platinum.[35] Daneel's measurements
were unreliable, but Jaroslav Heyrovsky, of Czechoslovakia, used a polarographic
method involving mercury to measure amounts of oxygen.[36] This was used
clinically by some investigators in anesthesia, including Henry Beecher, of
the Massachusetts General Hospital, who reported on it in 1942.[37] However,
the mercury electrode was difficult to use, and attention was switched back to
platinum.

To study oxygen tensions and metabolism in nervous tissue, Detlev Bronk
used a platinum electrode covered with a semipermeable membrane.[38] After the
war, Clark endeavored to monitor oxygen tension in his laboratory, but by 1952
he realized that to prevent the "poisoning" of the electrode's platinum surface
some kind of coating was required.[39] He put together some glass, platinum, and
silver wire with a drop of potassium chloride and "a bit of polyethylene film."[40]
The result was the polyethylene-covered electrode that became so widely used
thereafter in measuring oxygen concentrations. Clark's triumph was the peak of
much investigation that had gone before, and it may not be greatly exaggerating
the degree of his achievement to state that blood-gas analysis is indeed one of the
most ubiquitous of clinically useful laboratory techniques[41] that are available to
the anesthesiologist. Apart from its enormous value in anesthesia and medicine
and surgery, the Clark electrode is an elegant example of one among the many
contributions that the plastics industry as well as chemistry made to monitoring
equipment.

Carbon dioxide tension (pCO₂) and blood acidity/alkalinity (pH). Attempts to measure the pCO_2 and the pH in blood also took time and effort. They were first calculated from the Henderson-Hasselbalch equation but, from 1924 onward, the manometric Van Slyke apparatus was used in measuring the pressure of blood gases, including carbon dioxide.[42] In 1932, Douglas and Havard constructed a glass electrode to measure pH,[43] but even then, there was little interest in sampling arterial blood, in part because a specialty of critical care medicine had not been even conceived. That interest came with the poliomyelitis epidemic in Copenhagen in 1952, when concerted efforts were made to measure pH and pCO_2. (see also chapter 11). Indeed, the management of the epidemic marks the transition of blood gas analysis from a physiological laboratory exercise to a clinical necessity.[44]

Because ventilation in many of the poliomyelitis patients was depressed, the pCO and pH had to be analyzed promptly before the ventilation was adjusted. Taking arterial samples, Poul Astrup formulated a new equilibration method to allow him to estimate the acid base balance. The basis of his method was as follows: he determined both the bicarbonate ion concentration and the pCO_2 by measuring the pH in the arterial sample, he equilibrated the sample with two gas mixtures of known pCO_2, and he remeasured the pH at each known gas tension.[45]

The practical development of the CO_2 electrode had begun in 1926, when Gesell and McGinty used manganese dioxide in making an electrode.[46] In 1954, Richard Stow described a pH electrode covered with a rubber membrane that allowed only carbon dioxide to pass through it.[47] This was not completely satisfactory, but in 1958, American anesthesiologist John Severinghaus produced the first clinically useful electrode.[48] He also made the first blood-gas analysis apparatus to incorporate electrodes for all three of the main components of blood-gas analysis.

Oxygen saturation and expired carbon dioxide partial pressure. Some of the anesthesia-related accidents that continued to occur in the second half of the twentieth century related to the frequency with which a patient's breathing could be jeopardized by mishaps associated with the breathing circuit on the anesthesia machine. In such cases, the blood and, eventually, the brain were inadequately oxygenated. A rise in the carbon dioxide would also characteristically occur in such incidents. Pulse oximetry and capnometry, which are crucial as monitors of oxygen and carbon dioxide as impending trouble, are therefore discussed together.

Pulse oximetry. The need to accurately determine oxygen saturation of blood in the operating room led to the monitoring of oxygen by pulse oximetry.

This came to be used universally in anesthesia and widely in other areas of patient care; it may well be one of the most significant technological advances in relation to the well-being and safety of patients during anesthesia, recovery, and critical care.[49] It is yet another example of one of the many contributions that electrical engineering and chemistry have made to anesthesia.

Pulse oximetry, introduced in the 1980s, shows how anesthesiologists continually apply technological advances to patient care. It soon became one of the standards of practice that is enforced in operating rooms, and it is required by hospital certification. Even so, despite the pervasive use of pulse oximeters, and their apparently obvious benefit, no study has yet positively demonstrated their utility.

The evolution of the pulse oximeter began in 1864. The substance that colors blood was found also to transport oxygen.[50] This substance was named hemoglobin. Its optical spectra were then studied.[51] In 1935, Mathes used a device and from the spectra measured the saturation of blood with oxygen.[52] During World War II, Glen Millikan and others transformed the device into an instrument to help the British study loss of consciousness in aviators during dogfights.[53] A prototype oximeter, applied to the ear, was first used in an operating room around this time, as McClure and colleagues endeavored to control anoxemia.[54] Oxygen saturation of the blood was the main focus of interest, basic research being carried out by Millikan,[55] Goldie,[56] and Squire.[57] The venous and capillary blood was squeezed out of the earlobe or the earlobe was warmed to arterialize it before measurements were made. That train of research was one way in which the saturation of oxygen in the blood could be measured.

However, pulse oximetry, as it is known in anesthesia today, originated in a different approach. The background of this was the study of blood flow using transmitted light, or photoplethysmography. This began in the 1930s, when the waveform of the pulse in a finger was analyzed by examining changes in the intensity of transmitted light.[58] In the 1970s, the Japanese physiological bioengineer Takuo Aoyagi became interested in measuring cardiac output by the dye dilution method. He knew both that ear oximeters had been used for dye measurement and that the transmitted light signal had pulsatile variations that were difficult to eliminate. Aoyagi attempted to cancel these variations by electrical means, but the cancellation was inconsistent. He concluded that this inconsistency could be related to changes in oxygen saturation. A eureka moment followed, and as Severinghaus and Honda have noted, "This failure of elimination of pulsatility in the dye curves led directly to pulse oximetry."[59] Aoyagi then measured only the pulsatile changes in the transmission of light through tissue in order to compute the arterial saturation; changes in light transmission at all wavelengths would be due only to the pulsatile variations of the arterial blood volume. His device was marketed in 1975, though its clinical value was not recognized until the early 1980s.

Capnography. Monitoring of carbon dioxide gives essential information about gas exchange and the adequacy of ventilation, and capnography became as universal in the operating room as oximetry. Two of the original methods of analysis are infrared analysis and Raman spectroscopy. They can also be used to determine partial pressures of anesthetic agents and nitrogen. Infrared analysis of gases in anesthesia, which depends on light energy absorbed by a gas, was derived from its use in respiratory medicine in the 1950s.[60] Raman spectroscopy, which depends on a shift in wavelength of light following re-emission of energy when ultraviolet light strikes gas molecules, was introduced to clinical anesthesia in the 1970s.[61]

Carbon dioxide tensions, which were of concern during the poliomyelitis epidemics of the 1950s, have highlighted the relationship between inadequate ventilation and hypercapnia (or hypercarbia; an abnormally raised blood pCO_2) and inadequate ventilation, and indeed the lethality of hypercarbia.[62] As a result, anesthesiologists became aware that knowing the pCO_2 of the blood of a patient in the operating room was essential, though a more immediate way to recognize hyper—or hypocarbia was to measure the carbon dioxide partial pressure in the expired air. This form of measurement was termed capnometry, while the graphic display became known as capnography.

In some respects capnography provided more crucial, and certainly more immediate, information than pulse oximetry. Capnometry and capnography constitute an anesthesia disaster early warning system,[63] for a sudden decrease in the expired carbon dioxide partial pressure to zero provides immediate, real-time information about an impending respiratory critical incident. Accidental intubation of the esophagus, complete disconnection or obstruction of the artificial airway, and malfunction of a ventilator may be signaled.[64] On the other hand, an increase in the expired concentration may signal the occurrence of carbon dioxide venous embolism, as in gynecologic laparoscopy.[65] It can also be useful in the initial diagnosis of malignant hyperthermia (dangerously high body temperature).

Problems in interpreting data. Monitors provide information, and that has to be interpreted by an anesthesiologist so that the appropriate action can be taken. What may be regarded as a negative or a positive result may, in fact, be only falsely negative or falsely positive. It was therefore necessary for anesthesiologists, as actuators, to learn how monitors, as the sensors, function and then how to interpret the data displayed in the context of the situation. Abnormal readings from a pulse oximeter, for example, should make an anesthesiologist suspect poor perfusion and low blood pressure before a fault in the sensor is considered. Similarly, after the trachea of a patient whose heart has stopped is intubated, the reading of carbon dioxide tension in the end-expired (end-tidal) air must be interpreted with caution since it could arise from the presence of the tracheal tube in the stomach and its becoming inflated. Again, the absence of carbon dioxide in the end-tidal air could be consistent with a tube placed correctly in the trachea in a patient whose heart has stopped and is therefore producing no carbon dioxide.

Intravascular Pressure

Indirect, noninvasive forms of blood pressure measurement by the sphygmomanometer continued to be topics of research in the second half of the twentieth century, and one line of study yielded a device that permitted noninvasive monitoring of the blood flow and pressure in a finger.[66] The Finapres purported to measure noninvasive pressures continuously, but because it did not provide vascular access for blood sampling, it was still only possible to measure the arterial pressure intermittently. However, an automated device was introduced in 1979.[67] Even so, with noninvasive techniques, it was difficult to measure the pressure in patients with arrhythmias.

Such noninvasive methods of pressure measurement were, however, not satisfactory in detecting the fast-moving changes in the anesthetic or surgical care of patients undergoing heart surgery. It became necessary to measure the arterial pressure continuously and in real time by inserting devices into arteries and veins. Measurement of pressures in major vessels such as the internal jugular or the subclavian vein and the pulmonary artery were considered essential to good management, both in anesthesia and, by extension, in critical care. Catheterization of peripheral arteries, the pulmonary artery, and central veins became part of standard care in patients undergoing major surgery. Since the invasive technique is common to direct measurement of pressure in these various vessels, evolution of intravascular monitoring will be discussed in a single section.

Intra-arterial pressure. In 1947, Edward Lambert and Earl Wood, at the Mayo Clinic, used a manometer attached to a resistance wire strain gauge to measure intra-arterial pressure.[68] In this technique, stretching or contraction of a wire leads to changes in electrical resistance, which is detected by a

Wheatstone bridge. At this time, it was necessary in determining the pressure directly to incise an artery and insert a rigid metal needle, but other technical advances helped to make the intra-arterial technique accessible. One technique was to introduce a catheter *through* a needle that lay temporarily in the artery and to leave the catheter in the artery as the needle was withdrawn.[69] Another was to use a needle that was covered with plastic, such as the Rochester needle.[70] An important advance was made in 1953 by Sven Seldinger, of Stockholm, who inserted a wire through a needle nick in the arterial wall and then threaded a catheter *over* the needle into the artery before withdrawing the needle.[71] Only a relatively small needle was needed. A final advance was made in 1961 by Per-Olof Barr, also of Stockholm, who publicized the technique of puncturing the radial artery with a Teflon-covered needle, the needle being withdrawn after the catheter had been threaded into place.[72] It then became routine for anesthesiologists to monitor the arterial pressure beat by beat and in real time, and not only for patients undergoing heart surgery.

Pulmonary arterial pressure. In 1929, Werner Forssmann, a surgical trainee in Germany, introduced a catheter via the left antecubital vein in his arm into his own right atrium.[73] Measuring the pressure in the right side of the heart continued to be important in cardiac operations. In 1953, Lategola and Rahn devised a catheter with an inflatable balloon at its tip[74] for work in dogs, and it did not become common in clinical practice until 1970.[75] Catheterization of the pulmonary artery and, indeed, monitoring of the cardiovascular status of anyone who was critically ill then became a reality. The pulmonary catheter revolutionized cardiovascular monitoring.[76]

Central venous pressure. The steps in measuring the central venous pressure were relatively simple compared with those in measuring the pulmonary artery. The Seldinger technique paved the way, and in 1969, English and colleagues described percutaneous catheterization of the internal jugular vein.[77] Monitoring of the central pressure via the internal jugular, or often the subclavian, vein then became more frequent, together with radial artery monitoring, than almost any other form of invasive monitoring.

Risk/benefit ratios in invasive vascular monitoring. Invasive monitoring is sometimes difficult and potentially harmful. Complications such as pneumothorax, venous air embolism, arterial puncture, and cardiac tamponade had to be considered, and physicians began to look more closely at the indications for invasive monitoring. Aids such as ultrasound were used to facilitate placement of catheters.

Standards, Selection, and Outcome Assessment of Monitoring

Progress in monitoring in the second half of the twentieth century was only one aspect of progress in anesthesia, for changes in society's expectations of medicine, from the 1960s on, had a profound influence on medicine in general and on anesthesia and monitoring in particular. As medicine changed, so did society's expectations of it, and what society expected of anesthesia was not any different. The growing emphasis on the importance of professionalism and accountability for all physicians, anesthesiologists included, reflects this. Nor is it any coincidence that the great explosion in monitoring instrumentation came about at the same time of a liberalization of society, or that the incorporation of monitoring occurred when society expected anesthesiologists, like all physicians, to be accountable for their actions. In the 1950s, when a patient died under anesthesia, especially if this was not expected, it was often passed off as an accident. No longer. Because of the remarkable progress in science and technology that characterized the second half of the twentieth century, anesthesiologists were expected to be able to guide a patient safely through anesthesia or, if this did not occur, to be held accountable for their actions. The importance attached to monitoring can therefore be seen in this context.

Three general aspects of monitoring are relevant. One is the finding by Cooper and his colleagues, noted briefly earlier, that the leading cause of serious anesthesia accidents is human error.[78] Cooper presented the problem the situation quite baldly: most (82 percent) of the preventable mishaps involved human error; but at the same time, such information concerning the actual causes of the mishaps could stimulate the motivation and resolve to take specific corrective action.

A second aspect of monitoring in this context is the investigation that was launched in 1985 by a group of anesthesiologists who concluded that formulating minimum standards for monitoring during anesthesia would lead to improvements in anesthesia care.[79] They argued that adherence to certain minimum standards of anesthesia care would reduce the incidence of serious morbidity and of mortality associated with anesthesia. Notably, this was an initiative launched by professionals themselves. The standards, known as the Harvard Standards, were promptly adopted by the House of Delegates of the American Society of Anesthesiologists.[80] The impact of these standards was profound: monitoring became universal in the practice of anesthesia. Indeed, anesthesiologists took the lead in medicine in developing standards that would enhance the quality of health care.

The investigation that led to the Harvard standards is another indication that anesthesiologists were in the forefront of concerns about standards of patient care. They were consistent with Cooper's findings because an analysis of litigation claims had shown that most anesthesia mishaps were actually preventable and that monitoring would do much to prevent them. Though the standards, listed in table 10.2, were essentially minimum standards and revolutionary in being promulgated as standards for all anesthesiologists to consider following, the objectives in publishing them were hardly revolutionary. They were to improve patient care, to enhance detection of relatively low-frequency events, to provide a means for objective evaluation, and to establish a precedent.

Table 10.2. Harvard Standards, minimal monitoring*

Anesthesiologist or nurse anesthetist in operating room
Measurement of arterial blood pressure, heart rate each 5 minutes
Continuous display of electrocardiograph

For ventilation, at least one of the following recommended:

continuous palpation or observation of breathing bag auscultation of breathing sounds monitoring of respiratory gas or expiratory gas flow

For circulation, as near continuous monitoring as possible of one of the following:

pulse palpation
intraarterial pressure
pulse plethysmography/oximetry
ultrasound peripheral pulse

When mechanical ventilator is used:

detection of disconnection of any breathing component, plus audible alarm when alarm threshold is exceeded

Oxygen analysis in breathing system with low-limit alarm (American National Standards Institute standard Z.79.10)

Readily available means of measuring patient's temperature

*After document by J. Eichorn, J. Cooper, D. Cullen et al., Standards for patient monitoring during anesthesia at Harvard Medical School, *JAMA* 1986; 256:1017-20.

Yet a third aspect of the concern of anesthesiologists at this time is evident in an investigation by anesthesiologists of closed-claims malpractice insurance files in 1989. Some 31 percent of negative outcomes were thought to have been preventable by additional monitoring; if the monitoring had combined pulse oximetry and capnography, approximately 93 percent of mishaps could be regarded as preventable.[81] These results were apparent solely as a result of anesthesiologists themselves acting professionally in the best interests of patient safety, and thus being accountable to society.

In the context of accountability, a larger study of mishaps in general, conducted later by the Institute of Medicine, also must be noted. Thousands of patients, it was reported, die each year in the United States from deaths from misadventure, mostly by means of adverse drug reactions or even frank error in administration.[82] Even if just anesthesia accidents are considered, and even if it is accepted that the death rate is relatively low—the risk of death directly attributable to anesthesia in the last decades of the twentieth century was estimated to be about 1 in 10, 000[83]—the cumulative total of serious morbidity and mortality over many years and in many countries would be huge. Therefore, it is reasonable to consider whether monitoring is indeed sound from the public health point of view, as well as from that of anesthesia. A number of questions are pertinent. For example, has monitoring beneficially affected the outcome of anesthesia? Some questions are cynical: Do monitors do any good? And, is all they do distract the practitioner? Two other questions are these: Are minimum standards sufficient? And, should an anesthesia practitioner use the minimum number of monitors or more than a minimum? In addition, hospitals had to decide whether they should purchase only a minimal array of monitors or look for more. A great deal of debate was held about such matters. To give a sense of these debates, the discussions that concerned pulse oximetry and outcome of anesthesia and selection of monitors will be reviewed.

Does pulse oximetry improve the outcome of anesthesia?

The Aoyagi device for pulse oximetry was marketed in 1975, and its value was beginning to be recognized in the 1980s. It was clear that hypoxemia could be recognized when a pulse oximeter was used,[84] and use of this monitor soon became universal. Yet Canadians Peter Duncan and Marsha Cohen, among a number of other investigators, concluded in 1991 that its effectiveness still had to be demonstrated.[85] In other words, there was no *statistical* proof that pulse oximetry affected the outcome of monitored anesthesia.

Many anesthesiologists, therefore, thought that a large, controlled, and prospective study would answer the question of outcome. However, it could not be answered by even a large Danish study in which one group of patients was monitored with a pulse oximeter and another group was not. No fewer than 20, 802 patients were enrolled. The results, which were published in 1993,[86, 87] led the authors to conclude that though pulse oximetry could facilitate detection of hypoxemia and was associated with a decrease in the rate of myocardial ischemia, it did not seem to affect the overall rate of postoperative complications. What the study did do was, instead of answering the question of outcome, to set the stage for further debate.

Even that debate was not conclusive, though it is instructive to summarize the main points taken by two protagonists in one debate: John Eichorn, one of the Harvard pioneers but who had moved to the University of Mississippi department, on the one hand, and Frederick Orkin, of Dartmouth Medical School, on the other.

Eichorn's argument[88] was as follows: Prior to the Danish study, anesthesiologists had held that pulse oximetry was "a good thing.". It had attained a de facto standard of excellence. The Danish study failed to reveal significant reduction in the incidence of serious postoperative complications, though a reduction in the incidence of cardiac arrest from 12 cases among the 10, 490 nonmonitored patients to 8 in the 10, 312 monitored patients was suggestive. One problem was to show even a hypothesized moderate benefit of pulse oximetry as being "huge," for anyone who demands scientific proof on the basis of $P<0.05$ would not find it in studies that are less than huge. What is required is to make use of alternative definitions of "truth," such as consensus reached by many anesthesiologists, and to recognize that pulse oximetry is one of several factors that have improved anesthesia care in recent decades. In Eichorn's view, pulse oximetry had become a standard of care regardless of studies such as the Danish one.

Orkin, together with Duncan and Cohen, provided a different perspective. They described this in an editorial,[89] which was published along with Eichorn's. They agreed that soon after its introduction, pulse oximetry had become an integral part of anesthesia care, and that it was generally believed that the detection of hypoxemia it permitted would serve as an early warning of the possibility of serious anesthesia complications. However logical this seemed intuitively, they stated that the validity of the hypothesis had not been demonstrated; it was speculative at best. In addition, over the previous four decades—thus antedating the introduction of pulse oximetry—anesthesia-related mortality had begun to diminish. Now came the Danish study, which showed that pulse oximetry had no apparent effect on patient outcome. Orkin agreed that this study was not large enough to track outcome, for 500, 000 to 1.9 million patients in relatively good health would be required to rigorously demonstrate any efficacy of oximetry on outcome. Orkin and his colleagues referred to points made in 1991 earlier by his two coauthors concerning a slightly different argument.[90] As Eichorn had argued in 1989, prior to the Harvard Standards, the rate of major intraoperative accidents was 0.16 per 10, 000 cases, whereas afterward it was 0.031—a 5.22-fold improvement.[91] In addition, R. L. Keenan reported in 1989 that after pulse oximetry had been adopted, there had been no cardiac arrests attributable to hypoxemia in 31, 000 anesthetics, compared with a rate of 0.67 per 10, 000 from 1969 to 1985.[92] However, these data were not thought to be statistically significant. To make the matter more problematic, there was no basis on which to decide what extent of desaturation is unacceptable. Orkin, Cohen, and Duncan finally concluded that since the true benefit of pulse oximetry is difficult to establish, the possibility of harm should not be overlooked.

In the same year that Eichorn and Orkin presented their arguments, the role of monitoring as assessed from an analysis of closed malpractice insurance claims was discussed.[93] The consensus was that pulse oximetry would have prevented 322 injuries or deaths, or 93% of the total number of complications deemed preventable. This was yet another point to be pondered.

How much should be monitored?

If complete patient safety is the ideal goal of anesthesia, it would seem optimal to use a monitoring device to obtain a record of *each* of the bodily functions that can be monitored. However, this was thought neither feasible nor, in actual practice, necessary. In setting up the original Harvard Standards, the anesthesiologists thought it wise to promulgate *minimum* standards that could be realistically achieved. Even so, some anesthesiologists concluded that more than a minimum was required, while others sought an array that seemed logical.

In 1986, Frank Block argued that anesthesiologists did not monitor enough.[94] He recommended routine monitoring as follows: for breath and heart sounds; blood pressure; ECG; neuromuscular block when any muscle relaxants were given; inspired or expired oxygen fraction; oxygen saturation by pulse oximeter or transcutaneous oxygen tension; the respiratory carbon dioxide waveform; finger pulse plethysmography; respiratory flows and pressure; inspired and expired concentrations of nitrous oxide, volatile anesthetic agents, and nitrogen; oxygen consumption; carbon dioxide production; cardiac output, noninvasively; EEG; evoked potentials; and temperature. This was a large menu. To some extent, Block's opinion was shared by Jack Moyers who, in 1988, asked whether monitoring does indeed affect patient safety.[95] He regretted that there had not always been available monitors for "patient betterment," because the technology of the day made for better practice and better teaching.

At the same time, Boston anesthesiologist Ellison Pierce, a leader in patient safety, held that, while maximum patient safety was the goal and while monitoring instruments had significantly reduced the incidence of anesthetic mishaps, other factors should not be forgotten.[96] Even for high-risk patients, invasive monitoring, accompanied by aggressive treatment, could "considerably" decrease postoperative morbidity and mortality. Similarly, anesthetic mishap resulting in major disability or death could, with relative ease, be eliminated. However, other measures such as effective education and supervision, installation of up-to-date equipment, repeated examination of human error factors, and attention to vigilance by the practitioner should not be forgotten in considering the larger question of how to lessen anesthesia morbidity and mortality.

In view of the difficulty in rigorously attempting to validate monitoring by outcome assessment, it might not seem that a theoretically complete array of monitors is always warranted. By 1988, even Block had become more selective.[97] He noted that every mishap (except for acid-base imbalance) could be detected at a "high level" by one or more monitors. Therefore, one could eliminate those monitors that provided no high-level information, such as the stethoscope and evoked-potential method, and cardiac output instruments. One would also remove those high-level monitors that gave information that was provided by another monitor giving high-level information. The definitive list was as follows: pulse oximeter with quantitative plethysmograph; integrated capnograph, oxygen and nitrogen analyzer; agent-specific halometer; mass spectrometer/Raman scattering and perhaps infrared monitors; autosphygmomanometer; ECG; thermometer; transcutaneous oxygen and carbon dioxide tension monitor; and neuromuscular twitch monitor, plus, as "highly recommended," continuous blood pressure measurement by the finger method.

*   *   *

By 2006, the consensus was that in anesthetic practice, monitoring standards, and use of monitoring devices, had done much to reduce the incidence of adverse events, especially serious disability and death. Monitoring devices helped anesthesiologists achieve complete patient safety. This aspect of monitoring, with the knowledge and technological progress associated with it, had, of course, changed enormously in the 160 years since Henry Bigelow wrote in 1846.[98] The essential purpose of monitoring, however, had not.

Monitoring has been a vital part of the practice of anesthesia, in many ways reflecting the progress, and the refinement, of anesthesia. A review of its development suggests that it will continue to enhance the progress of anesthesia. It is likely to be used in quite remarkable ways: use of automated anesthesia records for trending together with access to previous medical records; supervision of anesthesia in multiple operating room or anesthetizing locations, allowing for telemedicine and remote care; interpretation of evoked responses and of transcranial Doppler studies; blood-glucose concentrations; development of closed-loop feedback systems, to eliminate the human as actuator, including neuromuscular block (concept of servo-anesthesia); and use of alarms, such as false alarms, smart alarms, and ergonomics (i.e., monitor placement, display, audio signals, and noise overload), all overriding human factors. Despite this, the concept remains that the monitor is only as good as the actuator, so that education will be required in order to interpret readings and malfunctions.

Chapter 11

ANESTHESIA AND INTENSIVE CARE

Intensive care has much in common with the practice of anesthesia, and anesthesiologists were involved in it even before it emerged as a separate medical specialty in the 1960s. Anesthesiologists have a natural understanding of intensive, or critical, care because in the operating room, they routinely support the respiration and the circulation of their patients, which is often the essence of intensive care. In the operating room, they induce coma and muscular paralysis, monitor their patients' condition, assess changes in blood-gas and electrolyte concentrations, and take corrective action when necessary. All that is part of intensive care as well. Anesthesia and intensive care touch at many points, so that a discussion of the history of intensive care is appropriate in a history of anesthesia.

The origins of intensive care are twofold: care of surgical patients in the recovery room and care of poliomyelitis patients whose respiratory muscles were paralyzed. As it evolved, intensive care, like anesthesia itself, was influenced by developments in many other fields. The development of intensive care owes much in particular to anesthesiology, biochemistry, biotechnology, electronics, engineering, internal medicine, nursing, space research, and surgery. In this chapter, the evolution of intensive care will be reviewed, and intensive care in three subspecialties will be discussed in order to emphasize certain points in the history of intensive care.

Antecedents of Intensive Care

Patient Care in the Recovery Room

A key concept of intensive care is placing in one locale patients with various surgical and medical problems that require similar therapies. The concept originated in two developments. One was the planning of the enlargement of the infirmary in Newcastle, England, in 1801. Two five-bedded rooms were to be put aside for the care of those patients who were dangerously ill or who had undergone a major surgical operation.[1] The other development was a statement in 1863 by Florence Nightingale, who noted that in some hospitals, "a recess or small room [led] from the operating theatre in which the patients remain until they have recovered . . . from the immediate effects of the operation."[2] Thus one antecedent of intensive care, and of the intensive care unit (ICU), is the postoperative recovery room.

A recovery room next to the operating room of the Johns Hopkins Hospital was opened in July 1923 for Walter Dandy's neurosurgical patients. Thus Dandy might be regarded as being the originator of the ICU.[3] His recovery room and ICU was staffed twenty-four hours a day with special recovery room nurses. This marked the beginning of careful attention to airway care, temperature control, circulatory monitoring, and fluid and electrolyte balance. Other postoperative recovery suites were the combined recovery room and ICU in the surgical hospital of the University of Tübingen directed by Martin Kirschner, who reported on it in 1930,[4] and the post-anesthesia recovery room that John Lundy inaugurated at the Mayo Clinic in 1942.[5] In general, therefore, the ICU concept grew as patients with similar surgical problems were logically placed in one geographic area. This made for efficiency and safety in patient care, and for economy.[6] Recovery rooms became more common in the 1940s because many nurses left for military service.

The similarity in intensive care of patients in the operating room and of patients in the ICU[7] is another factor, for the ICU environment is in many respects familiar to anesthesiologists. The ICU is designed to enable health care staff to perform tasks that have a common purpose and require similar equipment. Some of the problems treated there are similar to those treated surgically, and some of these problems are often solved by use of anesthetic knowledge and techniques, such as tracheal intubation and ventilation and sedative and even paralytic drugs.

Also relevant is the view that patients with similar pathophysiological disturbances are best treated by individuals who have special knowledge and skills. These include anesthesiologists. Concentrating therapeutic expertise in one locality is efficient and logical and good use of specialized health care resources. This was recognized as early as 1898, when Pierre-Constant Budin, a Paris obstetrician, recommended a special department for "weaklings" so premature infants might be looked after more effectively.[8]

Care of Patients with Respiratory Disturbances

The idea of a dedicated area where special knowledge and skills were applied influenced the treatment and the nursing care of patients with poliomyelitis or disorders of respiration. In poliomyelitis, the depressed respiration requires intensive care, and it was the initiative of Danish anesthesiologist Bjorn Ibsen (fig.11.1) in 1952 in applying his anesthesia-related knowledge and skills to the care of poliomyelitis patients that was the true beginning of what would become known as intensive care.

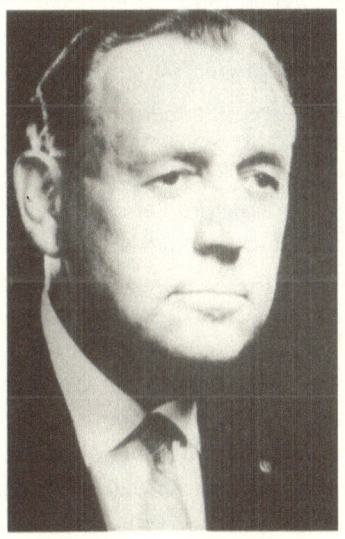

Fig.11.1. Bjorn Ibsen (1915-2007)

Bjorn Ibsen graduated from the University of Copenhagen in 1940. Earlier that, Ibsen gave anesthetics in a small provincial hospital, using a bag filled with 100 ml ether, a mouth opener, and tongue forceps. Anyone was permitted to give an anesthetic, and luxuries such as oxygen and suction facilities were not on anyone's shopping list. Things were little less primitive in the hospital in Jutland, where Ibsen worked next, and by the time he had worked his way up to the Rigshospitalet in Copenhagen, he realized that anesthesia was vital to success in surgery. Ibsen decided to learn more about anesthesia, which he did during a year at the Massachusetts General Hospital under Henry Beecher. He returned to Copenhagen with new ideas about anesthesia, and his approach to anesthesia was furthered by attendance at a World Health Organization course given by Ralph Waters and Stuart Cullen. Then, in 1952, Ibsen was consulted regarding the management of patients with paralytic poliomyelitis, in many of whom treatment with the iron lung was failing. He advised that patients be ventilated with positive pressure through a tracheal tube. This turned the situation around and demonstrated what anesthetic techniques could do for patients with respiratory failure. Ibsen gave a clear demonstration of the potential that anesthesia had outside the operating room. (Photograph by permission of *American Journal of Respiratory and Critical Care Medicine*, fig.4 in 1998;157:S114-122.)

Ibsen's innovative approach in Copenhagen came about as follows. From 1929 until the early 1950s, patients with bulbar poliomyelitis were provided respiratory support in units supplied with the Drinker tank respirator,[9] or the iron lung. Though these units did provide intensive care, the arrangement had disadvantages. Nursing was difficult, respiratory support was not always adequate, and in the immobilized patient, an increased tension of carbon dioxide in the blood (hypercarbia, hypercapnia) often occurred. That last problem was lethal during the serious outbreak of poliomyelitis in Copenhagen in 1952, which affected nearly three thousand patients,[10] and which overwhelmed the available facilities. Initially, the iron lung was used in treating patients with respiratory paralysis, but twenty-seven of thirty-one patients who were so treated died. At that point, Ibsen was asked to help reverse this dismal trend. Immediately recognizing the basic problem, he radically changed the way the patients were treated. Thinking in anesthesia terms, he advocated tracheal intubation and artificial respiration, at first by hand via a Waters to-and-fro soda-lime canister (see fig.7.24) and a breathing bag and, later, by means of mechanical ventilators.[11] Those methods were customary in the care of some surgical patients, so Ibsen recruited all the Copenhagen anesthesiologists, medical students, and anesthesiologists from other countries who were studying in the World Health Organization Anesthesiology Center in Copenhagen to work in four-hour shifts in order to ventilate the patients. He also asked C. G. Engstrom, in Sweden, to bring his ventilator to help in the management of the epidemic.

This therapeutic innovation wrought a sea change in the treatment of bulbar poliomyelitis, and it inaugurated modern intensive care. Ibsen's contributions also show how a single anesthesiologist could shape intensive care—and redirect the thinking in anesthesia and medicine in general that led to the widespread adoption of mechanical ventilators.

The significance of Ibsen's initiative cannot be exaggerated. Patients in a tank respirator died mainly because depressed breathing caused hypercarbia and because secretions blocked the respiratory tract; moreover, the existence of hypercarbia was masked by the normal pink skin color that oxygen administration deceptively maintained. The critical need in management, therefore, was to ensure adequate ventilation. Accordingly, the carbon dioxide concentrations in the blood had to be monitored, and appropriate equipment and analytical methods had to be found. Measurement of arterial blood-gas concentrations was from then on a routine part of intensive care—as, of course, were many other special investigations in ICUs in due course.

Ibsen's innovative therapy was soon shown to be beneficial: fewer patients were dying. In an article in the *Lancet* in 1953, Ibsen showed that respiratory inadequacy could, and should, be managed according to simple principles of anesthesia.[12] So could other medical conditions besides poliomyelitis, in which the respiratory center or the respiratory musculature is affected. These include chronic obstructive pulmonary disease, myasthenia gravis, Guillain-Barré syndrome, myelitis, barbiturate poisoning, potassium depletion, head injury, and tetanus. A basic therapeutic principle applied to the management of all these disorders: if a disease impairs respiration, it should be treated according to established principles of respiratory therapy. This principle came to be applied to the intensive care of any organ insufficiency, and is a basic one in critical care.

Developments in Surgery

Developments in surgery were antecedents of intensive care. Chest surgery became more common in the 1930s, and anesthetists made increasing use of ventilators, especially as use of cyclopropane and curare became widespread. Ventilators were commonly used during the Second World War, and then in the 1950s on, with the Copenhagen poliomyelitis epidemic in 1952 and the frequency of heart surgery in the latter 1950s making their use essential. Well-known ventilators include the Air-Shields, Beaver, Bennett, Bird, Blease, Dräger, Engstrom, Jefferson, Manley, Monaghan, Morch, and Radcliffe.[13] As a result, surgeons and anesthesiologists became accustomed to using ventilators, both in the operating room and in the ICU.

The value of intensive, or critical, care was confirmed by military experience, as in the conflicts in Korea, Vietnam, Afghanistan, and Iraq. Triage and specialized care in forward hospitals benefited the care of soldiers with hemorrhagic shock, sepsis, and acute renal failure, quite apart from injury of vital organs. Intensive care improved the management of trauma and burns. Early treatment near the scene of injury and removal of the patient to a tertiary care center having an ICU then became general in civilian practice also.

The increasingly complex surgical operations of the 1950s onward also made care in ICUs necessary. The practice, however, took time to establish. Even as late as 1953, patients in some centers sometimes went straight from the operating room to their private room or the surgical ward,[14] but this was obviously not satisfactory, especially after heart surgery, so heart surgeons at first kept their critically ill patients in recovery rooms. That, however, increased the work of the recovery room nurses. The use of special nurses was a partial solution, particularly as in the early period of cardiac surgery, ventilators were not standard equipment in post-anesthesia recovery rooms. Gradually, a core of full-time nurses with intensive care experience developed, and in time, some ICUs were dedicated to the care of surgical patients.

The Growth of ICUs

Care of surgical as well as medical patients in ICUs thus became standard practice beginning in the late 1950s and early 1960s. In the United States, the first ICU staffed around the clock by full-time physicians was located in the Baltimore City Hospitals,[15] though priority in the world as whole was claimed by the Gentofte Hospital in Coopenhagen, where a unit was opened in 1953.[16] Many different specialties besides general surgery and internal medicine—such as pediatrics, respirology, and cardiology—made use of ICUs, and care of the critically ill in an ICU became accepted as "a modern necessity."[17] It was soon clear that ICU care was beneficial: the mortality of ICU patients was lower than in patients with similar conditions treated in other part of the hospital.[18] This resulted from a number of factors: ICU direction by a full-time intensivist,[19, 20, 21, 22] staffing by specially trained and skilled nurses,[23] an effective and appropriate protocol,[24] and effective coordination between physicians and nurses.[25]

In the last quarter of the twentieth century, intensive care attracted much attention, in education and research, as well as in clinical practice. Embracing a great deal of medicine, ICUs were suited to the treatment of many different conditions, and specialties like pediatrics and cardiology developed ICUs of their own. While the clinical successes of ICUs are obvious, with function restored in critically ill patients, ethical issues became more critical as patients often seemed to be kept between life and death by sophisticated technological aids. As Ibsen put it in 1975, "At the beginning of intensive therapy it was a problem to keep the patient alive—today it has become a problem to let him die."[26]

Intensive care has evolved as the physicians who have seen its essential value overcome a variety of challenges. To illustrate some of the variations in the evolution of intensive care and in the approaches to care of different types of disorders, three types of ICUs will be discussed: pediatric ICUs, respiratory ICUs, and coronary care ICUs.

The Pediatric Intensive Care Unit

The origins of intensive care of infants and children go back to the second half of the 1940s.[27] It developed as five areas of medicine that were established in the 1950s grew: neonatology and newborn intensive care, adult respiratory intensive care, pediatric general surgery, pediatric cardiac surgery, and pediatric anesthesiology.

The first ICU dedicated to pediatrics was opened in 1955 in Gothenburg, Sweden; though in 1903, Julius Hess had established a center for the care of premature infants at Chicago's Michael Reese Hospital. These early initiatives illustrate the human virtue of giving special care to the weaker brethren—even if it sometimes was honored more in the breach. A second pediatric ICU was opened, in Stockholm, by Hans Feychting in 1961, before the trend to adult ICUs had become widespread.

Many pediatric anesthesiologists took leading roles in directing pediatric ICUs from the start. Among them were Ian McDonald and John Stocks in Melbourne (1963), Jackson Rees in Liverpool (1964), Jack Downes in Philadelphia (1967), Stephan Kampschulte in Pittsburgh (1969), James Gilman in New Haven (1969), David Todres in Boston (1971), and Alan Conn in Toronto (1971). The leading role that pediatric anesthesiologists played was a result of their everyday concerns with airway and cardiopulmonary control, which are so frequently the main concerns in ICUs as well.

Mastery of the fundamental knowledge and technology base and of technical skills was an essential, as it was in the development of adult ICUs. After the Second World War several anesthesiologists established this base of knowledge and skills and techniques, including Robert Smith in Boston, Margaret van Deming in Philadelphia, Digby Leigh and Ronald Stephen in Montreal, Robert Cope in London, as well as Rees and Conn.

However, the knowledge base that was necessary for pediatric intensive care to formally develop had to include the broader field of pediatrics itself. Basic research in several areas built up this knowledge: neonatal physiology, including the maternal, fetal, and transitional circulation; blood group abnormalities; fluid and electrolyte metabolism; temperature control; and neonatal asphyxia and such conditions as the respiratory distress syndrome.

Pediatric anesthesiologists also helped to build up some of the knowledge. In 1953, Virginia Apgar, of New York, described a method of evaluating the condition of the neonate immediately after birth.[28] Known as the Apgar score, it proved of great and lasting clinical value (see also chapter 14). In 1959, Arthur Bull, working with South African pediatrician Patrick Smythe, showed that neonates with tetanus could be treated in adult fashion by tracheostomy, neuromuscular block, and mechanical ventilation,[29] and showed that ventilation of the neonate was feasible. In 1963 and 1964, anesthesiologist Paul Swyer and Maria Delivoria-Papadopoulos and Henry Levinson, in Toronto, ventilated premature newborns suffering from severe asphyxia of respiratory distress syndrome.[30] Another advance by an anesthesiologist was continuous positive airway pressure,[31] which George Gregory used in treating infants with respiratory distress syndrome beginning in the 1970s.

Surgical concerns also influenced the development of ICU care of infants and children. After World War II, pediatric surgery comprised a wide variety of operations, including those encroaching on vital areas such as the thorax and cranium. Advances in cardiac surgery were, of course, particularly dramatic, and some of those are noted in chapter 14. Operations for congenital lesions like esophageal atresia and tracheoesophageal fistula lack the drama of heart surgery, but results of surgery for those conditions also were improved by intensive care.

By the end of the 1950s, multidisciplinary ICUs had standardized the care of infants and children of all ages.

Critical care continued to develop. In 1981, a section on pediatric critical care was formed within the Society of Critical Care Medicine; and in 1987, a committee was struck by the American Board of Pediatrics with a view to offering certification in this sub-subspecialty.[32] In fifty years, pediatric intensive care had developed to a remarkable degree, and pediatric ICUs continued to provide areas where critically ill infants and children could receive highly specialized care.

The Respiratory Care Unit

Pediatric ICUs deal with children with a wide variety of pathophysiological conditions, both medical and surgical. In contrast, attention in respiratory ICUs is focused primarily on one: respiratory insufficiency.

Before the poliomyelitis epidemic in Denmark in 1952, the term *respiratory insufficiency* traditionally conjured up visions of asthma, pneumonia, and chronic lung disease on the one hand, and of heart failure on the other. Treatment was based on oxygen therapy and drugs that, apart from morphine for sedation, were largely inefficacious. Ibsen's innovative treatment for poliomyelitis changed that picture—for poliomyelitis itself, with the visions of cohorts of patients dying in "iron lungs," but also for conditions besides lung and heart disease with respiratory insufficiency.

Several things became clear after the poliomyelitis pandemic of the early 1950s. One was the fact that respiratory insufficiency, if not treated promptly according to the principles of respiratory care (which are common to anesthesia care), was frequently lethal. The earlier form of poliomyelitis treatment underlined the inefficacy of respiratory support in a tank or a cuirass respirator, the danger of lack of recognition of hypercarbia (even if oxygen is administered), and the danger of less than vigorously clearing the airway of secretions. In Denmark from 1934 to 1944, when cuirass respirators were being used in the treatment of patients with respiratory insufficiency and bulbar disease, among seventy-six patients, the mortality was 80 percent.[33] After the poliomyelitis outbreak, when tracheostomy and positive-pressure ventilation were instituted, it was reduced to 40 percent, and to 26 percent late in the epidemic.

However, ventilator treatment was not free of danger.[34] In the early days, disconnect alarms were not built into the ventilator system, and a break in the connection between the ventilator and the paralyzed patient might not be noticed if a nurse was not present. And in those days, there were no units in which full-time one-to-one nursing coverage was the standard of care. More than one patient died in such circumstances.

Physicians concerned about the treatment of respiratory insufficiency, therefore, stressed the need for units staffed over twenty-four hours by dedicated coverage by nurses and specialist physicians. Respiratory units were established soon after the 1952 poliomyelitis epidemic, one of the first respiratory units being at Oxford's Radcliffe Infirmary.[35] That unit concentrated on poliomyelitis and neurological disorders such as lower motor neuron disease. Such conditions present problems that are not common in other diseases, and the necessary treatment is highly specialized, as, for example, with tetanus.[36] Hence the rationale for treatment in a special unit.

After the 1952 poliomyelitis pandemic, many respiratory care units began to deal with cases of bulbar poliomyelitis. However, following universal use of the Salk vaccine, poliomyelitis virtually vanished in the Western world, and respiratory units dealt with many other diseases in which the respiration was affected.[37, 38, 39, 40] Over the next decades, much was learned about respiratory insufficiency. Clinical practice benefited from sound new ways of preventing and treating acute respiratory insufficiency, while research has established a firm knowledge base and teaching has spread ideas about optimum care of the patient with respiratory insufficiency.

The Coronary Care Unit

As critical care developed as a special field, the increase in knowledge and technological sophistication made it a dynamic one. It began in a small way, adhering to simple founding principles, and evolved into refined practices that greatly benefited patient care. This dynamic aspect of evolution is evident in the approach to intensive care as formulated by cardiologists, and the evolution of coronary care units (CCUs) illustrates this point.

Just as drowning stimulated resuscitation in the eighteenth century, so in the twentieth century, coronary heart disease honed the practice of intensive care. Just as resuscitation was developed in order to save lives in the eighteenth century, so coronary intensive care was developed to save lives in the twentieth. How did this come about?

With the lessons that were learned in the evolution of cardiopulmonary resuscitation, or CPR (see also chapter 13), Cleveland cardiac surgeon Claude Beck, who had defibrillated a boy in 1947, was justified in saying, even in dramatic terms, that "the veil of mysteries is being lifted from heart conditions, and the dead are being brought back to life."[41] This veil was lifted higher, and the belief that the dead were being brought back to life confirmed, by the experience that was gained from coronary intensive care.

In the 1940s and 1950s, many "heart attacks" were fatal. Because surgeons like Beck would not tolerate high mortality rates in conditions they were treating surgically, it was logical that internists and cardiologists should not accept death rates that were associated with passive management. So they became more aggressive in managing acute myocardial infarction and other diseases.[42] CCUs were then introduced. Their value is apparent for the estimate suggesting that in the United States, they saved nineteen thousand lives each year and were responsible for approximately 13.5 percent of the decline in mortality from coronary disease between 1968 and 1976.[43] The history of CCUs shows how, in just a few decades, attention that was focused on a serious epidemiological problem greatly diminished it—to say nothing of the extension of life among countless individuals.

How the incidence of sudden death from acute myocardial infarction might be reduced was asked by Desmond Julian in Edinburgh soon after modern CPR practice was introduced in 1960 (see also chapter 13). Because neither open-chest and defibrillation nor closed-chest compression and defibrillation seemed entirely satisfactory, Julian and his colleagues considered a more global approach.[44] They argued that many cases of cardiac arrest associated with acute myocardial ischemia could be treated successfully if all medical, nursing, and auxiliary staff were trained in closed-chest cardiac massage, and if the cardiac rhythm was monitored by an electrocardiogram linked to an alarm system. Appropriate apparatus would not be prohibitively expensive if the patients were admitted to special intensive care units. Such units should be staffed by suitably experienced people over twenty-four hours.[45]

Julian's concept was then widely applied in the monitoring of myocardial infarction patients. CCUs were established in the next two years in Kansas City,[46] Philadelphia,[47] and Toronto,[48] and soon in virtually every community hospital in North America.[49]

Since cardiac arrest is frequently preceded by serious arrhythmia, continuous EKG monitoring was initially emphasized in CCUs. This was the first principle of CCU management. The second was CPR, which had just been formulated. A third was to place cardiac drugs and specialized monitoring and resuscitative equipment near patients. Two other key principles included the admission of patients with similar medical diagnoses such as acute myocardial infarction to a special coronary care facility, and their care by nurses who were specifically trained in coronary care and in recognizing serious arrhythmias and who were authorized to initiate resuscitation on their own should a physician not be immediately available. The importance of this focused approach cannot be exaggerated. The CCU has been regarded as "the single most important advance in the treatment of acute myocardial infarction."[50]

As technology developed, CCUs became more expensive, and their efficacy was questioned. At first, the mortality in CCU-treated patients didn't seem much lower than that of those treated in other parts of the hospital, but as CCU management became more finely tuned, mortality did seem to decrease. The mortality among patients with acute myocardial infarction who were treated in a regular ward was found to be 26 percent, as opposed to 7 percent among those treated in the CCU.[51] One estimate showed that CCUs save approximately twenty thousand lives each year in the United States, and accounted for some 13 percent of the decline in mortality from coronary disease between 1968 and 1976.[52]

*   *   *

The development of intensive care owes much to the development of anesthesia, of anesthesia subspecialties, and of resuscitation medicine, which, as noted in chapter 13, is closely related to anesthesia. It also paralleled the development of medicine. Though these various branches of human endeavor have been shaped by the extraordinary role of technology, they also indicate the intensive way in which challenging medical and surgical conditions became managed. In both these respects, anesthesia has had a central place.

Chapter 12

Anesthesiologists and Pain Management

Pain is as old as humankind, and over the centuries, numerous types of healers endeavored to relieve it using various regimens. After the advent of anesthesia in 1846, those healers included anesthesia practitioners. At first, they relieved pain just in surgical patients in operating rooms, though occasionally, chloroform[1] and ether[2] were used in the treatment of various medical conditions. Interest in the treatment of pain grew in the twentieth century, along with a growing interest in nerve blocks; and after World War II, anesthesiologists were more active in managing pain relief in patients outside the operating room. They helped women in labor, cancer patients, and patients with chronic pain that was caused by a variety of conditions. Pain medicine became a subspecialty within anesthesia. Today, anesthesiology and pain management are closely linked.

The pain-relieving role of anesthesiologists outside the operating room, however, came relatively late in the development of anesthesia. In the nineteenth century, practitioners did not even make use of morphine specifically to obtund pain in their surgical patients, relying on inhalational agents to achieve analgesia, as well as hypnosis and muscle relaxation; and after cocaine was introduced in 1884,[3] it was surgeons and not anesthetists who seized on this new anodyne. Not until after the First World War did anesthetists begin using local anesthetics, first as part of the anesthetic technique and much later for the separate purpose of relieving pain outside the operating room. Even before the Second World War, few anesthetists spent much time on the separate treatment of pain outside the operating room. That began to change only after the war when, fortuitously, new local anesthetic drugs and opioids were developed. Then the practice of anesthesia began to include the practice of pain medicine. Therefore, in this chapter on anesthesia and pain management, the emphasis will be on the ways anesthesiologists managed pain from 1946 onward. First, however, the treatment of pain up to the end of World War II will first be summarized.

Early Concepts of Pain and Its Management

The Legacy of René Descartes

René Descartes, the French philosopher and mathematician, put forward ideas on pain in 1664,[4] and for the next three centuries, they influenced ideas on pain management. Pain impulses were thought to be transmitted unchanged from the periphery or the viscera along specific pain fibers to a pain center in the brain, where the pain was perceived. The so-called specificity theory of pain engendered the belief that tissue injury activated pain receptors and that pain impulses sped up a specific spinal pathway to the brain, and after cocaine analgesia was discovered, it seemed logical to inject local anesthetics near nerves, or even by surgically cutting them. The governing concept was that of a one-to-one relationship between injury and the resulting pain.[5]

This concept of pain and of its treatment can be illustrated by the work of George Crile, a Cleveland surgeon, early in the twentieth century. He formulated the principle of anoci-association,[6] according to which the onset of pain and accompanying surgical shock could be prevented by infiltrating the operative site and its nervous supply with local anesthetic before performing a scheduled surgical operation. New York and Johns Hopkins surgeon William Halsted was another surgeon who used cocaine in this manner.

Though a few anesthetists did have some concerns about pain in their surgical patients at this time, none followed the examples of surgeons like Augustus Bier and Rudolph Matas in relieving pain with cocaine or its successors (see chapter 4). New York anesthetist James Tayloe Gwathmey, for example, expressed concern about pain in surgical patients, but wrote in the context of premedication. This, he wrote, eased immediate postoperative pain, as well as reassuring nervous patients, reducing the necessary dose of anesthetic, lessening the amount of mucus in the throat, and diminishing the liability to shock; it also gave the patient "a happier exit from the influence of the anesthetic."[7] Even this leader of American anesthesia failed to make use of cocaine or procaine specifically to relieve pain.

Concepts of Pain and Its Management after World War I

A new perspective on pain became apparent in the 1920s with the work of
the French surgeon Gaston Labat. As noted in chapter 4, he taught regional
anesthesia at the Mayo Clinic in 1921 and 1922 before moving to New York.
He showed anesthetists, as well as surgeons, how to use nerve blocks to treat
pain in various disorders and in the postoperative state. Labat emphasized
variations in patients' sensitivity to pain and stated that "with the combined
narcotics it is possible to equalize the different expressions of pain and bring
them down to the lowest convenient term."[8] As founding president, in
1923, of the original American Society of Regional Anesthesia, when he was
practicing in New York, Labat spread the word about regional anesthesia in
the management of pain.[9]

     In the 1930s and 1940s, physicians used a number of agents and
techniques in treating pain, in addition to local anesthetic drugs and standard
nerve blocks. Swertlow, in 1926, injected alcohol into the upper thoracic
part of the sympathetic chain to relieve the pain of angina pectoris,[10] and
J. C. White reported similar treatment in 1928.[11] In 1930, René Leriche,
another surgeon, described the treatment of causalgia (phantom limb pain)
by injecting procaine.[12] In the following year, Archile Dogliotti, the Italian
surgeon, reported injecting alcohol into the subarachnoid space to relieve
the pain of cancer and other conditions.[13] In Liverpool, England, in 1934,
Robert J. Minnitt devised a self-administration technique for women to use
nitrous oxide and air during labor.[14] Among those physicians who sought to
add pain management to their duties in anesthesia can be added John Lundy
and R. Charles Adams at the Mayo Clinic. Lundy gave sodium thiopental
in patients with migraine and with metastases,[15] injected alcohol around the
fifth cranial nerve to treat trigeminal neuralgia[16] and intrathecally to relieve
cancer pain.[17] Adams used sodium amytal, as well as morphine, to treat
patients with cancer pain.[18]

     Evidently, the belief that pain, as the consequence of tissue damage,
could be treated by directing specific attention to its perceived nervous
origin still flourished up to World War II. However, a few anesthetists who
used nerve blocks did take a new approach by setting up clinics specifically
to facilitate the management for that purpose. They included Philip
Woodbridge in 1930,[19] Henry Ruth in 1934,[20] and Emery Rovenstine and
H. Wertheim in 1941.[21] The concept of the pain clinic took hold, and
it was more fully developed by John Bonica after the end of the Second
World War.

Postwar Developments in Pain Relief

The Development of Multidisciplinary Pain Clinics

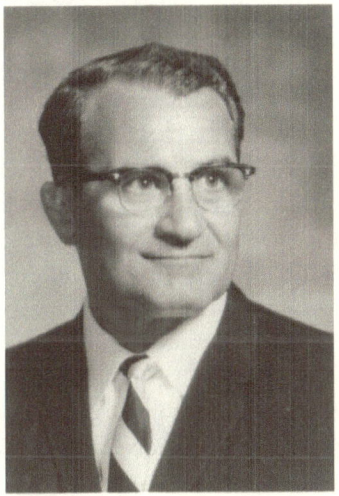

Fig. 12.1. John Bonica (1917-1994)

John Bonica was born on an island off Sicily. His family moved to New York in 1928. His father died in 1932, and Bonica shined shoes and sold newspapers and fruit and vegetables to fund his education; and as a student in Marquette University School of Medicine, he wrestled professionally as the Masked Marvel and Johnny "Bull" Walker. An eighteen-month residency gave him credibility when he was appointed to head up anesthesia in the Madigan Army Medical Center in Fort Lewis, Washington during the war. There, Bonica became interested in regional block and in pain relief. He developed his interest and his skills further when he became director of anesthesia in Tacoma, Washington. He set up a residency training program and a clinical research program in regional pain relief. Bonica was also interested in regional anesthesia in obstetrics. As founding professor and chairman of the anesthesia department at the University of Washington in 1960, he opened a multidisciplinary pain clinic. Bonica played an enormous role in pain medicine, writing the key textbook *The Management of Pain* and serving as founding and honorary president of the International Association for the Study of Pain. In his work on pain, Bonica demonstrated a dimension of the role that anesthesiologists play outside as well as in the operating room.

As an anesthesiologist in the United States Army in World War II, John Bonica (fig. 12.1) saw many patients with painful conditions. Though nerve blocks for conditions such as causalgia often helped, in more complex problems of pain, they did not. Because the sparse information about chronic pain in the medical literature was widely dispersed, Bonica was handicapped when working on his own. Even consultation with colleagues in other specialties was time-consuming and inefficient. However, group meetings with his colleagues were much more productive. He would present cases for discussion in the traditional manner, and the insight he thus gained led him to develop the team concept of the management of chronic pain.

After the war, Bonica put his ideas into practice. The multidisciplinary pain clinic was one outcome of his thinking.[22] Advice and recommendations from more than a single physician would be part of a therapeutic plan. Bonica realized that pain was more than a local, organic disturbance, and that it was a symptom of a disorder or distress in a patient as a whole individual. He stressed the inadequacy of pain relief, which he attributed in part to a lack of understanding of the mechanism and nature of pain. Bonica and others who were concerned about the treatment of pain concluded that physicians looking after medical patients did not know as much as they should about the treatment of pain. The treatment of pain was inadequate, even in hospitals.[23] Conventional ideas failed to fully explain the nature and transmission, as well as the treatment, of pain, while the group meetings of Bonica and his colleagues were fruitful. The discussions that Bonica had with his colleagues in group meetings furthered his convictions, and the concept of the multidisciplinary and interdisciplinary team for the management of chronic pain arose.

In 1946, Bonica formed a multidisciplinary facility at the Tacoma General Hospital in Tacoma, Washington.[24] His team comprised an anesthesiologist, a neurosurgeon, an orthopaedist, and a psychiatrist, each with a special interest in the management of pain. Each specialist gave a slightly different viewpoint on a patient's problem, and discussion yielded consensus on diagnosis and treatment; no longer was the patient seen through one pair of eyes. Nerve blocks remained a central part of the anesthesiologist's work, but the psychotherapeutic perspective and the emphasis on rehabilitation made up for what an anesthesiologist working alone could not provide.

Bonica's concept proved sound, and over the next few years, similar clinics were founded elsewhere. In the United States, F. A. D. Alexander at the Veterans Administration Hospital in McKinney, Texas, started one in 1947[25] and W. K. Livingstone and F. Haugen inaugurated another at the University of Oregon in Portland in 1951.[26] In England, where the first pain clinic was set up by B. G. B. Lucas in 1947,[27] neurosurgeons and neurologists frequently shared the work with anaesthetists, and they too considered the whole patient, an approach that lay at the heart of the multidisciplinary concept. J. Penman, for example, writing on the treatment of chronic pain as a result of his experience with 275 patients with tic douloureux, advised that "doctors who relieve such should study the personalities of their patients before treatment, try to pick out those who are attached to their pain and be ready to deal themselves with subsequent emotional disturbance."[28] Multidisciplinary clinics enhanced the management of patients with chronic pain.[29]

Many pain clinics were organized and run by anesthesiologists. This was logical, for their training, knowledge, and skills gave anesthesiologists an unrivalled command of some of the more important modalities of pain management. As Seattle anesthesiologist Brian Ready pointed out in 1988, anesthesiologists are familiar with the pharmacology of analgesics, they customarily provide pain relief in the postoperative period, they are knowledgeable about pain and its transmission, and they are skilled in using techniques of intervention such as nerve and epidural and subarachnoid blocks.[30] Pain clinics greatly expanded the role of anesthesiologists in managing pain.

Bonica's experience with chronic pain made him the leader in this new field. He provided sound advice. He stressed the need for physicians who treated patients with chronic pain to remember that nerve blocks were not necessarily the only diagnostic and therapeutic tools, and he warned against anesthesiologists being cornered into the role of a technician who was expected to do no more than perform a technical procedure. His work ultimately led to the founding of societies and journals that were directed to stimulating the growth of knowledge about pain, such as the International Association for the Study of Pain (IASP), founded in 1974, and *Pain*, which began publication the following year.

Bonica realized that part of the problem was the lack of knowledge about the management of pain, and in his magnum opus of 1953, he endeavored to correct this. His seminal textbook, *The Management of Pain*,[31] was a comprehensive volume that filled some of the voids in the knowledge about pain that had hampered management. It corrected assumptions that weakened the approaches that so many anesthetists took to the treatment of pain and stimulated an interest in pain and its mechanisms and treatment. Bonica was followed by numerous other anesthesiologists in devoting themselves to pain relief and conducting studies of pain and analgesia.

The Understanding and Treatment of Pain in the 1960s and 1970s

Further progress in the understanding of pain was made in the 1960s and 1970s. New ideas were developed about pain and its management, and these influenced anesthesiologists in their approach to the relief of pain.

As Ronald Melzack, a Montreal psychologist, noted, the Cartesian view of injury, pain impulses, and a pain center, followed by treatment directed at what was thought to be the site of the cause, was simplistic and also erroneous.[32] Newer ideas were needed. While interest in modalities such as acupuncture and marijuana was maintained, in the scientific environment of the twentieth century, greater interest was generated by the innovative theory of the gate control of pain, which Melzack and his colleague Patrick Wall proposed in 1965.[33]

The gate theory, discussed below, renewed interest in the study and treatment of pain, but anesthesiologists found that their day-to-day management of pain in the operating room was influenced more by three other advances in the management of pain. The first was the development of new local anesthetic agents. The second was the introduction of patient-controlled analgesia (PCA), which, under the supervision of anesthesiologists and nurses, enabled patients themselves to be responsible for pain relief. The other advance, which originated in research by neuroscientists, was the practice of administering opioids centrally, or neuraxially, by subarachnoid and epidural injection. Progress with respect to opioids is discussed in chapter 9, and therefore, only the points that bear on day-to-day pain management with local anesthetics and opioids are considered here.

The Gate Control Theory of Pain

In emphasizing the need for the multidisciplinary approach to the treatment of chronic pain, Bonica was ahead of his time in believing that his patients suffered pain not simply from a physical cause. W. K. Livingston, in a book on pain mechanisms in 1943,[34] and W. Noordenbos, in another in 1959,[35] realized with Bonica that pain did not result from a wholly organic cause of pain. Pain occurs in a number of ways. It may occur in a bone that is obviously broken, but it may also occur, as causalgia, in a limb that had been amputated and is no longer part of the body. In contrast, pain may be surprisingly absent, as in the wounded or lobotomized individuals. However, none of the mechanisms that had been proposed up to then could explain all the various aspects of pain; and none could integrate all the various clinical, physiological, and psychological findings that might characterize the occurrence of pain. It was such inconsistencies and inadequacies in the management of pain that led to the formulation of the gate control theory of pain.

The gate control theory was a forward step because the ideas of Melzack and Wall on modulation of inputs in the spinal cord and on the dynamic role of the brain with respect to pain processes explained the contribution of factors that affected pain such as psychological therapy and acupuncture. They emphasized, as others had not, the role of the central nervous system in the perception of pain. Their theory marked a paradigmatic shift in our understanding of pain.

Simplified, the basis of the gate control theory of pain is as follows. Pain impulses are transmitted from the periphery to three systems in the spinal cord: the substantia gelatinosa of the dorsal horn of the spinal cord, the nerve fibers in the cord that project toward the brain, and the first central transmission (or T) cells in the dorsal horn of the cord. The substantia gelatinosa acts as a gate control in modulating afferent patterns before they can influence the T cells, the afferent patterns in part activate selective brain processes that influence the gate control, and the T cells stimulate mechanisms that are responsible for response and perception. Whether pain occurs is determined by the interactions among these several systems. The "gate" may be closed by the activity of non-nociceptive cells and inhibits further transmission of impulses up to the pain-perceiving brain, or if the "army" of pain impulses is strong enough, the hypothetical gate is opened to allow them to pass up to the brain and so effect action if this is warranted.

In essence, pain is thought of not as a single ring of a central bell, but as an ongoing process. Nor is the action all one-way, for the brain may transmit impulses peripherally to close the gate if this appears to be necessary. The gate control theory was an advance because it moved attention, and explanations, away from purely peripheral factors to a consideration of the brain and the dorsal horns of the spinal cord as essential components in pain. The emphasis on central nervous systems in the gate control theory meant that pain would no longer be thought of in terms of peripheral factors; central factors are important as well.

For anesthesiologists, the gate control theory explained much about pain that was not understood before, but it did not affect their practical management of pain in the way that Bonica's concept of multidisciplinary pain clinics did. Similarly, the three other developments of this period did make a great deal of difference to their daily work.

New Local Anesthetic Agents

Swedish chemists and pharmacologists, in association with the pharmaceutical industry, followed up on the successful synthesis of lidocaine in 1943[36] by synthesizing several other local anesthetics. Beginning in the 1950s, improved methods of studying the physiology of nerve conduction made it possible to evaluate the effects of local anesthetic agents on isolated nerves.[37] New agents that were used included chlorprocaine in 1952, mepivacaine (1956), prilocaine (1959), bupivacaine (1963), and etidocaine (1971).[38] Ropivacaine followed in 1991.[39] The availability of so many more local anesthetic drugs, together with the newer understanding of nerve transmission and how that might be blocked, now made it possible for anesthesiologists to vary the management of pain, to treat pain more effectively, and to perform regional nerve blocks more efficiently.

Patient-Controlled Analgesia (PCA)

In the same year that Melzack and Wall enunciated their new concept, Philip Sechzer conceived the idea of permitting patients to control the analgesic regimen themselves.[40] He was interested in applying operant conditioning techniques to measuring pain and pain relief, and it was a logical extension of this idea to permit a patient in pain to press an analgesic-demand button to obtund the

pain stimulus by means of an injection of morphine or meperidine.[41] It was also
an extension of the principle of self-administration analgesia that Minnitt had
formulated for women in labor in 1934.[42] Indeed, neither the idea of patients in
pain taking the responsibility for self-medication nor the idea of patients receiving
frequent doses of opiates was new in the 1960s. In 1952, obstetrician T. N. A.
Jeffcoate and his Liverpool colleagues introduced the practice of continuous
analgesia with relatively large doses of meperidine,[43] and in 1963, B. B. Roe
showed that small intravenous doses of opioids gave more effective pain relief,
and at lower total dosage, than did conventional intramuscular regimens.[44]
What was new was the ready application of the idea to clinical practice using
a computerized delivery system that made for precision and safety. Sechzer's
patient-controlled analgesic-demand apparatus in 1966[45] initiated an approach
to postoperative pain that anesthesiologists eventually came to used in virtually
all major hospitals.

Other physicians besides Sechzer had conceived similar ideas at about this
time, though for practical reasons, they did not begin to publish until the 1970s.
In 1970, Liverpool obstetrician James Scott described a patient-controlled
technique with intravenous morphine to relieve the pain of labor.[46] In 1970
also, anesthesiologist W. H. Forrest and his colleagues described a more complex
piece of apparatus, though using the same principle of self-administration.[47]
And in 1971, Michael Keeri-Szanto, an anesthesiologist in London, Ontario,
gave an account of apparatus that was designed to provide demand analgesia
in postoperative patients.[48] Sechzer gave a fuller report in 1971,[49] and in 1976,
Cardiff anesthesiologist J. M. Evans and his colleagues published a report of a
digitally controlled pump and syringe that would deliver meperidine on demand
by labor patients.[50] PCA was then accepted very quickly.

Patients, as well as anesthesiologists, welcomed PCA. The results favored the
technique. Typical were the conclusions about PCA of Jane Ballantyne and her
colleagues that were published in 1993.[51] They looked at many publications and
compared the results in fifteen randomized controlled trials. Patients preferred
PCA to conventional methods of administering analgesic drugs and the degree
of pain relief was superior to that of conventional analgesia; there was a trend,
though it was not statistically significant, to shortening of the hospital stay in
PCA patients. PCA became an integral part of the anesthesiologist's management
of pain.

Neuraxial Administration of Opioids

The injection of opioids (i.e., substances having pain-killing activity that are
related to opiates such as opium and morphine) into the epidural space or the
subarachnoid space (i.e., the neuraxial approach) is a pain-relief technique that
is very much in the anesthesiologist's domain. Of all physicians, anesthesiologists

have the greatest expertise in the technique. Since a full discussion of the history of opioids research and use is provided in chapter 9, only those points bearing on pain management will be noted here.

Morphine was first given intrathecally in 1901,[52] but interest in morphine and opioids in neuraxial block grew out of research into opioid peptides and analgesia in the 1970s.[53] The essence of that research is that morphine and various opioids induce analgesia by acting at certain parts of the brain and spinal cord, that this effect is mediated by the presence of opiate receptors, and that, remarkably, the body is capable of making its own opioids.[54, 55, 56, 57] Once analgesia by means of neuraxial block was established, it became an important part of the anesthesiologist's approach to pain management.

Anesthesiologist Michael Cousins has given a good account of how opioid and non-opioid drugs were developed in anesthesia.[58] Initially, anesthesiologists achieved neuraxial block for relief of pain by injecting local anesthetic agents into the epidural space. This was first done by Fidel Pages, of Madrid, in 1921,[59] and the technique gradually became more common, particularly after World War II. Two representative practitioners in this period were Bonica, in Seattle,[60] and Philip Bromage, in Montreal.[61] However, not a great deal of objective documentation was gathered before 1970, though more recently several studies suggested beneficial effects in postoperative patients.[62, 63]

The research on opioids on the nervous system that was carried out in the early 1970s gave anesthesiologists a new understanding of how pain could be relieved by injecting opioids into the neuraxis. Particularly significant for Cousins were the reports of Snyder and Pert on opiate receptors in 1973,[64] of Hughes on endorphins in 1975,[65] and Akil on naloxone, a narcotic antagonist, in 1976[66] (see chapter 9). Other key steps in the path that led to the clinical use of opioids in anesthesia were those of Duggan and his colleagues, who confirmed in 1976 that morphine directly affected pain-stimulating activity in the dorsal horn of the spinal cord,[67] and of Yaksh and Rudy at the University of Wisconsin, who showed in the same year that the analgesic action of analgesics was mediated by a direct action on the spinal cord.[68] All this provided more evidence that the body managed pain centrally rather than peripherally. Then in 1979, Cousins and his group in Adelaide reported work that suggested a spinal site of action for meperidine that was given by epidural injection.[69] Also in 1979, J. K. Wang and his colleagues at the Mayo Clinic reported relief of pain by the intrathecal injection of morphine in eight patients with cancer pain,[70] and M. Behar and coworkers in Jerusalem announced their initiative of injecting morphine into the epidural space to relieve severe chronic pain in ten patients.[71] These accounts all validated the neuraxial use of opioids by anesthesiologists.

For anesthesiologists, the neuraxial administration of opioids was tailor-made for the relief of pain. It soon became part of the practice of anesthesia, particularly in the treatment of acute pain of surgical patients, of women in labor, and of patients with chronic pain in pain clinics and cancer units. Because the knowledge of the action and effects of intraspinal opioids grew in leaps and bounds, anesthesiologists rapidly learned about this new dimension of pain relief. They were able to provide pain relief that was based not just on powerful analgesia but on analgesia that was selective and on a low incidence of side effects. As it became part of anesthetic practice, adverse consequences of the intraspinal administration of opioids became progressively less of a concern, and it was generally agreed that neuraxial analgesia with opioids was superior to that given systemically.

*   *   *

Anesthetists have been concerned about obtunding pain since the days when anesthesia was a craft. At first, their activities were confined to the operating room; but they soon realized that pain could be relieved by the agents that they were familiar with, both for surgical patients and for others in pain. As the knowledge of medical science grew, anesthesiologists found new ways of treating pain, and these took them out of the operating room to other parts of the hospital. They relieved the pain of women in labor and of patients with chronic pain due to a multiplicity of conditions; and in moving to pain clinics, anesthesiologists went outside the hospital. The value of this work is impossible to quantify, but it is considerable for anesthesiologists and their professional status. In relation to just the use of regional anesthesia for postoperative pain relief, Daniel Moore estimated that of the 25 million persons who underwent surgery in 1989, 6 million suffered severe to very severe pain, and 3 million had moderate to severe pain.[72] According to Moore, if it were possible for anesthesiologists to help only a small proportion of those patients, this type of service, like the direct provision of good obstetric analgesia, would afford them an unusual opportunity to interact with the patient more closely and more frequently and for a longer period of time than is possible in the usual visit after a surgical operation. Moore's observations provide another illustration of how anesthesia was becoming integrated into health care.

For patients, the value of pain relief also is impossible to quantify, as is the potential for value in terms of pain relief, even though an examination of numbers indicates that it surely exists. Chronic pain disables an enormous number of individuals. According to one estimate, in 1985, in the United States, over 4 billion workdays were lost as a result of chronic pain at a cost to the economy of $55 billion.[73] Only a fraction of that burden can be lifted by pain treatment, which leads one to conclude that valuable as the work on pain relief by anesthesiologists has been, it has been no more than a drop in the ocean, and that the potential for such work will continue to exist.

Chapter 13

Anesthesiologists and Resuscitation

Anesthesia and resuscitation have much in common, in both their history and practice. For example, the primitive resuscitation kits of the eighteenth century were progenitors of devices such as tracheal tubes that eventually came to be standard anesthesia equipment; in turn, the oral airways and the tracheal tubes that anesthetists use daily became part of the standard equipment of ambulance paramedics on resuscitation calls. That is true of more complex equipment such as ventilators: anesthesiologists use them daily in operating rooms and in caring for victims of sudden cardiac and respiratory collapse. Anesthesiologists too, particularly in the second half of the twentieth century, carried out key research that enhanced the understanding of resuscitation, and they taught the principles and practice of cardiopulmonary resuscitation (CPR) to health care personnel and to lay persons.

The close relationship between the theory and practice of resuscitation and of anesthesia is evident in the history of the practice of both, and for this reason, the history of resuscitation is discussed in this history of anesthesia.

Broadly, the term *resuscitation* refers to procedures that are aimed at restoring life in someone who has suddenly and unexpectedly collapsed. While sudden collapse may result from hemorrhage, trauma, or septic shock, in this chapter, the term will be restricted to the management of sudden and unexpected arrest of the heart or cessation of lung function, as in a life-threatening heart attack. The essence of resuscitation lies in three practical measures: restarting the arrested heart, restoring the heart's normal rhythm, and supplying oxygen to the lungs. Running like threads through the history of resuscitation, they are, to some extent, based on technical knowledge, but because lay persons have always been likely to be the first at the scene of a collapse, public education is another important element of resuscitation. There is, therefore, both a social and a health-care context to resuscitation, and both further illustrate the expanding role of anesthesia in health care.

The Ancient Lineage of CPR

Though the modern ideas and practice of CPR came to fruition just over fifty years ago, the basic elements are ages old. In fact, none of the principal methods of CPR—artificial ventilation, heart massage, and defibrillation—originated recently. Mouth-to-mouth ventilation was known in ancient Egyptian and biblical times; tracheal intubation was known in the ninth century; cardiac massage to restore the action of the heart, with the chest open or closed, was known in the seventeenth century; and electric shock dates from the eighteenth century. If cooling to protect brain function is also considered, it too is by no means recent, for cooling the body (hypothermia) was known to Hippocrates.

CPR may seem modern, but that is because the elements were periodically forgotten or rejected and rediscovered much later—a phenomenon that is common to medicine, including anesthesia. Rediscovery and later application of the properties of a drug or technique, and a delay between recognition—even dim recognition—of a phenomenon and its application often explain this. Also relevant to the history of CPR, and to anesthesia, is the fact that the time and circumstances must be right for progress to be made.

CPR itself also continues to evolve, and this is another aspect of the history of resuscitation. The basis for the modern practice of CPR was established by studies beginning in the 1950s that combined artificial respiration with artificial circulation,[1] and the ABC mnemonic (for *A*irway, *B*reathing, and *C*irculation) that was established in the 1960s seemed to settle the priorities in resuscitating someone in an acute emergency. That seemed to cap the many efforts to the protocol for resuscitation readily understandable by the lay public. However, changing circumstances frequently mean that protocols have to be changed; and in 2005, new ideas led to a revision of the priorities. The mnemonic ABC was reversed in 2005 to become the new one of CBA (for *C*hest compression, *B*reathing, and *A*irway).[2] Nor is that all. In 2007, greater emphasis in first-response actions came to be placed on the chest-compression component and less on the rescue breathing component.[3] That is, evolution has changed the practice of resuscitation medicine, just as it has the practice of anesthesia.

Resuscitation in Ancient Egypt and the Bible

Since resuscitation means restoring life to someone who has seemingly just died suddenly, correct treatment must be urgent and immediate. Since the first individual to reach the victim is a lay person, the role of the lay public has long been prominent in accounts of the history of resuscitation, and many of the oldest accounts of resuscitation, even though some may be mythical, give graphic descriptions of lay persons resuscitating victims.

In ancient Egypt, for example, Isis is said to have restored life to her brother Osiris by lying on him after their brother Seth had attacked him.[4] The Bible tells of Elisha's resuscitating a boy with a headache who then became unconscious by lying over him.[5] Interesting though these accounts are, the mechanism of recovery is not clear. It is only a possibility that Isis used mouth-to-mouth respiration; and with Elisha, the warmth of his body or the tickling of his beard (since the boy is said to have sneezed seven times on recovering) may have led to recovery. However, the account of the action of the midwife Puah seems more credible. She breathed into a baby's mouth to make it cry,[6] and so does seem to have definitely performed mouth-to-mouth respiration. That was the start of a long tradition of mouth-to-mouth breathing by midwives.[7]

Table 13.1. Some lay resuscitation techniques

Yelling, shouting, making loud noises
Slapping, hitting
Rubbing
Warming, including use of ashes, hot water
Stretching the tongue
Inflating the lungs with bellows
Placing smelling salts under the nose
Tickling the pharynx with a feather
Fumigating the mouth, rectum with smoke
Rocking the victim on a barrel or horse
Inverting the body: pressing and releasing the chest

Lay persons carried the banner of resuscitation for centuries, using quite unsophisticated methods (table 13.1). Only the limits of the human imagination made the list shorter than it might have been. The techniques included stimulation of the victim's nervous system by yelling, crying, and other loud noises, plus slapping, hitting, and whipping, and sometimes the gentler technique of rubbing or the rougher one of stretching the rectum; placing the victim on top of a barrel or a horse, for reliance on the effect of motion; stimulation of the upper airway by salts under the nose or a feather in the pharynx, or stretching of the tongue; fumigating the mouth or rectum with tobacco; inversion, with chest pressure to aid expiration and release of pressure to aid inspiration; and the bellows, which may have done no more in some cases than inflate the mouth.

Physicians had no more than a passing interest in resuscitation until a body of basic knowledge had been acquired, beginning in the sixteenth century, and until society was urbanized and industrialized, as from the eighteenth century.

Early Theoretical and Practical Knowledge

Sixteenth Century: Andreas Vesalius and Tracheostomy

One of the clearest descriptions of resuscitation was given in 1543 by Andreas Vesalius. He performed experiments on pigs and dogs. He wrote that

> life may in a manner of speaking be restored to the animal, an opening
> must be attempted in the trunk of the trachea, into which a tube
> of reed or cane should be put; you will then blow into this, so that
> the lungs may rise again and the animal take in air. Indeed, with a
> slight breath in the case of this living animal the lungs will swell to
> the full extent of the thoracic cavity, and the heart becomes strong
> and exhibits a wondrous variety of motions.[8]

Vesalius was describing tracheostomy and artificial ventilation, which became part of resuscitation beginning in the eighteenth century, but he also referred to the benefit to the heart of restoration of ventilation.

Seventeenth Century: Studies of Heart and Lung Function

In his book on the motion of the heart of 1628, William Harvey noted the interdependence of the respiration and circulation, which is central to resuscitation, as it is in normal health. He observed that a dove's heart that had been stilled by lack of blood flow was restored to action by direct manual stimulation. After the heart had stopped pulsating and when the auricles too were motionless, Harvey placed a warm finger, moistened with saliva, directly on the heart, whereupon "under the influence of this fomentation it recovered new strength and life, so that both ventricles and auricles pulsated, contracting and relaxing alternately, recalled as it were from death to life."[9] Harvey unconsciously foreshadowed the introduction of direct cardiac massage in the nineteenth century, another element of resuscitation.

Harvey was mainly interested in the heart, but as is noted in chapter 1, the Oxford virtuosi, under Robert Boyle, added fundamental knowledge about respiration, the lungs, the heart, and the blood. Their work was primarily academic, but one case in Oxford shows how resuscitation was performed in clinical practice in the seventeenth century. A young woman named Anne Green was sentenced to be hanged on December 14, 1650, because it was thought, incorrectly, that she had murdered her newborn babe, who was actually stillborn.[10] The attempt to hang her was bungled, and Anne was left suspended, supposedly for half an hour. To put her out of her misery, her friends thumped on her chest and jerked her legs up and down. Thought to be dead, she was taken in a coffin to the house of Dr. William Petty, who, as Reader in Anatomy, was permitted to acquire the bodies of executed persons and to dissect them.

When the coffin was opened, however, Anne apparently took a breath, and her throat rattled. Petty, together with Thomas Willis (later an authority on anatomy of the nervous system), decided they should attempt to resuscitate rather than dissect her. They pried open her mouth and poured cordial down her throat, which they also tickled with a feather. They rubbed her limbs, placing heating plasters on her chest, administered a warming enema, and put her to bed, ordering a woman to sleep with her to keep her warm. After twelve hours, Anne began to speak; after two days, she could remember everything except for the execution and the resuscitation. And after one month, she appeared to have fully recovered. She even married, had three children, and lived for another fifteen years.

Progress in the Eighteenth Century

The Humane Societies

Life provided more leisure in eighteenth-century Europe, and winter pastimes included skating on frozen canals and rivers. In Holland, drowning and near-drowning became common, and some people learned how to resuscitate the victims. As experience of resuscitation of drowning victims grew, so did the practice of resuscitation. But deaths persisted; in 1767, for example, some 400 drowning deaths were reported from Amsterdam.[11] Efforts were made to prevent such deaths, and the Society for the Recovery of Drowned Persons was formed that same year. That evidently helped, for in 1771, the Society claimed to have saved the lives of 150 drowning victims. Other societies followed suit: Venice and Milan in 1768, Paris in 1771, London (the Royal Humane Society) in 1774, and Philadelphia in 1780.[12] Physicians now began to become much more actively involved in resuscitation and took a prominent part in the efforts of the humane societies.[13]

Drowning was not the only reason for resuscitation in the eighteenth century. In the era of the Industrial Revolution, work-related injuries sometimes called for resuscitation. Thus, one asphyxiated miner was resuscitated by William Tossach using the ages-old mouth-to-mouth technique.[14]

The humane societies recommended several resuscitation techniques,[15] though they were much fewer than those that were used by lay persons down the ages (see table 13.1). However, it is likely that only aspiration of the mouth, warming, and mouth-to-mouth respiration were truly effective.

Artificial Ventilation

By the eighteenth century, two of the main elements of CPR were in place, albeit in somewhat primitive condition. They include techniques of ventilating the lungs and using electric shock to restart the arrested heart.

Several natural scientists were interested in ventilation in this period. Stephen Hales, for example, put its study on an objective footing: he carried out rebreathing experiments on himself in 1733,[16] and he wrote of using large bellows to ventilate crowded public spaces in 1743.[17] But others ventilated the lungs to resuscitate patients. John Fothergill in 1745 reported the successful application of mouth-to-mouth ventilation,[18] Benjamin Pugh in 1754 recommended an "air-pipe" to help resuscitate neonates,[19] and surgeon and anatomist John Hunter in 1755 operated a double-chambered bellows, with one chamber filling the lungs and the other removing air.[20] His bellows was the first device to deliver positive and negative pressure in assisted ventilation. Hunter's account, which was not published until 1776, when there was greater general interest in resuscitation, emphasizes the interdependence of the respiratory and circulatory systems, and the deleterious effects of delay in resuscitative action.

Hunter made two other useful observations. First, when he stopped working the bellows, the heart's action gradually faded, and then ceased to move; second, when he used the bellows again "the heart again began to move, at first very faintly, and with long intermissions; but by continuing the artificial breathing, its motion became as frequent and as strong as at first." Repeating the process in the same dog to see what would happen, he found that when he stopped inflating the lungs with the bellows, the heart became "extremely turgid with blood, the blood in the left side becoming as dark as that in the right, which was not the case when the bellows were working."[21] Hunter also suggested that electric shock might be helpful in victims requiring resuscitation.

Several other individuals realized that the lungs of the unconscious victim should be ventilated. Resuscitation kits were made available in the eighteenth century, among which one of the most practical was that prepared by Charles Kite, of London.[22] He suggested that the chest wall of the victim be actively moved. If there was any "impediment," a "crooked tube," bent like a male catheter, was to be introduced through the mouth or nostril into the glottis, with the proximal end attached to a blowpipe. Kite also suggested intravenous stimulants and electric shock.

Alexander Monro II, of Edinburgh, also advocated tracheal intubation for resuscitation. According to William Cullen, Monro suggested using a male catheter.[23] The Danes John Herholdt and Carl Rafn in 1796 recommended the simpler mouth-to-mouth techniques, as well as electric shock, across the chest and warming the victim.[24]

The Use of Electricity

Electric shock, which was then a novelty, constituted the second front of progress in resuscitation in the eighteenth century. It was first used clinically in 1774.[25] An attempt to reproduce the "nigh-miraculous effect in rendering strength and consequently life" that Giovanni Bianchi had observed in 1756[26] was made in London in 1774. The victim was young Sophia Greenhill, who was "to all appearance dead" after falling from a window; the resuscitator was a London surgeon named Squires.[27] Evidently, Sophia was not "dead" enough for the morbid state to become mortal; twenty minutes are said to have elapsed before Squires applied a shock, and a further few minutes passed before a second shock through the thorax elicited "a small pulsation" and before the girl began to breathe. But all turned out well, whether or not the use of electricity here was the restorative agent.

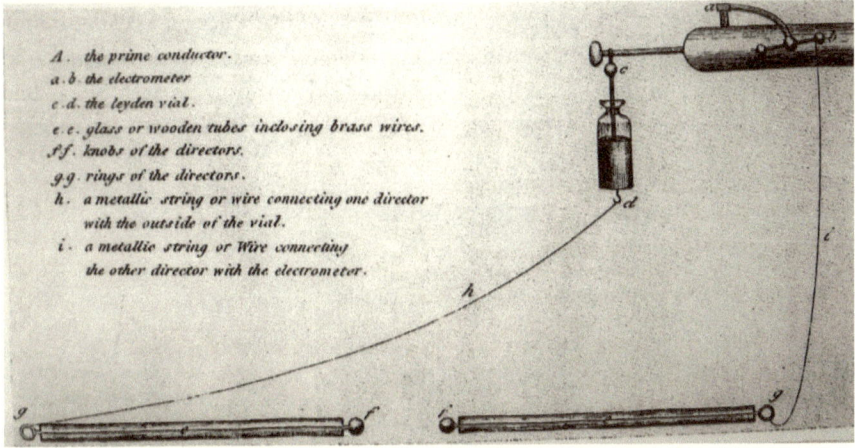

Fig. 13.1. Charles Kite's apparatus of 1788 for use of electricity in resuscitation, regarded as prototype of defibrillation. (Source: C. Kite, *An Essay on the Resuscitation of the Apparently Dead* [London, 1788], note 18, opposite p. 192.)

Many such accounts indicate that electric shock was not a primary form of treatment. Hunter at first thought that it might be tried when other methods had failed.[28] Later, he concluded that it *should* be tried when other methods failed, adding—significantly in view of twentieth-century developments with defibrillation—that "it is probably the only method we have of immediately stimulating the heart." However, practitioners continued to have faith in the use of electricity. Among them, Kite was a visionary, and his apparatus for the safe use of electricity in resuscitation[29] (fig. 13.1) suggests a close relationship of his device to the defibrillators that were introduced in the twentieth century.

Developments in the Nineteenth Century

Interest in electric shock was maintained in the nineteenth century. In 1815, James Curry claimed that experience had shown that it was one of the most powerful of stimulants, capable of exciting contraction in "the Heart and other muscles . . . after every other stimulus has ceased to produce the least effect."[30] Elaborate details of the technique of electroresuscitation were provided by Richard Reece in 1824. His graphic sketch of the apparatus shows a bellows through which air could be passed through a silver cannula in the larynx, a metal tube in the gullet, a galvanic battery linked to an esophageal conduit, and a wire that made contact "particularly about the regions of the heart, the diaphragm . . . [and] the neck"[31] (fig. 13.2).

The value of applying electric shock to restore heart action became better understood later in the nineteenth century. Less well understood was the value of new methods of ventilating the lungs and of the important step of cardiac massage, both of which were actually introduced in the nineteenth century.

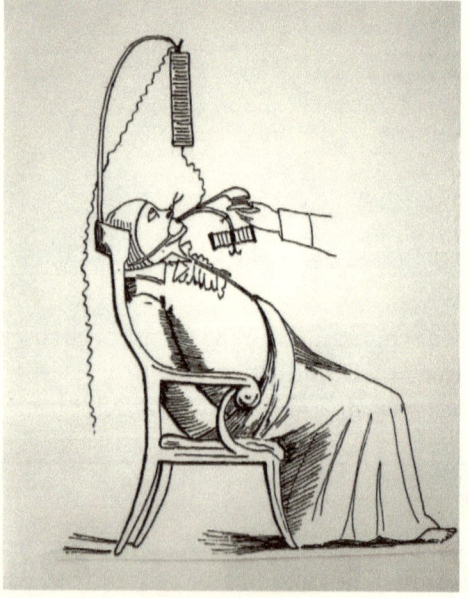

Fig. 13.2. Illustration of measures for resuscitation, 1824. Patient is seated in "reanimation chair"; nostrils clamped, ears plugged, ventilated via bellows and silver cannula in larynx, metal tube in gullet to convey "ether or any other stimulating fluid that may be thought proper." Victim completes electrical circuit of one wire from galvanic battery to esophageal conduit and second that contacts various parts of body. (Source: R. Reece, *Medical Guide for the Use of the Clergy, Heads of Families, and Junior Practitioners in Medicine and Surgery* [London: Longman, Hurst and Company, 1824].)

Wider Uses of Electric Shock

The advent of anesthesia, and reports of death and misadventure associated with it, stimulated interest in the power of electricity to resuscitate persons in a state of suspended animation. In 1851, the French Academy of Sciences discussed a suggestion that operating rooms be fitted with electrical apparatus. The academy recommended that "collapse" under ether or chloroform be treated by electropuncture of the head and spine, or by discharges through moist sponges on the chest wall.[32] Doctors in hospitals felt obliged to install electrical equipment. Electric shock was also advocated for drug poisoning. In the United States, William Channing wrote a book about the medical uses of electricity.[33] Such was the great interest in the resuscitative power of electricity. It was even used to confirm death: anyone whose body failed to react to an electrical discharge was formally considered to be dead.[34]

Not until toward the end of the century, however, was the role of electricity in restoring action of the heart clearly understood. Only then could electric shock be used rationally in resuscitation. Two events are important. One is the suggestion by Scottish physician John MacWilliam in 1889 that a "quivering movement" of the walls of the heart was a cause of fatal cardiac arrest[35]—the rhythm disturbance that Hoffman showed in 1912 to be ventricular fibrillation.[36] The second piece of significant research is the demonstration in dogs by Prevost and Batelli in 1899 that ventricular fibrillation could be reverted by means of alternating electric current.[37]

Manual Methods of Artificial Respiration

Though well founded theoretically, resuscitation by electric shock had disadvantages. One was that it was difficult to apply without delay. The appropriate apparatus was seldom at hand when someone had to be resuscitated outside hospital, and transportation of the patient to the site of the apparatus took time. Therefore, methods that inflated the lungs were sought. However, the mouth-to-mouth technique made people uncomfortable, and the bellows were not always applied promptly and did not inflate the lungs rather than the mouth. London surgeon Benjamin Brodie argued that the heart would stop two or three minutes after breathing ceased, and then no method was of value,[38] while Leroy d'Etiolles showed that overdistension of the lungs by the bellows was sometimes fatal in animals.[39] Warmth seemed to be the only efficacious and harmless method.

A different approach was that of English neurologist Marshall Hall. The drawbacks of current methods of resuscitation led him in 1856 to develop a manual method of ventilation.[40] The victim's body was placed prone to facilitate expiration (which might be enhanced by pressure on the back) and in the lateral position to facilitate inspiration. The position was changed sixteen times each minute. He claimed to generate tidal volumes of 300-500 ml/min.

Marshall Hall's method was followed by others in the next eighty years. The methods of Silvester (1858),[41] Howard (1877),[42] Schafer (1908),[43] Nielsen (1932),[44] and Eve (1932)[45] are the best known. Each had its proponents and opponents, and so in 1951, Archer Gordon and colleagues studied the Silvester, the Schafer, the Nielsen, and a hip lift-back and a hip roll-back method.[46] Tidal volumes and arterial saturation were analyzed for each in six groups of subjects (including anesthetized and curarized volunteers, conscious volunteers, postoperative patients, and patients with intracranial disorders), as well as energy expenditure in the operators. The study indicated that the Schafer prone pressure method should be replaced with a more efficient one, and that a modified Holger Nielsen method should be recommended for general use. But later that decade, it was the age-old mouth-to-mouth technique that received the seal of approval.

Cardiac Massage

Often ignored in the history of resuscitation is the Hungarian surgeon Janos Balassa, who reported the technique of compressing the anterior wall of the chest in 1858.[47] Balassa did that after performing tracheotomy in a woman with tuberculous laryngitis. He rhythmically compressed the chest in order to stimulate breathing, but the woman had no pulse, though it returned, as did her respiration, after the chest was massaged.

In 1858, then, Balassa seems to have practiced the technique of *closed-chest cardiac compression*. Clinically, closed-chest compression was also performed in 1891 by Friedrich Maass, of Gottingen, in association with Franz Koenig,[48] but it was more often used in laboratories. In 1878, for example, its use was reported from Rudolf Boehm's laboratory in Dorpat, Germany, after it was noticed that compression of the chest was making the blood spurt out of the incised carotid artery.[49] As a clinical technique for resuscitation, however, closed-chest cardiac massage lay fallow for three-quarters of a century, despite the fact that noted surgeons like George Crile publicized it.[50] It is not clear why this was so. It may be that opening the chest and directly massaging the chest seemed the logical approach, and of course, the significance of defibrillation, with the chest open and, later, with it closed, was not understood until research on ventricular fibrillation began to bear fruit in the 1930s. And closed-chest compression did not emerge as an important component of CPR until 1960.

In the meantime, the technique of open-chest cardiac massage was introduced as a technique for restarting the heart. The first to do this was the Italian physiologist Moritz Schiff, in 1874.[51] He did so in animals who were made pulseless by chloroform. The first person to do it successfully in humans was Norwegian Kristian Ingelsrud in 1901.[52] After that, open-chest cardiac massage gradually became a standard emergency measure in cases of cardiac arrest, especially in operating rooms.

The Modern Era

The history of the modern era of resuscitation began immediately after the Second World War. It was then that anesthesiologists began making important contributions to resuscitation medicine; so did electrical engineers, surgeons, cardiologists, and physiologists. All furthered the two components of ventilating the lungs and restoring the action of the heart that had been initiated earlier, but some added the vital one of restoring normal rhythm to the heart by means of defibrillation. In that way, these components were put together in one "package" in the form of CPR in 1961. In due course, measures to protect the brain (the cerebral component) and to prioritize massage of the heart and early defibrillation were added.

Mouth-to-Mouth Ventilation

One day in 1946, during an epidemic of poliomyelitis in Minneapolis, medical resident and later anesthesiologist James Elam found himself in a hospital corridor that suddenly became the scene of frenetic activity. Noticing that a child on a gurney was blue in the face, Elam acted immediately and decisively. Almost without thinking, but remembering what he had read the night before about mouth-to-mouth ventilation of the newborn, he wiped secretions from the child's face, put his mouth over the nose, and inflated the lungs with his own expired air. After four breaths, the child turned pink.[53] This was not only small relief to him but a giant step forward for humankind. Now anyone, anytime could resuscitate a victim of sudden collapse. All that was required was to blow into the lungs of someone whose respiration had failed and to thump on the chest if the heart had stopped. That quantum leap in management marks the beginning of the modern era of CPR.

Elam resuscitated the child with his own expired air at a time when there was a theoretical and a practical basis for resuscitation by artificial ventilation. The techniques of artificial ventilation from the 1930s on, new drugs—including muscle relaxants in the 1940s and early 1950s—and thoracic surgery and blood-gas analysis in the 1950s had all made anesthesiologists familiar with acute abnormalities of the airway. Elam's initiative in 1946 was important because it provided insight into the management of the pulmonary aspects of resuscitation—just as Bjorn Ibsen's initiative in 1952 did in the management of the pulmonary aspects of poliomyelitis[54] (see also chapter 11)—but it had to be validated in terms of homeostatic parameters. Only in that way could the mouth-to-mouth technique be part of the standard approach to resuscitation and have universal application.

In a key article in 1954, Elam argued that mask-to-mouth or mouth-to-mask ventilation was the ideal emergency procedure for artificial ventilation.[55] It was quite straightforward. The necessary equipment was absurdly simple: a regular anesthetic-type face mask, or a handkerchief as a filter if the mouth-to-nose technique was preferred. The technique was simple too: the operator, who could tell immediately if the lungs were being inflated, automatically exerted sufficient inflating pressure to provide adequate air delivery, since the operator tended to compensate for changes in airway resistance and lung compliance. The artificial ventilation rapidly raised the victim's alveolar oxygen tension, and the gas composition in the lungs was equally rapidly returned to normal.

Elam's efforts impressed another anesthesiologist, who immediately realized the need for formal and intensive research into resuscitation. This was Peter Safar (fig. 13.3), of Baltimore City Hospital, who later made some of the greatest contributions to resuscitation medicine. Safar met Elam in a crucial encounter in October 1956. As Safar said, it was the birth of modern resuscitation.[56] Safar switched from clinical and educational interests to long-term resuscitation research,[57] which encouraged other anesthesiologists to conduct research into resuscitation. Three of them, besides Safar, included Elam in the 1950s and 1960s, Eugene Nagel in Miami in the 1960s and 1970s, and Roger White, of the Mayo Clinic, in the 1980s and 1990s.

For his part, Safar first set about validating Elam's initiative. He formulated a three-part plan: to study the mechanisms of soft-tissue obstruction in the upper airway, to compare ventilation volumes produced by traditional methods of resuscitation with those of mouth-to-mouth ventilation, and to determine the feasibility of mouth-to-mouth ventilation by lay persons. He was extraordinarily productive: his first article on resuscitation after meeting Elam was published in 1957, on the mouth-to-mouth airway, which he wrote himself.[58] His last article on resuscitation, which he wrote with several coauthors, was published in 2000.[59] In the intervening years, he wrote many papers with other physicians, the following being just a sample of key papers in the early years. With Elam, he wrote on manual artificial respiration versus mouth-to-mouth ventilation;[60] with Lourdes Aguto-Escarraga and F. Chang, on upper airway obstruction in the unconscious patient;[61] with Escarraga and Elam, on a comparison of the mouth-to-mouth and the mouth-to-airway methods with chest-pressure arm-lift methods,[62] and with S. Morikawa and J. DeCarlo, on the influence of the head-jaw position on the patency of the upper airway.[63]

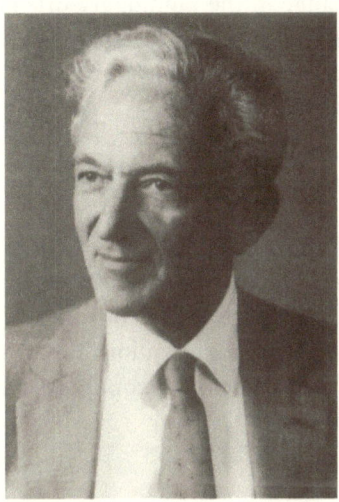

Fig. 13.3. Peter Safar (1924-2003)

Peter Safar was Viennese. He grew up when the Nazi menace loomed, and he worked in a labor camp in Bavaria in 1938. He enrolled in the medical school in the University of Vienna in 1943, graduating in 1948. Awarded a surgical fellowship at Yale, he realized that surgery would not advance without having improved life support that is provided by anesthesia. After working in Robert Dripps' anesthesia department in Philadelphia, Safar joined the anesthesia department at Johns Hopkins University Hospital in 1954, but later set up an academic department in the Baltimore City Hospital. His earlier interest in resuscitation was furthered in 1956 by meeting James Elam. The direction of Safar's career then changed; he began to develop the field of resuscitation medicine, both in the academic setting and in the community. After William Kouwenhoven, James Jude, and Guy Knickerbocker demonstrated the value of closed-chest cardiac massage and defibrillation, Safar emphasized the respiratory component and the cerebral component in resuscitation. After moving to Pittsburgh in 1961, Safar established a multidisciplinary critical care program. Like Bjorn Ibsen, Peter Safar demonstrated how anesthesia came to be of enormous benefit in areas outside the operating room: Ibsen, in the care of respiratory failure; Safar, in the care of individuals requiring resuscitation.

The research by Safar and his colleagues demonstrated some simple points. For example, just tilting a person's head backward would ensure patency of the airway; and while manual ventilation techniques up until then had failed to aerate the lungs sufficiently, mouth-to-mouth ventilation did. Moreover, anyone could be taught the mouth-to-mouth method. Safar's work on the airway in adults was complemented by Archer Gordon's in children.[64] Such studies were sufficiently convincing, despite some resistance based on dislike on esthetic grounds, to bring about a radical change in the pulmonary-oriented methods of artificial ventilation. By 1958, the mouth-to-mouth technique had been endorsed by the American Medical Association, and was recommended wherever and whenever pulmonary resuscitation was required.[65]

Cardiac Resuscitation

It took longer to establish the cardiac element of CPR; its development stretched over a period of a century. The cardiac package had three components: closed-chest massage, open-chest massage, and defibrillation. The package was more complex than that of pulmonary resuscitation, and intensive technical research and development were required before it could be generally accepted.

Ventricular Fibrillation and Defibrillation

The role of ventricular fibrillation in cardiac arrest and of defibrillation in resuscitation was understood much more gradually than was that of cardiac massage, even though the chest lay open to permit cardiac massage to be applied, both in laboratories and in operating rooms. The arrhythmia was first described by Karl Ludwig in 1850,[66] when a galvanic or a faradic current was passed through a dog's heart. Its clinical significance was better understood after MacWilliam reported in 1889 that "the cardiac pump is thrown out of gear" by what he called "fibrillar contraction,"[67] and after Prevost and Batelli had arrested a dog's fibrillating heart with countershocks applied to the myocardium with both AC and DC electricity.[68]

Realization of the full significance of ventricular fibrillation was delayed, in anesthesia as in resuscitation. In anesthesia, its significance in relation to cardiac arrest of the triad of ventricular fibrillation, *light* chloroform anesthesia, and adrenalin in a patient's blood was not understood until Goodman Levy demonstrated it in 1911.[69] In resuscitation, the significance of ventricular fibrillation as the usual cause of cardiac arrest, and of defibrillation as a principal modality of treatment, was not apparent for many years after that. It was not even apparent when electrical engineer William Kouwenhoven, in Baltimore, and his colleagues Orthello Langworthy and Donald Hooker in 1933 showed that alternating current (AC) could induce ventricular fibrillation[70] and that ventricular fibrillation in dogs could be *corrected* by a current of greater intensity and—what is more remarkable—with the *chest closed*.[71] The second of those reports, however, was published in an engineering rather than in a medical journal and was not noticed by physicians.

Clinically, the value of defibrillation was first recognized only when Claude Beck defibrillated a boy's heart in the operating room, with the chest open, in 1947.[72] Beck's experience with cardiac arrest was crucial to later developments in the understanding of defibrillation. Beck, who worked in Cleveland and knew of the work on cardiac rhythm of Cleveland physiologist Carl Wiggers, as well as Kouwenhoven's work, had first seen a case of cardiac arrest nearly twenty years earlier. As he witnessed a case of intraoperative cardiac arrest, he was astonished to see that it was managed not by physicians but by a *fire department rescue squad*, which, moreover, used clumsy oxygen-powered resuscitators, and that not until fifteen minutes had elapsed after the arrest.[73] Beck understood, but others did not, that it was not surgical injury but an electrical disturbance that is the usual cause of death in coronary heart disease, and that ventricular fibrillation during surgery was not necessarily fatal.[74] He saw the need to treat ventricular fibrillation for what it was: a surgical emergency. He also saw the need for every hospital to equip itself with a resuscitation team, and one was established at University Hospital, where Beck worked.

Beck's success of 1947 encouraged Kouwenhoven to continue his work in developing an open-chest defibrillator in this period when *open-chest* massage seemed the right and logical way of getting the heart to beat normally again. Kouwenhoven persisted, and by 1951, the Hopkins model of defibrillator became available.[75]

Defibrillation as a definitive therapeutic maneuver. Defibrillation, as performed originally by Prevost and Batelli, then by Hooker and his group, and later by Beck, consisted of shocks given by AC. The next step, in the 1950s, was to perfect defibrillation so that it could be used readily, promptly, and effectively. Meetings between the team of Wiggers and Beck with Kouwenhoven facilitated the development of the latter's AC defibrillator. Kouwenhoven's team showed that Prevost and Batelli had been correct in 1899, and they proceeded to develop an AC defibrillator suitable for use in hospitals by 1951, and a defibrillator for closed-chest use by 1957.[76]

Defibrillators designed by Paul Zoll[77] and Bernard Lown,[78] both of Boston, were other key advances. Zoll was interested in external countershock for patients with heart rhythm abnormalities and acute myocardial infarction, though this did not need heart massage. He developed an AC defibrillator in 1955. He confirmed the efficacy of external countershock, noting that externally applied electric countershock was immediately effective, safe, and clinically feasible. Lown sought to design a technique to meet certain requirements: instant and consistent control of the ectopic mechanism, avoidance of depression of normal cardiac pacemaking and myocardial contractility and of prolongation of conductivity within the heart, lack of damage to vital tissues, and simplicity of operation. Lown considered that the AC defibrillator sometimes caused serious arrhythmias and was not entirely safe. A DC defibrillator would be better: it was based on instant depolarization during a safe part of the cardiac cycle, it was simple to use, was effective, and had no side effects. Because it was portable, it broadened the applicability of defibrillators.

The 1960s: The CPR Package Comes Together

The modern form of CPR, therefore, came together only as several components— cardiac and respiratory—were integrated. Representative of that integration and its applicability by lay and professional persons alike were two groundbreaking events. The first occurred in 1960, when Kouwenhoven, James Jude, and Guy Knickerbocker published the seminal article on closed-chest cardiac massage.[79] The second occurred in the following year, when Safar emphasized the need to add the respiratory elements of airway alignment and expired-air ventilation to the Kouwenhoven-Jude-Knickerbocker technique.[80] Thus did the modern approach to CPR finally take shape.

The ideas of the Kouwenhoven team originated in a key observation that Knickerbocker made in 1958. A Fellow in Kouwenhoven's laboratory, he noticed that the weight of heavy defibrillator paddles on a dog's chest increased the intra-arterial pressure.[81] Study of methods of moving the blood by massaging the intact chest led the team to develop a safe and effective way of massaging the heart without having to open the chest. Clinical testing followed. The method reportedly was successful in resuscitating twenty patients. In three of these patients, defibrillation was applied by an AC device; and in thirteen others, artificial ventilation was carried out simultaneously with the closed-chest massage. They also reported the details of four cases of cardiac standstill and one of ventricular fibrillation.

The reintroduction of closed-chest cardiac massage was highly significant. This is evident in the words of the concluding paragraph of their groundbreaking article of 1960:

> Closed-chest cardiac massage has been proved to be effective in cases of cardiac arrest. It has provided circulation adequate to maintain the heart and the central nervous system, and it has provided an opportunity to bring a defibrillator to the scene if necessary. Supportive drug treatment and other measures may be given. The necessity for a thoracotomy is eliminated. *The real value of the method lies in the fact that it can be used wherever the emergency arises, whether that is in or out of the hospital*"[82] [italics added].

In other words, cardiac massage could be performed by anyone, anywhere.

Safar's contribution was significant because the article of 1960, important as it was, described only part of the CPR package and only part of the new practice of CPR. As Safar noted, it "took ventilation and oxygenation for granted."[83] That part had been of interest to Safar and his group following his crucial meeting with Elam in 1956. Safar, therefore, combined the work of the Kouwenhoven team with the work of his own group on ventilation. It was this, as summarized in an article of 1961,[84] that completed the CPR package. Safar also did much to bring back the lay public fully into CPR.

Although in this account the work of a number of individuals has been discussed, a great many others have made valuable contributions to the practice of resuscitation. A detailed account of those other figures—especially from the United Kingdom, Germany, the Scandinavian countries, and Russia—is provided in the book titled *Resuscitation Greats*.[85]

Out-of-Hospital Resuscitation

Anesthesiologists began to become actively involved in CPR outside the hospital toward the end of the twentieth century. The contributions of some, like Safar, were unique and seminal. Others, like Eugene Nagel in Miami and Roger White in Rochester, Minnesota, made valuable contributions in their own communities. Their work added to that of cardiologists like Leonard Cobb in Seattle.

Out-of-hospital resuscitation is an important aspect of public health. Sudden cardiac arrest outside the hospital is a major problem in the United States and in other parts of the developed world. In 1998, among United States residents aged thirty-five years or older, there were 719,456 such deaths from cardiac disease; and of these, 456,076 were considered to have been sudden, unexpected, and natural due to a cardiac cause.[86] (Sudden cardiac death was taken to be a death that occurred in an individual either out of the hospital or dead on arrival in the emergency room, with the cause of death being reported as heart disease.) Since ventricular fibrillation, the precipitating cause of the collapse,[87] is associated with a high mortality in communities where there is no access to early defibrillation—survival may be less than 10 percent[88]—and since rapid access to defibrillation reduces the mortality of sudden cardiac death,[89] defibrillation is the key to modern resuscitation, especially in the community setting. For these reasons, emergency medical services (EMS) grew up in communities around the need for efficacious out-of-hospital resuscitation.

Emergency medical services did not exist in the 1950s. What sparked their development is debated. Safar, who moved to the University of Pittsburgh in 1961, attributed it to the coalescence of several opportunities that were seen to be lifesaving.[90] Military experience had shown that helicopter evacuation of wounded and their prompt attention in forward hospitals facilitated resuscitation, and anesthesiologists and trauma surgeons in civilian life, particularly in Europe, began to apply the life-support measures known in the operating room, outside the operating room, and even outside the hospital. Guidelines for community-wide EMS systems were formulated, beginning in Pittsburgh in the 1960s. Soon, the public began to demand EMS.

Eugene Nagel took a slightly different view. He pointed to a revolution in the 1960s that transformed emergency care in civilian life. It started with an electrical engineer's accidentally discovering closed-chest cardiac massage during experimentation on defibrillation techniques.[91] Both the public and the medical community then realized that their efforts in the field could reverse apparent death. The revolution that Nagel referred to was the transformation from simple first aid to sophisticated prehospital emergency medical care.

Safar worked in Pittsburgh on delivery of emergency care by ambulance personnel; Nagel, in Miami on delivery by fire rescue personnel. For both, and for the other individuals who stressed the importance of rapid delivery of emergency medical care such as Mayo Clinic anesthesiologist Roger White, what was important was to train paramedics so that they could administer sophisticated life support measures and be in constant radio touch with a physician. A 2003 study from the Mayo Clinic illustrates some of the points underlying the philosophy of emergency medical care for victims who were resuscitated from a condition of sudden death.[92] The population studied consisted of two hundred patients in Olmsted County, Minnesota, who had sustained ventricular fibrillation out of the hospital and were treated by defibrillation after being found to be pulseless. Those admitted to hospital and survived were compared with those who were admitted to hospital and who did not survive. The main factors for the seventy-nine survivors as compared to the sixty-three nonsurvivors who reached the hospital alive were these: a younger age, a larger ejection fraction, a shorter interval between the 911 call and the first shock, a higher proportion of bystanders who witnessed the arrest and performed CPR, and a lower proportion who required epinephrine (adrenalin). It was also concluded that the quality of life among the survivors was similar to that of the general population. A second study from the Mayo Clinic showed that early defibrillation (as a result of reduced call-to-shock time) was a key factor in survival.[93]

Innovations in the Twenty-first Century

The practice of CPR continued to evolve. In 2007, a new approach was described,[94] which was considered to be of the "utmost importance."[95] Chest compression only was recommended, *without rescue breathing*. Chest compression without ventilation was found preferable in attempts by bystanders to resuscitate individuals in whom an out-of-hospital cardiac arrest was witnessed. Aside from the general dislike of performing mouth-to-mouth rescue breathing on a stranger, mouth-to-mouth respiration has the serious drawback that even when performed adequately, it actually takes up time that would be better used in maintaining the circulation to the heart muscle and the brain.

As Arthur Sanders and Gordon Ewy noted in 2005, one problem was that many health care professionals did not perform CPR according to published guidelines.[96] They urged improvement in the quality of "real-world CPR." Ewy had earlier summarized the new approach to CPR, pointing out that, every time a "rescue breath" was given, chest compression had to be stopped, thus interrupting vital flow of blood to the heart and brain.[97] This would be damaging because aside from recovery of heart function, restoration of adequate circulation in the brain is critical to satisfactory neurological recovery. Ewy invoked a further change of mnemonic to CCR, for *cardiocerebral resuscitation*, which, if fully followed, makes hypothermia logical as a means of protecting the brain.[98]

It is likely that the components of CPR will continue to evolve. There is much interest in correct and timely use of the 911 system to summon emergency aid, and of automated external defibrillators.[99] These too will be developed in order to enhance survival of out-of-hospital cardiac arrest.

*   *   *

The purpose of resuscitation has remained the same over the centuries: to restore life to someone who has suddenly and apparently died. This was customarily done by a lay bystander, and until the eighteenth century, physicians were inclined to believe there was not much they could add to the simple measures that had been taken up to then. As drowning and industrial accidents became more common, physicians realized that they could, indeed, add much to resuscitation practice. With the advent of anesthesia and the danger of cardiac arrest under chloroform in particular, anesthesiologists became interested in resuscitation. As their knowledge of the problems of acute heart and lung disturbances grew, and as it became clear that their technical skills could be applied to resuscitation practice, a number of anesthesiologists were able to influence the understanding of resuscitation so that it too became a specialized field itself. As a result, to paraphrase Peter Safar, the science, reason, and compassion that underlie resuscitation comprise "a positive force in our striving to give more and more humans a chance to live full human lives."[100]

Chapter 14

THE CONTINUING EVOLUTION OF ANESTHESIA THE DEVELOPMENT OF SUBSPECIALTIES

The recognition of anesthesia as a specialty in the latter 1930s marked its coming-of-age, but the complex that was the art and science of anesthesia continued to evolve. Progress was notably rapid after the Second World War, many factors being responsible. Among them: new anesthetic drugs and techniques; advances in medicine and surgery; innovations generated by experiences in military medicine; developments in fields such as biochemistry, molecular science, and genetics; the rapid changes in the fields of technology of computers and electronics; and the many applications of the plastics industry. All these factors affected the practice of anesthesia, but they also contributed to changes related to the expanding role of anesthesia in intensive care, pain medicine, and resuscitation medicine. Yet another sign of the evolution of anesthesia was the emergence of subspecialties in anesthesia, with which this chapter is concerned.

Recognition as a specialty took ninety years; the formal acknowledgment of subspecialties followed after only another thirty years. The factors that brought about that development were different from those that led up to the specialty recognition of anesthesia as a whole, and in this chapter, the emergence of five subspecialties is considered in order to illustrate some of the factors that led to subspecialization and to enhance our understanding of specialization in medicine in general. The subspecialties that will be discussed are obstetric anesthesia, paediatric anesthesia, geriatric anesthesia, neuroanesthesia, and cardiothoracic anesthesia.

Factors in the Development of Subspecialization

Immediately after World War II, most anesthesiologists were generalists, for the standard surgical operations were well established, and few of them were particularly complex or specialized. However, this began to change as innovative heart operations, followed by operations on the lungs and brain, pushed back the frontiers of surgery. Anesthesia developed in parallel; sometimes it even led the way.

Heart surgery had begun to develop just before World War II. Patent ductus arteriosus was corrected in 1938, and coarctation of the aorta and congenital pulmonary stenosis,[1] in 1944. But surgery could not progress in the absence of refinements in anesthetic management. Consider the surgical correction of pulmonic stenosis—first performed by Alfred Blalock, of Baltimore. That opened a new chapter in surgery, but the anesthetic technique for the operation, which was performed on very sick children, also marked a new chapter in anesthesia. The cases were reported by Merel Harmel and Austin Lamont in 1946.[2] Anesthesiologists soon developed techniques for other complex procedures that were introduced after the Second World War, including operations within the chest and skull such as those for tracheoesophageal fistula and brain aneurysms. The approaches that anesthesiologists devised for these procedures were often challenging, indeed.

By a process of division of labor, these new operations on the heart and lung and brain, which broached new surgical frontiers, tended to attract anesthesiologists with the skills and knowledge and interest that were appropriate to such challenging anesthesia care. As the surgery became more specialized, so it bred "subspecialist" anesthesiologists who somewhat naturally sought the company of others doing the same work, and subspecialty societies and journals appeared. Anesthesia for surgery of the heart and brain may have been seemed to be full of drama and excitement, but a similar division of labor and subspecialty growth was occurring in other branches of anesthesia that seemed more grounded, such as obstetric anesthesia and geriatric anesthesia. The result was that by the last quarter of the twentieth century, subspecialty work occupied a significant part of the practice of anesthesia.

The development of subspecialization in the latter part of the twentieth century was, however, not an entirely new development. Earlier in the twentieth century, anesthetist S. Griffith Davis had worked with Harvey Cushing in neurosurgery in the United States.[3] In Canada, Charles Robson was the first anesthetist to be appointed full-time to pediatric anesthesia,[4] and in England, after the First World War, Ivan Magill and Stanley Rowbotham worked with plastic surgeon Harold Gillies in anesthetizing patients with faciomaxillary injuries.[5] However, those individuals constituted a very small and widely dispersed group, and no special organizations, such as subspecialty societies, grew up around them. That was different in the later part of the twentieth century, when there were many more subspecialists and when the value of subspecialty societies as a matrix in which subspecialties could grow was more generally recognized. Hence subspecialty anesthesia did not really emerge until the last quarter of the twentieth century.

Subspecialization was a consequence of the logical belief that anesthesia care would be optimized if managed by a practitioner with special knowledge of a particular field. In general, there are advantages to division of labor, but there are disadvantages also. The principal advantage is that a body of specialized knowledge and technical skills develops, and in anesthesia, as in medicine in general, appropriate use of specialized knowledge is frequently essential, even vital. If knowledge is the sine qua non for development of a specialty, it is just as important, or even more important, for development of a subspecialty. Against that may be set the disadvantages of fragmentation of interests,[6] and a separation of the subspecialist from the wider field of the general practice of anesthesia. At the same time, subspecialization also leads, as Cushing implied,[7] to increased knowledge in a particular area. And in anesthesia, special knowledge is obviously essential for the care of patients with other conditions besides heart or brain disorders. The youngest infants and the oldest adults, for example, are frail and fragile; and women in labor present their own physiological and pharmacological challenges to anesthesiologists. Special skill, even dexterity, is another factor: some anesthesiologists are better suited physically than others to handle infants a day or two old, especially in performing procedures such as venipuncture and tracheal intubation, while others are better able, temperamentally or otherwise, to deal with the stresses of anesthesia for cardiac surgery.[8, 9]

Table 14.1. Anesthesia subspecialty societies*

American Academy of Pain Management
American Academy of Pain Medicine
American Pain Society
American Society of Critical Care Anesthesiologists
American Society of Interventional Pain Physicians
American Society of Regional Anesthesia and Pain Medicine
International Association for the Study of Pain
International Society for Anaesthetic Pharmacology
International Trauma Anesthesia and Critical Care Society
Pediatric Cardiac Intensive Care Society
Society for the Advancement in Geriatric Anesthesia
Society for Ambulatory Anesthesia
Society of Neurosurgical and Critical Care
Society for Pain Practice Management
Society for Pediatric Anesthesia
Society of Cardiovascular Anesthesiologists
Society of Critical Care Medicine
Society of Neurosurgical Anesthesia and Critical Care
Society of Obstetric Anesthesia and Perinatology
Society for Technology in Anesthesia

*U.S.- or international-based

Subspecialization in the modern era dates from the 1960s. As the need for a subspecialty was recognized, each subspecialty formed a professional society (table 14.1). Some societies were associated primarily with anesthetic practice in the operating room, and these are considered further in this chapter. Other prominent subspecialties were associated with critical care and pain medicine, as discussed in chapters 11 and 12. The initiating factors varied, but they can be traced in the evolution of the five subspecialties that are now considered.

Obstetric Anesthesia: 120 Years of a De Facto Subspecialty

The evolution of obstetric anesthesia illustrates the complexity and the length of the gestation of subspecialties. Anesthesia for childbirth is, in fact, one of the oldest of subspecialty topics, for Edinburgh obstetrician James Young Simpson articulated some of the complex problems of obstetric anesthesia after he gave ether to a woman in labor on January 19, 1847.[10] Yet not until 1968 was the Society for Obstetric Anesthesia and Perinatology (SOAP) founded. But the founding of SOAP did confirm the existence of what had been a de facto subspecialty for over a century.

Interest in the subspecialty was limited at first; in 1969, "only a handful" of anesthesiologists stated that they had a special interest in obstetrics.[11] This is surprising in view of Simpson's concerns of 1847. Of ether, he thought that it would be necessary "to ascertain its precise effects, both upon the action of the uterus, and of the assistant abdominal muscles; its influence, if any, upon the child, whether it has a tendency to haemorrhage or other considerations; the contra-indications peculiar to its use; the most certain modes of using it; the length of time it may be employed, &c."[12] He was perceptive, for those points remained relevant as part of the cognitive basis for the development of obstetric anesthesia.

The early history of anesthesia in obstetrics has been reviewed by anesthesiologist and historian Donald Caton.[13, 14, 15, 16] Of the factors influencing the thinking about subspecialty development in anesthesia, the most significant were the physiological and pharmacological problems associated with pregnancy, the application of regional techniques of anesthesia, and the need to assess the condition of the accompanying patient, the neonate.

The Physiology and Pharmacology of Pregnancy

Some of the problems of the Simpson era persisted into the twentieth century. For many years, the knowledge of pregnancy and labor was minimal. Many physicians had only a sketchy understanding of a woman's bodily responses to pregnancy, and even less of the responses to drugs in pregnancy or labor. Placental function and the effects of drugs on it were enigmatic, as were physiologic and pharmacologic responses in the fetus and newborn, and the mechanism of postpartum hemorrhage and infection.[17]

Resolving these problems was not easy. One approach was for anesthesiologists with a special interest in obstetric anesthesia to get together and discuss the problems; that was how SOAP was formed. Though research was desirable, this was difficult because little competent research had been conducted into either pregnancy or obstetric anesthesia. All that took time, and answers did not come easily. For example, even today, the precise effects of epidural anesthesia on labor are still being debated.[18]

Regional Anesthesia in Obstetrics

Most of the uncertainties about regional anesthesia, however, were worked out without delay, and its use in expert hands was soon found to be efficacious and safe. It was long favored in obstetric anesthesia. In the first half of the twentieth century, local anesthetics were frequently given by local infiltration; by paracervical, paravertebral, and caudal block; and by subarachnoid and epidural block.[19] Subarachnoid block, the commonest form of regional anesthesia in obstetrics, was used first by Kreis in Germany in 1900 for operative vaginal delivery.[20] It was popularized in the United States by George Pitkin's description of the hyperbaric technique in 1928[21] and by John Adriani's advocacy of saddle block in 1946.[22]

Regional anesthesia in obstetrics was a rational alternative to inhalation anesthesia, and it was a focus around which obstetric anesthesia was specialized. John Cleland, of Oregon, in 1933, described the sensory innervation of the birth canal and reported on lumbar paravertebral and caudal block.[23] Robert Hingson and Waldo Edwards, of New York, advocated continuous caudal block in 1942.[24] It was furthered by neuraxial block, which resulted from the injection of opioids or a local anesthetic into the subarachnoid space or the epidural space, or even into both. In the combined technique, two needles are used: subarachnoid injection of fentanyl via a narrow needle lying within and beyond a larger epidural needle provides analgesia immediately, while injection of a local anesthetic like bupivacaine into the epidural space provides analgesia for longer.[25]

The Apgar Score for Neonatal Assessment

Despite the popularity of regional anesthesia, up to the early 1950s, drugs for control of labor or to relieve pain were still given by intramuscular injection. They included sedatives such as potassium bromide, chloral hydrate, paraldehyde, and bromethol; the analgesics morphine and meperidine; barbiturates such as Nembutal and Seconal; and inhalation agents such as cyclopropane and trichloroethylene, in addition to ether, chloroform, and nitrous oxide.[26] However, drugs sometimes adversely affected labor and, eventually, the fetus and neonate. Obstetricians tended to refer to abnormalities in nonspecific terms; *neonatal apnea*, *oligopnea*, and *neonatal asphyxia* were used by obstetricians. Moreover, they never described any measurements that objectify such conditions. Such a semantic fog hindered communication and understanding. Nor were physicians clear about the effects of drug therapy, including anesthesia in the newborn, for well-conducted studies had never assessed them.

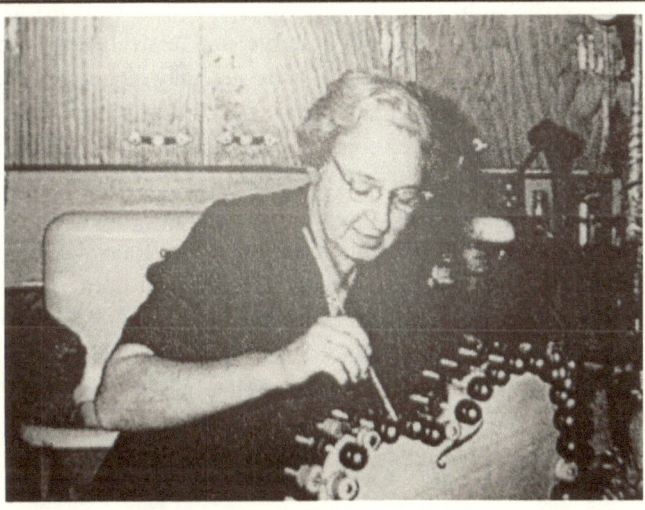

Fig. 14.1. Virginia Apgar (1909-1974)
Virginia Apgar's birthplace was Westfield, New Jersey. Scholarships and various jobs helped her study at Mount Holyoke College, and she enrolled in New York's Columbia University College of Physicians and Surgeons and graduated in 1933. The prospects for a woman to practice as a surgeon being dim, Apgar decided to train in anesthesia. She did so with nurses at Columbia Presbyterian Hospital for a year and took six months with Ralph Waters in Madison and further training with Emery Rovenstine in New York. In 1938, she became director of anesthesia at Columbia. In 1939, when Emanuel Papper was named professor at Columbia, Apgar, also as a professor, took up obstetric anesthesia. Asked how she would evaluate the condition of a newborn baby, Apgar replied that she would rate heart rate, respiratory effort, muscle tone, reflex irritability, and color. She published a report on her ten-point scoring system in 1953, but in 1962, the system became known by the acronym APGAR, for appearance, pulse, grimace, activity, and respiration. Apgar did not rest on her laurels: she obtained a degree in public health, studied genetics and birth defects. She was a professor at Cornell University, assisted the March of Dimes (formerly the National Foundation of Infantile Paralysis), and learned how to fly and make stringed instruments. In 1994, her stature was deservedly honored on a postage stamp. (Photograph courtesy Dr.Selma Calmes.)

This changed after 1953, when Virginia Apgar (fig. 14.1), in New York, published a groundbreaking paper on a method of evaluating the newborn infant.[27] The 1953 version of the Apgar score was the original version, because in 1962, Denver pediatrician Joe Butterfield modified it by cleverly using the letters in the name of Apgar to make an mnemonic acronym: *A* for appearance or color, *P* for pulse or heart rate, *G* for grimace or reflex irritability, *A* for activity or muscle tone, and *R* for respiratory effort.[28] The score was very influential, for physicians, understanding these terms clearly, could now numerically (and objectively) assess the condition of neonates. The outcome of neonates whose mothers had just been anesthetized, for example, for Cesarean section by different techniques could be compared. The scores were generally higher for subarachnoid anesthesia than for general anesthesia. Physicians could also score the condition of the neonate, and this facilitated comparison between anesthetic and obstetric regimens. The Apgar score made the condition of the newborn infant the new standard for evaluating obstetric (and anesthetic) management.[29]

A scientific approach to anesthesia for obstetrics followed Apgar's work. By 1953, there was more interest in basic aspects of obstetric anesthesia as a special field of interest. As a result of other advances in medicine of the 1950s and 1960s, such as measurement of anesthetic gas concentrations and blood-gas concentrations, anesthesia for obstetrics entered a new phase.

Pediatric Anesthesia: Needs of Infants and Children

Reports of children who were anesthetized are also among early records in the history of anesthesia. Four years before Morton demonstrated the ability of ether to induce anesthesia, Crawford Long, on July 3, 1842, gave ether to "a negro boy."[30] He did well. Because children generally did well when anesthetized, it is ironic that the first person to die under chloroform anesthesia was a child. On January 28, 1848, fifteen-year-old Hannah Greener died within minutes of receiving chloroform, even before the scheduled removal of a toenail was begun.[31] Hannah did not die because she was a child, but because she dreaded the surgical experience; a combination of fright, a high concentration of adrenalin in the blood, and a low blood level of chloroform sensitized her heart to a lethal arrhythmia. The fact that it took some sixty years to find the reasons for the lethality of this combination[32] underlines the importance of research in progress. It also justifies the development of specialization.

In children, the 'window' of normal and acceptable responses to anesthesia and surgery tends to be smaller than in adults, and a cascade of potentially critical events may appear sooner and progress more rapidly. Physicians with special knowledge and experience of anesthesia in children were therefore welcomed when they decided to give full attention to the field. Beginning in about 1940, it was clear that anesthesia for some operations, particularly in neonates, called for clinical understanding and technical skills, including human and manual skills and dexterity. Some individuals managed anesthesia for tiny infants with conditions such as tracheoesophageal fistula, omphalocele, congenital diaphragmatic hernia in neonates, and congenital cardiac abnormalities better than others. Anesthesiologists who practiced such demanding work, moreover, found it intensely satisfying.

Specialty organizations and journals soon arose. In 1966, anesthesiologists from the United States and Canada formed a section on pediatric anesthesiology, and a separate organization for pediatric anesthesiology was established in the United Kingdom. In North America, the founding of the Society for Pediatric Anesthesia (SPA) in 1986 was further evidence of the de facto existence of the subspecialty and of the need to foster pediatric anesthesiology clinically, educationally, and academically. Though this society was founded years after the special skills of individuals dealing with children were first recognized, pediatric anesthesia had, in fact, been moving toward a subspecialty for some time. The process evolved in three phases.

Stage I: Prior to 1937

Up to World War II, special knowledge or equipment was not used in anesthesia in children. Anesthesia was often induced with a handkerchief or a gauze mask impregnated with ether or sprayed with ethyl chloride. Tracheal intubation and monitoring devices were infrequent. The child was regarded as a small adult, though some physicians did realize that children differed anatomically and physiologically from adults. Articles on special problems in anesthesia were uncommon, and the first English-language textbook on anesthesia for children did not appear until 1923.[33]

None of this is surprising, for the specialty of pediatric surgery did not emerge until well into the twentieth century. In North America, it originated in the work of Boston surgeon William Ladd in 1917. He answered the call to work with children in Halifax, Nova Scotia, who had been injured in the devastating explosion of an armament ship in the harbor. Their "awful plight" made him decide to switch from gynecology to pediatric surgery. Later, he said that Halifax was the birthplace of pediatric surgery.[34]

Other events advanced pediatric anesthesia. One was the appointment in 1919 of Charles Robson as chief anaesthetist to the Toronto Sick Children's Hospital,[35] a full-time position that was similar to Robert Cope's in London.[36] Robson's expertise, including his use of endotracheal intubation, showed the benefits of full-time anesthesiologists to progress in this field, just as expertise in anesthesia as a whole confirmed the logic of specialty recognition of anesthesia in the 1930s.

Drugs and techniques also influenced the development of anesthesia for children as a special field. Cyclopropane, introduced in 1930, was valued for inducing and maintaining anesthesia in children, largely replacing ether, but skill was needed for its administration. Skill was also required for tracheal intubation, though it was made easier by technical innovations, which themselves greatly improved the administration of anesthesia in younger children. An example of this is the elegant simplicity of the T-piece designed by Philip Ayre, of Newcastle, in 1937. To help him anaesthetize children with harelip and cleft palate—from which he himself suffered—Ayre added a T-shaped connection to the tracheal tube,[37] and so made the management of respiration easier for him and less stressful for his patients. The T-piece reduced equipment dead space and prevented hypoventilation. Simple though this concept was, it demonstrates the priceless value of concentration of thought that only comes with subspecialization. Ayre's idea was one of many that periodically advanced anesthesia.

Stage II:1937-1960

Pediatric anesthesiology evolved rapidly after World War II, when anesthesiologists had to solve new problems, especially for anesthesia for complex surgical procedures. Digby Leigh, of Montreal, is an exemplar. In 1938, after training with Ralph Waters in Madison, he joined the staff at McGill University and became director of anesthesia at the Montreal Children's Hospital. In 1947, Leigh moved to Los Angeles, where, like Ayre, he recognized the need for special equipment for children, notably a non-rebreathing valve[38] and an infant circle filter.[39] With Kay Belton, he published *Pediatric Anesthesia* in 1948.[40] Also active in the United States were William McQuiston in Chicago, Robert Smith in Boston, Herbert Rackow in New York, and Margo Deming in Philadelphia.[41] All shaped the evolution of the subspecialty.

Other textbooks—by Robert Smith,[42] Clement Smith,[43] Helen Taussig,[44] and William Nelson[45]—added to the knowledge base of anesthesiologists interested in pediatric anesthesiology. Journal articles also fueled its growth, partly by fostering clinical investigation. Specific problems, such as tracheal abnormalities following endotracheal intubation[46] and slowing of the heart after succinylcholine was injected into infants and children[47] were discussed. Research was encouraged by the increased interest in pediatric anesthesia; topics of inquiry included the nature of endotracheal tubes[48] and the newborn's response muscle relaxants.[49]

Innovations in drugs and techniques continued to stimulate progress. In Liverpool, England, Jackson Rees combined nitrous oxide with curare and adapted the so-called Liverpool technique for use in children.[50] Rees also modified the T-piece by adding an expiratory tube and a breathing bag so he could control ventilation. Halothane, introduced in 1956, was a welcome addition to, and then replacement for, ether and cyclopropane. Halothane was neither pungent nor inflammable, like ether; induction of anesthesia was rapid and not stressful, and it did not require a tightly closed breathing system, like cyclopropane.

Between 1937 and 1960, a consensus was reached on most aspects of anesthesia for children. By 1950, its practice was delineated, at any rate in terms of concepts and techniques.[51] The future for excellence in anesthesia for children looked bright.

Stage III:1960-2000

Even if perfection was not attained between 1960 and 2000, progress was significant. Four aspects of anesthesia are notable. The first concerns drugs. The fluorinated inhalational agents, short-acting opioids, and rapidly acting muscle relaxants were potent and efficacious, and had few side effects. The second relates to anesthesia equipment, which was more sophisticated. Third, monitoring devices gave information that was more precise and of a broader range of information. And fourth, by the 1960s, anesthesiologists were beginning to understand the physiological and pharmacological basis of anesthesia in infants and children more clearly. Anesthesia was more precise than ever before.

Clinical practice was enhanced by the research into pediatric anesthesia that began in the 1960s. For example, it had not always been clear whether anesthesia was adequate or not,[52] and because research in children was honored more in the breach than the observance, information was often grossly lacking. Thus before 1969, there were no studies of the pulmonary exchange of anesthetic agents in infants. That was rectified that year[53] and, incidentally, confirmed what Snow had observed in 1858.[54] Other areas of research interest include the minimum effective doses of halothane,[55] the minimum alveolar concentration and the higher halothane requirement in infants than in adults,[56] pulmonary mechanics in infants and children,[57] use of curare in children,[58] and neuromuscular transmission in neonates.[59] Specially designed machines for ventilation of infants and children were introduced, and the concept of positive end-expiratory pressure in improving respiratory gas exchange became better understood.[60]

As in other aspects of anesthesia, progress in areas besides anesthesia itself contributed. Adult respiratory intensive care, neonatology and neonatal intensive care, pediatric general surgery, and pediatric cardiac surgery all furthered progress in anesthesia for infants and children[61] Thus, in the century and a half since Long anesthetized a boy in 1842, many factors determined the way pediatric anesthesia evolved as a subspecialty. Yet the subspecialty existed in de facto form long before it became a recognized entity with, for example, the founding of the SPA in 1986. However, the fact that pediatric anesthesiologists were successful in gaining recognition as subspecialists cannot be doubted. Textbooks on pediatric anesthesia abound, research proliferates, specialty journals flourish. Opportunities for training in pediatric anesthesiology are available, and all residency programs in North America require a period of training in pediatric anesthesia. The subspecialty thrives.

Geriatric Anesthesia: Some Formative Imperatives

Interest in anesthesia for the elderly also dates from the early years of anesthesia. A patient's age has always been known to influence the effects of anesthesia,[62] but two questions of definition are pertinent. First: who is "old"? In contrast to our ready recognition of infants and children, whom we have no difficulty in defining in terms of years, our conception of who is old varies widely from person to person, as it has, indeed, from period to period. Old age once meant older than forty; later, sixty-five; later seventy-five; today, even some eighty-year-olds do not seem "old." This reflects the second question related to definition: how do we define the physiological effects of aging? After all, those effects seem to be "peculiar" to the older person only in becoming more evident with age, even though those effects may have begun in the same individual at a younger age. Those questions bring up a third: how can geriatric anesthesia be a subspecialty when such factors are not clear-cut? While, certainly, there are good reasons for regarding geriatric anesthesia as a subspecialty, they do not seem to be as firm as those regarding pediatric anesthesia, for example.

Interest in anesthesia for the elderly grew in the second half of the twentieth century, though organizations intended to foster concentration of thoughts and energies on it as a special field did not develop until late in the century. In the United Kingdom, the Age Anaesthesia Association was not formed until 1987; in the United States, not until 2000 was the Society for the Advancement in Geriatric Anesthesia (SAGA) formed. Today there is great interest in geriatric anesthesia: the American Society of Anesthesiologists, for example, sends representatives to the Council for Surgical and Related Medical Specialties, and it has prepared a syllabus on geriatric anesthesia; and textbooks on geriatric anesthesia and fellowships in geriatric anesthesia are available. Even if it is not formally recognized as a subspecialty, it certainly is one de facto.

The formative aspects of geriatric anesthesia provide a further opportunity to analyze forces that have shaped the evolution of a subspecialty. The forces may be considered as imperatives, each being relevant to the question as to whether geriatric anesthesia is, or should be, a subspecialty.

The Demographic Imperative

In 1992, persons in the United States aged sixty-five or older numbered 32.2 million, or 12.7 percent of the population.[63] It is estimated that by 2030, those figures will be 70 million and 20 percent. The elderly segment of the population, proportionally, began growing rapidly in the twentieth century, being of the order of 2.5 percent annually.[64] In 1990, there were as many persons aged sixty or older as there were under the age of fourteen.[65] This trend is a continuing one. In the twenty-first century, persons aged eighty-five years or older will be the most rapidly growing segment of the population.[66] In terms of absolute numbers, in 1990, while there were 18.1 million Americans in the sixty-five-to seventy-four-year-old group, there were 10.1 million in the seventy-five—to eighty-four-year-old group.[67] Toward the end of the twentieth century, the implication for anesthesiologists was quite clear: more and more of their patients would be elderly.

The Physiological Imperative

Many of the physiological changes that occur as we grow older are adverse. The functional capacity of body organs, for example, steadily decreases with age. The greatest decrease in physiological reserves is in maximum breathing capacity, which falls to approximately 40 percent of the mean value at age thirty; the least, in conduction velocity in the heart, to approximately 87.5 percent.[68] The significance for anesthesia—and an argument, perhaps, for recognition of geriatric anesthesia as a recognized subspecialty—is that, with age, the inadequacy of function of the more vital organs is such that even a minor stress during anesthesia or surgery may prove critical, or even fatal. The loss of function is, moreover, aggravated by disease of the organ or organs in which function is depressed.

The Pathological Imperative

The presence of a chronic disorder is a third imperative justifying geriatric anesthesia as a subspecialty. As anesthesiologist Ron Stephen showed in 1984, the health of most elderly persons is adversely affected by one or more chronic disorders that are potentially disabling.[69] These include high blood pressure, narrowing and blockage of the blood vessels (including the coronary arteries), kidney disease, heart enlargement and failure, obstructive lung disease, and diabetes. One or more of these will tend to aggravate the state of health that is already compromised by physiological impairment. Coexisting disease is a significant factor as far as perioperative morbidity and mortality are concerned,[70] and it is more significant than age, and also anesthesia.[71] In this context, English anaesthetist Tony Davenport's advocating the anesthesiologist as a perioperative geriatrician rather than as a geriatric anesthesiologist is logical.[72] Since some of the coexisting conditions affect many patients younger than those who are considered old, it may be preferable that the anesthesiologist taking care of an elderly patient has a broad experience of all types of adult cases. Nevertheless, the anesthesiologist with a special interest in the elderly may be more likely to preserve as far as possible the limited function that both physiological and pathological changes have wrought.

The Pharmacological Imperative

The way the body deals with drugs is also affected by age.[73] The decrease
in lean body mass and the total volume of water, and the increase in body
fat, are factors.[74] So are other physiological changes such as cardiac output,
clearance of drugs by the liver and the kidney, and the minimum alveolar
concentration in the lungs. The initial concentration of a drug after being
injected is relatively greater, since its initial concentration depends partly on
the volume in the body's central compartment. The way a drug is redistributed
to peripheral tissues and is eliminated is another factor, as is clearance by
the liver or the kidney. When an anesthetic agent is inhaled, its action is in
part determined by the minimum alveolar concentration, and this decreases
steadily with age. While the body deals with different drugs in different
ways, elderly patients do require smaller drug doses. This does not, on its
own, justify geriatric anesthesia being regarded as a subspecialty; but rather,
it is evidence of a further aspect of knowledge that is unique to anesthetic
care of the elderly.

The Surgical Imperative

The fact that today more surgical patients are elderly—in whom physiological,
pathological, and pharmacological problems loom large—has an impact on
the practice of anesthesia. Many are octogenarians and nonagenarians, with
progressively severe physiological and pathological problems. Prior to the
1960s, surgeons did not like operating on the "elderly," but improvements
in various aspects of medical care, including anesthesia care, changed that.
Now more than one million persons in the United States are ninety years
or older,[75] and surgery on nonagenarians is no longer uncommon. Between
1975 and 1985, for example, Mark Warner and his colleagues at the Mayo
Clinic reported that 224 nonagenarians were operated on 319 times.[76] This
is remarkable, but so is the fact that 92 percent of those patients were able
to leave the hospital alive. Even so, since the various preoperative problems
are magnified with age, anesthesiologists will have to make every effort to
make anesthesia care as meticulous as possible. A case could therefore be
made that subspecialization, by directing thoughts and energies toward
ways of delivering meticulous care, is one way in which the very best of
anesthesia care can be planned. There is a great deal of knowledge on geriatric
anesthesia, and it is encouraging that despite the increased incidence of
chronic disease in the very elderly, these patients do appear to recover from
surgery so well.

Geriatric Anesthesia as a Subspecialty?

The foregoing observations make it understandable that an organization such as SAGA should have been formed specifically to improve the care of the older patient having surgery. What questions have been asked concerning recognition of geriatric anesthesia as a subspecialty?

One question is this: might subspecialization in geriatric anesthesia improve the outcome of the elderly patient undergoing surgery? Anesthesiologists Robert Jones and David Brown, of Houston, defined the goals of effective anesthesia care,[77] but in themselves, these goals are no different with respect to the elderly and younger adults. These goals are the following: to coordinate a patient's anesthetic management and postoperative requirements with the surgeon, to minimize the impact of the anesthetic and the procedure on the patient and subsequent hospital care, to provide appropriate and thoughtful care, and to return the patient to the accustomed lifestyle as soon as possible. Risk factors must be identified for each patient, and then the appropriate care determined. While these considerations in themselves are not an argument for geriatric anesthesia as a subspecialty, concentration of thought and energy along special lines on the part of dedicated personnel must improve the chances for favorable outcome.

Another question: how are anesthesia-related complications, both obvious and subtle, best avoided?[78] Obvious complications include hypoxia, hypoventilation, cardiac arrest, hypoperfusion, hypertension, and hypothermia and hypothermia. Subtle ones, more difficult to define, include ischemia (poor blood supply), cognitive impairment, and continuation of effects of anesthetic agents into the postoperative period, both noninjurious and tissue destructive. While such complications are of concern in all patients, the elderly are at greater risk because they are less functionally able to deal with such stressors, for even a single complication may prove too much for the body, already impaired by age and disease, to deal with. Heightened awareness of such problems will diminish their gravity.

In answering these questions, one must consider the level of individual anesthetic care. If, as anesthesiologist Davenport argued, the "allowance for carelessness" is to be regarded as a factor in anesthetic care of the elderly,[79] differences in competence among individual anesthesiologists may be vital. Evidence does show that differences, sometimes injurious, do exist. One study on complications associated with coronary artery bypass operations provides suggestive evidence.[80] The study concerned a relationship between new episodes of myocardial ischemia (diminished blood supply to the heart muscle) before heart bypass was started and myocardial infarction (a "heart attack"). Such a relationship did exist, but it was also found that this relationship occurred more frequently in the patients who were anesthetized by one particular anesthesiologist: the varying rates of ischemia during anesthesia among anesthesiologists reflected their varying skills in managing patients. Although this study was not concerned with aging and anesthesia, it does suggest that competence of an anesthesiologist is an important factor in outcome of surgery and anesthesia. Similar conclusions were reached in a second study of the role of the anesthesiologist as a "risk factor."[81] Among anesthesiologists caring for patients with coronary artery bypass operations, one was significantly "worse" than others with respect to the criterion for postoperative myocardial infarction that they used (aspartate amino transferase concentration).

These two studies suggest that the "skilled administrator" is a factor with respect to outcome, though those studies did not specifically concern anesthesia and aging. Even so, they suggest that the degree of skill of an anesthesiologist would be important in the care of elderly patients in whom, like cardiac patients, the occurrence of adverse events might be serious enough to tip the balance toward a negative outcome. However, that, again, is not an argument in itself for formalization of a subspecialty of geriatric anesthesia, though it does provide one more point in favor of it.

Considered together, these various imperatives suggest that as of the end of the twentieth century, formative forces were moving geriatric anesthesia in the direction of a subspecialty. For the historian, the interest in geriatric anesthesia lies in its illustrating the nature of some of those formative factors.

Neuroanesthesia: Sharing the Brain

Anesthesia for neurosurgery is unique in that in the patient undergoing intracranial surgery, the brain is the specific target organ for both surgeon and anesthesiologist.[82] What one does may affect what the other is trying to do. However, anesthesia practitioners became well aware of the consequences of their practice and of their research on the work of their neurosurgical colleagues. All this, however, has influenced the development of neuroanesthesia as a subspecialty,

Although the origin of neurosurgery as a surgical specialty can be traced to 1919,[83] it was not until the 1960s that the seeds for neuroanesthesia as a subspecialty were sown. Until then, anesthesiologists were thought to be ignorant of the effects of anesthetic agents and techniques on variables such as cerebral blood flow and metabolic rates and intracranial pressure.[84] That does not mean that significant research had not been done. Intracranial pressure,[85, 86] controlled ventilation,[87, 88] hyperventilation and intracranial and systemic dynamics,[89] and cerebral blood flow[90] were studied earlier in the twentieth century.

A factor that stimulated the subspecialty development of neuroanesthesia was a meeting of the Commission of Neuroanesthesia on July 9, 1960. Sponsored by the World Federation of Neurology,[91] the conference enabled anesthesiologists from nine countries to consider how to advance teaching and research in neuroanesthesia. Groups in Philadelphia, Rochester, and Glasgow,[92] and also in Richmond (Virginia), San Francisco, Cleveland, Montreal, and London[93] were encouraged to extend the work of earlier researchers. New principles began to emerge.

Other early initiatives include the first two textbooks of neuroanesthesia, in 1964[94] and 1965,[95] and, in 1965, the founding of the Neuroanaesthesia Travelling Club of Great Britain and Ireland to further the development of neuroanesthesia as a subspecialty.[96] The founding of the Neurosurgical Anesthesia Society (later the Society of Neurosurgical Anesthesia and Critical Care in 1973 also enabled neurosurgeons and neuroanesthesiologists to share common interests).[97]

All these events shaped the development of neuroanesthesia as a subspecialty. This development affected neuroanesthetic practice, education, and research, but also anesthesiology in general. Thus, the development of neuroanesthesia as a subspecialty affirmed the validity of specialty status for anesthesia. Recognition of subspecialty status gives its practitioners a sense of professional identity that comes about with special attention to teaching and research, as well as clinical practice. That is not peculiar to neuroanesthesia, but the special nature of neuroanesthesia illustrates it clearly.

That special nature is apparent in relation to five principles in particular: regulation of brain volume and pressure, control of hemorrhage, protection of nervous tissue from ischemic and surgical injury, maintenance of prolonged anesthesia, and management of intensive care. Understanding the effects on the brain of variations in oxygen and carbon dioxide tensions and in the blood pressure continued to determine practice, and the development of engineering and electronics in numerous sophisticated monitoring instruments made precise measurements of these and many other parameters enhanced neuroanesthetic management. So too did guidelines for specific aspects of practice as developed by the Society of Neurosurgical Anesthesia and Critical Care.[98]

Subspecialty recognition—neuroanesthesia is recognized by the American Society of Anesthesiologists, for example—has stimulated education too. Several anesthesia textbooks on neuroanesthesia followed the very first two. Training positions burgeoned, from six in the United States and Canada in 1972 to sixty-four in 1989.[99] And research has continued to flourish, both in clinical and investigative aspects of the subspecialty. Nor has research been confined to established researchers: Jack Michenfelder noted that in 1992, there were twenty-five submissions for Young Investigator Awards and fourteen Starter Grant Applications.[100]

As a subspecialty, then, specialization of anesthesia for neurosurgery helped to refine the practice of anesthesia, not only in this area, but also in anesthesia in general. The benefits of subspecialization underlined the advantages of subspecialization. This is true of obstetric anesthesia and pediatric anesthesia as well, and also of cardiothoracic anesthesia.

Cardiothoracic Anesthesia: The Ultimate in Subspecialization?

The heart and the lungs are affected very quickly by anesthetic agents and by what the anesthesiologist does or does not do. Anesthesia may make a crucial difference to patients such as those with a diseased heart valve or in whom a whole lung has to be removed. It is essential to prevent, or at least minimize, a departure from what is a norm in such variables as the oxygen and carbon dioxide concentrations or the blood pressure, pulse rate, or large-vein pressure. Homeostasis (i.e., maintenance within acceptable limits of physiological variables) must be kept as close as possible to normal. The general principle of division of labor with respect to this subspecialty is perhaps more essential here than in any other anesthesia subspecialty. Subspecialization in cardiothoracic anesthesia was a logical development.

In practice, cardiac operations and thoracic operations are usually performed by different surgeons, and anesthesiologists interested in cardiothoracic work often divide up labor similarly. Still, because the heart lies within the chest, or thorax, certain problems are common to anesthesia for lung surgery and heart surgery. These problems had to be solved before cardiothoracic anesthesia could develop. This discussion will therefore be focused on the several issues concerning cardiothoracic anesthesia.

Prerequisites for Cardiothoracic Anesthesia

The first requirement for anesthesia for the heart and lungs was growth of specific knowledge about the physiology and pharmacology of the heart. For years, it was thought that the heart was too sensitive an organ to withstand surgical manipulation, but the removal of foreign bodies during the Second World War showed that the heart is actually quite robust.[101] Once this was understood, the way the heart responded to anesthesia and to surgery had to be learned, as well as ways in which the variations in the function of the heart could be kept within acceptable limits. As new surgical procedures were developed, so new approaches to anesthesia or modifications of established ones had to be devised. Thus innovations in surgery also added to the knowledge base of anesthesia.

Besides knowledge, another requirement was professionalism. As Harvard anesthesiologist Leroy Vandam observed, "Professionalism in any field entails study with consequent progress, the teaching and recruitment of others, interaction with the other branches of medicine, and devotion to the kind of investigation that solves its own problems."[102] Professionalism enhanced patient care, as well as the subspecialty of cardiothoracic anesthesia.

A third requirement concerned the availability of resources. There had to be enough patients with heart disorders that were surgically treatable and accepted as such in the contemporary health care environment, in which ethical and financial points must be considered. Enough specialist surgeons had to be available, together with a sufficiency of trained anesthesiologists to play their part. Similarly, technological resources had to be adequate: just as open-heart surgery, for example, required a heart-lung machine, so a cardiac anesthesiologist required technically appropriate equipment, whether a simple tracheal tube, a real-time analyzer for blood-gas concentrations, or a far more sophisticated monitoring device such as an echocardiograph.

Those prerequisites are general in nature. More specific were certain problems that had to be solved and questions that had to be answered. These indicate that many factors influenced the development of cardiothoracic anesthesia.

Issues in Cardiothoracic Anesthesia

Pneumothorax and its solution. Common to the safety of intrathoracic operations, whether on the heart or the lungs, is the solution to the problem of pneumothorax. When the chest is opened and if the lungs are not inflated, atmospheric air presses down on the surface of the lungs, and if this is not prevented, death follows. This was not appreciated when the first planned operation on the lung was performed in 1888. After experimenting on rabbits, H. M. Block, of Danzig (now Gdansk, Poland),[103] thought he was ready to operate on a woman with tuberculosis. However, she died after the operation; but so did Block, who committed suicide, because he was thought to have erred in performing such an operation. Probably, lung collapse and lack of oxygen caused the patient's death. Only after this problem was solved were doctors willing to give anesthesia for operations within the chest.

Ways of preventing the exposed lung from collapsing, therefore, were tested. At first, late in the nineteenth century and early in the twentieth, *negative* pressure was applied to the *exterior* surface of the lung, thus to "suck" it open.[104] But beginning in the latter part of the nineteenth century, some investigators tried applying *positive* pressure to the *interior* of the lung by rhythmically inflating the lungs. These methods were developed by surgeons, though, as noted in chapter 6, anesthetists did make use of tracheal insufflation, which kept the lungs expanded as oxygen and anesthetic gases streamed steadily through a relatively narrow tube in the trachea.

Not until 1919 did anesthetists come up with a made-for-anesthesia solution (see also chapter 6). In the van were Ivan Magill and Stanley Rowbotham, who found that inflating the lungs *rhythmically* with gases through a tube of wider bore was preferable to continuous-flow insufflation.[105] It was, in fact, this new practice of tracheal intubation, with the positive pressure it applied to the lungs, that solved the problem of pneumothorax.

Cuffed tubes to prevent soilage of the tracheobronchial tree. Simply placing a tube in the trachea and rhythmically inflating the lungs, however, was not enough to provide perfect operating conditions for the thoracic surgeon. An advance occurred when the tracheal tube was fitted with an inflatable cuff, for the tube fit tightly within the trachea and prevented secretions and blood from passing from the mouth and pharynx alongside the tube to the lungs. Tubes had been cuffed by Victor Eisenmenger in 1893,[106] but the type of cuff that was used in anesthesia was that of Arthur Guedel and Ralph Waters (see also chapter 6). They described that cuff in 1928,[107] dunking a dog in a tank of water to confirm the seal. A different step was Waters' designing the to-and-fro soda-lime canister in 1924, which facilitated absorption of carbon dioxide.[108] The device could be used—in cardiothoracic as well as general anesthesia—in children as well as adults.

Fitting a cuff on the tracheal tube was, however, only part of the solution. Although that did prevent blood and secretions passing from above into the trachea and lungs via the glottis, it could not prevent liquid matter passing from one part of the tracheobronchial tree, *within* the lungs, to another when a patient lay on the side for surgery on the lung lying uppermost. That was common when pulmonary tuberculosis was rampant. It became necessary to protect, or block off, the dependent, "good," lung so it would not be flooded with blood or secretions or pus from the other, "bad," lung. A special tube was passed so that one bronchus could be intubated, permitting so-called one-lung anesthesia. That type of tube—an endobronchial blocker—was described first in 1932 by J. Gale and Ralph Waters in Madison.[109] They took a fourteen-inch Guedel-Waters tube and fitted it with an inflatable cuff, molded in hot water so as to make a lateral curve. This was passed, by feel, so that the tip lay in the bronchus, with the cuff overlying the entrance to the *bronchus* of the diseased lung, which would thus be sealed off. This tube also minimized shift of the mediastinum by means of positive pressure and immobilized the operating field, and as well, it prevented the spread of potentially infective material into the trachea and other lung.

As noted in chapter 6, the Gale-Waters tube was the first of a long line of tubes that were designed over the next two decades to facilitate one-lung anesthesia. While the tubes performed as intended, their use emphasized two other points. First, by the 1920s, anesthetists were beginning to look seriously at the problems that would have to be solved if thoracic anesthesia was to be feasible; and second, the way was paved for thoracic anesthesia to become a subspecialty.

Could a beating heart be repaired? Chronologically, a second key advance came when surgeons realized that it was actually possible to operate on the heart. In 1896, for example, Ludwig Rehn, in Germany, repaired a heart that had been injured by stabbing.[110] He did this even before techniques for thoracic or cardiac surgery had been worked out. Just as solving the problem of pneumothorax marked the beginning of successful lung surgery, so Rehn's operating on the heart itself was the beginning of cardiac surgery. Though it is not known what anesthetic agents and technique were used, it was apparent also that anesthesia in heart cases was possible. Confidence was also boosted by Harken's later demonstration of the robustness of the injured heart.[111]

Mechanical ventilators in cardiothoracic anesthesia. Another stimulus to the development of both cardiac anesthesia and thoracic anesthesia was the introduction of mechanical ventilators. Originally, artificial ventilation of the lungs using negative pressure required bulky and expensive equipment, such as the iron lung, so devices generating positive pressure were more practical and efficient. At first, an anesthesiologist would rhythmically squeeze a breathing bag to inflate the lungs with each inspiration, but this function was later taken over by mechanical ventilators.

Many pieces of apparatus were constructed in the early years of the twentieth century. In Germany, they included those of Kuhn in 1905;[112] of Bernard Dräger, who in 1907 produced the Pulmotor,[113] which inflated the lungs rhythmically; and Arthur Lawen, whose 1910 device generated rhythmic artificial ventilation rather than constant pressure.[114] In the United States, surgeons N. W. Green and Henry Janeway designed equipment to provide automatic controlled ventilation for thoracic surgery,[115] though they tended to be cumbersome. In 1913, an apparatus of Janeway's assisted respiration by "merely accentuating the patient's efforts of respiration."[116]

Even the introduction of tracheal and bronchial tubes and ventilators was not followed immediately by widespread heart and lung surgery or by cardiothoracic anesthesia as a special field of interest. Events moved slowly. In the 1920s, for example, only two heart operations of note were performed. One was performed by Elliot Cutler, at the Peter Bent Brigham Hospital in Boston, who incised a stenotic mitral valve in 1923, though the patient died,[117] as did several others. The other operation of note was performed on May 6, 1925, at the London Hospital in England, by Henry Souttar, also on a woman with mitral stenosis. He clamped the left atrial appendage, inserted a finger into the auricle, and felt the expected stenosis of the mitral valve. He digitally dilated the orifice—a maneuver that, he said, "cannot be surpassed for simplicity and directness." Because the stenosis was less severe than he had anticipated, Souttar did not cut into the valve—which, as he said, "might only make matters worse by increasing the degree of regurgitation."[118] The patient recovered. This was the stuff of true surgical drama, but what of the anesthesia?

The anaesthetist was John Challis, whose services Souttar did not ignore—a mark of a great surgeon. The anesthesia consisted of premedication with morphine and atropine, induction with the ACE mixture of absolute alcohol, chloroform, and ether, and maintenance with ether administered by endotracheal catheter (possibly by insufflation), the patient breathing spontaneously.[119] Monitoring consisted of blood pressure recordings and, no doubt, by visual inspection and palpation of the pulse. By today's standards, astonishingly simple!

Those footnotes to history aside, thoracic surgery did not develop until the 1930s, and cardiac surgery not until the 1940s and 1950s. Why was there such a delay? There are several reasons. One concerns research. This ceased during World War I, and after the war, there was a shortage of funds for research, particularly in Germany. Another factor was the emphasis on artificial pneumothorax and thoracoplasty as treatments of choice for patients with pulmonary tuberculosis, rather than on surgical excision of lung tissue. Another factor was the need to control infection: the sulfonamides did not become available until the 1930s, and penicillin and streptomycin not until the 1940s. Problems in operating on the heart[120] also took time to be solved; not until the mid-1950s did open-heart surgery become a reality.

Although some ventilators were designed before World War I, progress in that field was slow also. In the interwar years, the only ventilator of note in this period was the Drinker iron lung,[121] which was used in the treatment of poliomyelitis victims and was not suited to anesthesia. Not until P. Frenckner in Sweden developed the Spiropulsator in 1934[122] was a ventilator with potentiality for use in the operating room. The Spiropulsator was used by Stockholm surgeon Clarence Crafoord, but it never caught on outside Sweden. The Spiropulsator, which could be driven by air, oxygen, or the "narcotic gaseous mixture," and whose timing mechanism was based on that of the device controlling the flashing of marker buoys, was, however, the first of a long line of ventilators that continued to be developed during the rest of the twentieth century.

Anesthesiologists were no faster in using ventilators in the operating room. A change in attitude, however, came in 1952, when Danish anesthesiologist Bjorn Ibsen provided a powerful argument for controlled ventilation. His own opinion was forged by his innovative use of tracheal intubation and positive-pressure ventilation during the catastrophic epidemic of poliomyelitis in Copenhagen in 1952[123] (see chapter 11). Any lingering objections to controlled ventilation and to ventilators faded.

These various developments did much to put thoracic anesthesia on a sound footing, and they provided an equally sound base on which cardiac anesthesia could eventually proceed.

Use of new drugs. Though constituting advances, new drugs are not always incorporated into practice with rapidity. Cyclopropane and curare illustrate this. Cyclopropane, introduced in 1930, was an inhalational agent, and therefore, physicians were, in general, familiar with its administration. The problem here, however, was that it depressed ventilation, in a way that the standby ether did not. Anesthetists therefore took time to get used to it. But because of this property, cyclopropane was well suited to cardiothoracic anesthesia. It could be given with a 100 percent concentration of oxygen and so was good for sick patients, and its respiratory depressant effect could be managed by manual compression of the breathing bag and by a mechanical ventilator when the use of mechanical ventilators became routine. However, cyclopropane was inflammable, and it was replaced after the nonflammable halothane became available in 1956. In its turn, halothane was replaced by the less biotransformable isoflurane beginning in the 1980s.

In a different category was curare (see chapter 5). Introduced in 1942, it was given by injection, and its paralyzing effect had to be counteracted by an antagonist drug. Ventilation was easy to control since it paralyzed the respiratory muscles, and because of their experience with cyclopropane, anesthesiologists felt no compunction in abolishing spontaneous respiration with curare. However, the fact that its effects lasted into the postoperative period was not understood at first. The problem came to a head in 1954, when Henry Beecher and Donald Todd published a report that blackened the good name of curare[124] by suggesting that it was toxic. The real problem was the failure to pharmacologically reverse the curare effects and the inadequate management of depressed ventilation in the meantime.

Once that problem was sorted out and principles of the use of curare and its successors clarified, it became clear that complete muscle paralysis was a boon for anesthesiologists, for it opened a new era in anesthesia. It also made many surgical operations easier and expedited the evolution of cardiothoracic anesthesia as a subspecialty.

Other anesthetic drugs that were introduced in the second half of the twentieth century, particularly halothane, isoflurane, succinylcholine, pancuronium, vecuronium, etomidate, and propofol further refined clinical anesthesia. At the same time, there was a resurgence of interest in one of the oldest of drugs, and a new way of using it was considered in anesthesia for heart surgery.

This drug was morphine. In 1969, Edward Lowenstein and his colleagues used it in a new way.[125] They found, in a group of heart surgery patients, that relatively large doses of morphine in the postoperative period seemed to have no adverse effects on the circulation. Would it be reasonable to use large doses in anesthesia for heart surgery patients? Lowenstein gave morphine, in a dose of 1 mg per kilogram body weight, to patients having surgery for aortic valve disease. He found the results "startling and pleasing." The cardiac output in the aortic-valve patients *increased*, and the systemic vascular resistance *decreased*.[126]

Lowenstein's study changed perceptions about the cardiac actions of opioids and set the stage for the eventual administration of larger doses of opioids.[127] Yet Lowenstein was at cross purposes with other anesthesiologists: they had, independently, begun to favor earlier removal of the endotracheal tube after heart surgery while Lowenstein was using morphine in high dosage precisely to enable patients to tolerate the presence of a tracheal tube. Although this use of morphine did not persist, Lowenstein'a paper on it, appropriately titled "The Birth of Opioid Anesthesia," did influence thinking about anesthesia. It directed the attention of anesthesiologists to using other opioids such as fentanyl and sufentanil as a new approach to anesthesia for heart surgery and, historically, it is an example of just one of many contributions that anesthesiologists have made to progress in heart surgery.

How should monitors be used? It is remarkable that in the early years, surgeons and anesthetists, despite the lack of monitoring devices, looked after their patients so well. For example, in 1912, Morriston Davies performed a right lower lobectomy for carcinoma,[128] and the patient survived the operation, eventually dying from a cause unrelated to anesthesia; and in 1918, Harold Brunn, of San Francisco, performed lobectomy in six patients without a single death.[129] Such results are remarkable because the only monitoring devices were the physical senses, the stethoscope, and the blood pressure cuff. (As noted in chapter 10, the electrocardiogram, though invented in 1903, was not used at all frequently until the 1960s.)

The same is true of monitoring in anesthesia for heart operations; it was minimal at first. For example, in anesthetizing an infant with patent ductus arteriosus in 1938, nurse anesthetist Betty Lank simply placed an alcohol-shrunken mask on the face, administered cyclopropane, and kept a finger, a la Clover, on the superficial temporal artery as a monitor.[130] It was a simplistic triumph. So was the minimal monitoring that Harmel and Lamont used in anaesthetizing the desperately sick children who underwent the Blalock operation for congenital pulmonic stenosis.[131] Their paper gives insight into what they could achieve, with a minimalist technique, in the extraordinarily exciting new field of cardiac anesthesia, interest in which must have grown enormously as a result. In contrast, beginning in the 1950s, monitoring became increasingly widespread and complex. The question then logically arises as to which body functions should be monitored, and to what extent. These questions are considered in chapter 10, and need not be considered further here, except to make the point that specialized devices, such as the V_5 electrocardiograph lead (introduced in 1976)[132] and transesophageal electrocardiography,[133] when used appropriately, did give valuable information that enhanced anesthesia management.

The cognitive value of journals and textbooks. Another stimulus to the development of cardiothoracic anesthesia as a subspecialty was provided by journals and textbooks. These facilitated communication and spread knowledge among anesthesiologists specializing in cardiothoracic anesthesia, and the journals that were specific to cardiothoracic anesthesia created a virtual image of the subspecialty.

Journal articles and textbooks not only advanced the subspecialty of cardiothoracic anesthesia but also provided a paper trail that we can follow in tracing its evolution. Some of the elements of that trail are evident in the work of physicians whose communications have already been noted in this section. Just a few of the others are the following "firsts" among significant publications: anesthesia for mitral commissurotomy in 1951 (Kenneth Keown, of Philadelphia),[134] anesthesia for patients with aortic insufficiency in 1955 (John O'Donnell, Thomas McDermott, of Washington),[135] the textbook of anesthesia for heart surgery of 1956 (Keown),[136] anesthesia for open-heart surgery (Ernest Gain, of Edmonton, in 1957),[137] and the the first paper on anesthesia for revascularization of the myocardium (Earl Wynands and colleagues, in 1967).[138]

The professional value of departments and societies. Cardiac anesthesia developed into a subspecialty as knowledge and experience, techniques and technology, and the pharmaceutical and engineering industries brought innumerable advances to bear. These, however, are mediated largely by universities and anesthesia departments. General residency programs and cardiac fellowship programs are crucial to the sound practice of cardiothoracic anesthesia, while research programs ensure the necessary growth of basic and specialized knowledge.

By 1972, the critical mass of cardiac anesthesiologists made it logical to found a society—the Association of Cardiac Anesthesiologists.[139] The membership was limited to only fifty, but that of its successor, the Society of Cardiovascular Anesthesiologists (SCA), was not. The membership of the latter society, founded in 1978, had grown to four thousand by 1994,[140] with international representation. Also indicating the vitality of cardiac anesthesia as a subspecialty is the publication, beginning in 1987, of the *Journal of Cardiovascular Anesthesia*. A section in the journal *Anesthesia & Analgesia* also publishes material written by members of the society.[141]

* * *

Why and how did subspecialties arise in anesthesia? Some of the reasons *why* are similar to those that led to specialization; others are not. The division of labor among individuals with differing skills is one similarity; the growth of knowledge and technology, the principle of optimizing anesthetic care, and the desire for autonomy among various groups of peers are others. But whereas specialization in general aims to improve the standard of anesthesia care for all patients, subspecialization aims to provide excellence of care by focusing attention on highly refined methods of practice. Indeed, subspecialization is, in effect, refinement of the art and science of anesthesia taken to the highest degree.

In the context of the process whereby anesthesia grew from craft to specialty, the phenomenon of subspecialization reflects two aspects of it. First, the process was indeed an evolutionary one: subspecialization is simply the logical outcome of specialization. Second, further subspecialization (sub-sub-specialization) is likely to continue as a trend, as anesthesia becomes ever more specialized. Thus, in a new and highly limited surgical field, where only a handful of surgeons will be competent—fetal surgery, for example—only a handful of anesthesiologists would have a similar degree of competence. Whether that is completely desirable is an open question.

As to *how* subspecialization came about, the long answer is by a combination of many factors, both individual and societal. Factors related to individuals vary depending on their presence at certain places at certain times and on their own vision and knowledge. Philip Ayre and Bjorn Ibsen exemplify this. Because of his own physical deformity, Ayre became interested in anesthesia for infants and children with harelip and cleft palate. He worked in a university that was known for excellence of pediatric care, and he had a vision of what anesthesia for children should accomplish, which his knowledge of anesthesia enabled him to bring to fruition. Ibsen too was knowledgeable, and he likewise had a vision of how certain patients should be treated. He understood why some poliomyelitis patients were dying, and he applied his knowledge and skills, honed in anesthetic practice, to initiate the correct solution to the problem.

Society too has had an influence on subspecialization, even if indirect. It condones the building of hospitals for special care, it funds research, and it is capable of making its approval or disapproval felt. Society has a deep interest in ethical issues also, and it is essential that knowledgeable anesthesiologists, by concentrating their thoughts along certain lines of inquiry, whether these concern brain death or rationalization of health care, enter a dialogue with society's representatives. Subspecialization implies appropriate use of knowledge, but responsibility also.

Chapter 15

CONCLUSIONS

A review of the history of anesthesia shows that it has developed by adapting to an evolutionary process. This process was a threefold one. First, anesthesia passed through a stage when it was a craft; then, a discipline; and finally, a specialty within medicine. Even after that, anesthesia continued to evolve, for subspecialties began to emerge from the 1960s onward. The process required that anesthesia adapt to changes in surgery and medicine that were frequently profound, and the transition that anesthesia made in itself indicates that it was successful in adapting to those many changes.

A second way anesthesia evolved is related to progress in its scientific basis and to new ways in which the knowledge and skills associated with anesthesia were applied. In the early years of anesthesia, empirical, or experiential, knowledge governed its practice. Anesthesia was a matter of pouring drops of a smelly liquid on a patient's face mask. That was how the main objectives of anesthesia, particularly the obtundation of pain and muscle relaxation, were achieved. Over time, a variety of agents with specific actions were used separately so that those objectives could be gained in specific fashion. The new drugs and techniques made the administration of anesthesia more precise, more accurate, and safer.

As the knowledge of anesthetic drugs grew, a new light was cast on the old question concerning the mechanism of anesthesia. Because there is still no certainty about this mechanism, the several theories of the mechanism of anesthesia have not been discussed in this history. However, as of the beginning of the twenty-first century, it is believed that it does not result from a unitary mechanism, as first thought, but from several different mechanisms. This shift of opinion, like other shifts such as those in critical care, pain medicine, and resuscitation medicine, as well as progress in the knowledge base, suggests that anesthesia will continue to evolve.

Anesthesia also evolved in a third way. As it matured and as its basic nature underwent changes, so its scope and nature changed. Initially, anesthesia was concerned primarily with abolishing the pain associated with surgery, and anesthetists worked almost entirely in operating rooms in performing work that was service-oriented. That began to change in the twentieth century, when anesthesiologists became involved in such activities as relief of pain in patients outside the operating room, as in women in labor and patients with chronic pain. It also became clear that the knowledge and skills of anesthesia were of value in other fields than surgery such as intensive care and resuscitation medicine. As a result, anesthesia came to participate more widely in providing health care in society. Surgeons, internists, obstetricians, pediatricians, oncologists, as well as physicians in the community had no hesitation in calling on anesthesiologists to provide specialized services that are highly valued. Today, anesthesia occupies a more central place in health care than it did when it was a craft.

These three aspects of change emphasize the evolutionary nature of the process whereby anesthesia evolved in the 150 years of its modern history. They form the background to a discussion on the principal evolutionary factors that a history of anesthesia yields. Here, four such factors are considered.

Positive and Negative Forces and Specialty Recognition

As anesthesia evolved, it became a medical specialty, but what were the main evolutionary factors in the process that led up to recognition of anesthesia as a specialty? Some were negative, particularly in the nineteenth century and early twentieth century; others were positive, such as those that moved anesthesia forward in the 1920s and 1930s. Let us look at these more closely, recalling that some of them have relevance to specialization in fields other than medicine.

Negative Forces Impeding Specialty Recognition

Originally, when anesthetists simply poured ether or chloroform on a face mask in order to present an immobile patient to the surgeon, anesthesia was a craft. Most individuals who administered anesthesia, some of whom had no appropriate qualifications, were concerned mainly with keeping a patient asleep and preferably immobile. Few were interested in the physiological changes that occurred during anesthesia, and even fewer studied the basic science and the clinical basis of anesthesia. As a result, in the first fifty years, little progress was made in this new field. Anesthesia *appeared* to be no more than a matter of pouring pungent liquids over someone's face, and for many physicians, this lacked interest. The practice of anesthesia was almost entirely built on an empirical basis in which there was very little science; moreover, for any one individual, the experiential basis of empirical knowledge was limited. Hence, Frederic Hewitt's decrying the lack of knowledge in anesthesia in 1896 and his implication that it had advanced very little in the first fifty years.[1]

Another negative force was the lack of fundamental research in anesthesia. The only exceptions to this early on was the research by John Snow on a wide variety of topics in the basic science and practice of anesthesia,[2] by Claude Bernard, which, however, was done only in animals,[3] and by Frederic Hewitt, which was limited to nitrous oxide and oxygen.[4] To this must be added another negative force: the lack of formal training in anesthesia in the nineteenth century. This lack is not surprising in view of the lack of a real and unique body of knowledge of anesthesia.

Not all the negative forces, however, were related to anesthesia itself. One was the condition of medical science, which was not well developed before the twentieth century. Physiology and pharmacology did not begin to have an impact on anesthesia until just before the First World War, when, for example, Samuel Meltzer and John Auer's work provided the scientific basis for insufflations anesthesia[5] and Henry Dale observed "the first hint" of the role of acetylcholine[6] that underlay some of the actions in the nervous system. Although chemistry was somewhat more advanced than the other basic sciences in the nineteenth century, such knowledge as there was on fundamental aspects of anesthetic drugs such as structure-activity relationships had no impact on the synthesis of anesthetic drugs until well into the twentieth century. Nor had anesthesia forged the close relationship either with pharmacology or the pharmaceutical industry that influenced its development in the twentieth century.

Another negative force was the absence of professionalism in anesthesia. This too was a late development even in the practice of medicine.[7] Professionalism implies the presence of individuals who have acquired knowledge by means of training and study and who desire to pass on that knowledge to others.[8] It is nurtured by the existence of universities, but university departments of anesthesia did not exist in the nineteenth century. If any physician did wish to take up anesthesia and learn about it systematically, there was no forum in which this could be done. Professionalism was central to the recognition of anesthesia as a specialty, but it took time for it to develop. The ground had to be made fertile. Much time and effort was also needed on the part of those individual anesthetists who had not only the credentials but also the vision that would take anesthesia beyond being a craft to a discipline and ultimately an autonomous specialty.

In the United States, yet another negative force was the lack of the tradition of physician-anesthesia, and with it an emphasis on research in anesthesia. In the United Kingdom, hospitals tended to appoint physicians to anesthesia posts earlier than they did in the United States. Snow, for example, worked freelance at several London hospitals. A physician was appointed chloroformist at London's St. Bartholomew's Hospital in 1852,[9] and Clover, Buxton, and Hewitt were all active in hospital practice. Anesthesia, and particularly physician anesthesia, was accepted as a part of medical practice quite soon after the advent of anesthesia. Physicians too were listened to when they made pronouncements about anesthesia. But in the United States, authoritative figures in anesthesia did not begin appearing until the beginning of the twentieth century; until then, surgeons were dominant. The absence of the tradition of physician-anesthesia meant that fewer physicians were attracted to anesthesia and there was less emphasis on research.

Nurse anesthesia was, and is, a feature of anesthesia in the United States, and made up a large proportion of all anesthetics given. Indeed, little of the outstanding surgical work in centers such as the Mayo Clinic could have been done in their absence. Some nurse anesthetists were experts in their field. For example, at the Mayo Clinic, Alice Magaw reported in 1906 on no fewer than fourteen thousand anesthetics that she had given without a single death.[10] The presence of nurse anesthetists is, perhaps, the most obvious difference in anesthesia practice between the United States and the United Kingdom; and historically, it does explain the absence of research in anesthesia in the United States in the second half of the nineteenth century in contrast to the situation in the United Kingdom, where physicians such as Joseph Clover, Dudley Buxton, and Hewitt, following the example of Snow, all maintained a level of inquiry into anesthesia.

One other negative force is peculiar to the United States. The two individuals who were best known for the introduction of anesthesia were dentists: Horace Wells and William Morton. Significant though they are in the history of anesthesia, Wells and Morton were "*only*" dentists—men who did not go about saving lives and who were often business-oriented, and so were not highly regarded, particularly by physicians, who did profess to save lives. Moreover, Wells committed suicide and departed the stage early, and Morton has been dubbed a "tarnished idol"[11] in light of his dubious practices in patenting ether and in trying endlessly to get recognition and compensation for what he termed his "discovery." That meant that physicians did not look on anesthesia in a particularly favorable light. In addition, the "ether controversy" did not reflect well on anesthesia.

Positive Forces in the Evolution of Anesthesia

Though negative forces impeded progress in anesthesia, and hence recognition as a specialty, in time, they were overridden by positive forces. What were they?

One of the most potent positive forces was the underlying desire for specialization. This, in fact, was of long standing. From Snow in 1852 onward,[12] a few physicians had emphasized the need for specialization in anesthesia. Hewitt called for it in 1896,[13] though he was thinking of specialism as full-time practice. In the United States, S. O. Goldan argued the case for specialism in 1901,[14] but he was more concerned about the independence of anesthetists from surgeons. James Tayloe Gwathmey, in 1916, also put the case for specialism, arguing that "the production of anesthesia . . . should fall into the hands of one who is giving himself entirely to that branch and loves it for its own sake."[15] Gwathmey was closer to the essence of specialization, for he referred to the "scientific" administration of anesthesia and to dedication to anesthesia as a vocation. Yet these various views about specialization lacked an all-embracing concept of a specialty. What had to be developed was not only excellence in patient care, which was based in turn on excellence in research and education, but also an effective umbrella organization that could create a matrix of professionals who were concerned about continuing growth of the art and science of anesthesia.

Positive forces began to predominate when anesthesia became a discipline as opposed to a craft in the first three decades of the twentieth century. Innovative ideas flourished: in the design of anesthesia machines, the research and development of a slew of new anesthesia agents for general anesthesia, the increasing use of local anesthetic agents, the development of techniques like regional blocks and endotracheal anesthesia, and the introduction of simple monitoring devices. All this gave anesthesia the momentum to progress beyond being a craft. The approach to anesthesia was more objective, even scientific. On a personal level, anesthesia as a discipline was apparent in the work of individuals like Walter Boothby,[16] Elmer McKesson,[17] and Dennis Jackson[18] in the United States and Cocky Boyle[19] and Ivan Magill[20] in England.

The stage of anesthesia as a discipline is significant because it laid a base from which the Everest of specialty recognition could be scaled. The achievements in anesthesia in this period were scientifically valid, which anesthetists' peers in medicine and surgery could see were specific to anesthesia and so justify specialty recognition. Just as important were the efforts that were made by certain individuals who fought hard for specialty recognition, who believed in the necessary ideal and who had the requisite momentum to keep the concept of anesthesia as a specialty alive. Those individuals include Ralph Waters,[21] Arthur Guedel,[22] and John Lundy[23] in the United States; Wesley Bourne[24] and Harold Griffith[25] in Canada; and Robert Macintosh[26] and J. Alfred Lee[27] in England. It was them whose dedication to anesthesia overcame the entropy of negative forces.

Just as, initially, some physicians were reluctant to accept the value of anesthesia when it was introduced, so some hesitated to accept the concept of anesthesia as a specialty. This was evident even in the highest reaches of the medical hierarchy. The view of one of the deans of the medical school at Harvard University illustrates this. Hearing that money had been set aside in 1917 for the endowment of the Henry Isaiah Dorr professorship of research in anesthesia, Dr. David Edsall deplored the endowment "in a subject in which it is unnecessary and undesirable . . . to have an actual Department of Anesthesia . . . [and] so narrow a subject that a good man would be hardly willing to tie himself down to that."[28] Edsall's statement shows what men of the ilk of Waters were up against. How, therefore, did they succeed? What did they do to achieve their goal of specialization?

The contributions of Waters may be considered here. Not only was professionalism evident in Waters, but several other virtues were apparent: the vision of a future for anesthesia, creativity and ideas with respect to both the theory and practice of anesthesia, the concept of integration of research and education into clinical anesthesia within a university, and the formation of an ordered and organized structure in anesthesia.

Waters' ideas are quite distinct from those of many other anesthetists early in the twentieth century, in whom the concept of specialization in anesthesia was much less developed. Consider, for example, those who were appointed as professors early in the twentieth century, such as T. S. Buchanan in New York, Orville Cunningham in Kansas, and L. Hardy in Iowa. As Yale anesthesiologist Nicholas Greene pointed out, they were essentially clinical directors of anesthesia departments rather than primarily as professors in university departments. They were concerned mainly about service. They lacked a systematic approach to education in anesthesia and the singularity of vision, the originality, and the scientific approach that was needed to make an impact on anesthesia on a national scale.[29] That makes Waters such a paragon. The same is true to a degree of Francis McMechan, who emphasized organizational aspects of anesthesia,[30] and of his contemporaries Boothby, McKesson, and Jackson, who, despite their unique contributions to anesthesia, did not create knowledge for the sake of knowledge but sought primarily to apply it.

Waters' achievements were of a different order. He managed to bridge the early period of anesthesia with the later, and his influence on the transition of anesthesia from discipline to specialty was profound. Again, Greene's observations are cogent.[31] When Waters went to Madison from Kansas City in 1927, and especially when he was appointed professor and head of the university department of anesthesia there in 1933, he had two unique qualities. The first was his fourfold vision of anesthesia: of excellence in clinical anesthesia, of teaching medical students anesthesia, of stimulating the development of graduate students in anesthesia, and of cooperative laboratory research.[32] The second was the talent and the intellect to take anesthesia beyond a "pragmatic, technical exercise" to a combination of activity that joined scholarly research with excellence of clinical care. In Madison, Waters envisioned a residency program and a research program that would yield results that were applicable clinically, and he contributed significantly to the literature of anesthesia. Not the least of his accomplishments was to encourage his younger contemporaries on both sides of the Atlantic and those he trained to spread his vision of anesthesia. All of them could then show their peers in surgery and medicine by their example that anesthesia had matured and was worthy of specialty recognition.

The work of Waters, then, was one of the most powerful forces that led to specialty recognition. Others contributed so that we may conclude that one of the most potent forces in specialization comprised the multitude of efforts of countless practitioners of anesthesia. In addition, many other forces facilitated progress in anesthesia, even though they are not discussed here. They include the innumerable contributions of basic sciences like chemistry and pharmacology, of industry comprising pharmaceutical and apparatus companies, of wartime experience, and of economic pressures.

The Influence of Science and Technology on Anesthesia

Also expediting the evolution of anesthesia were the many advances in science and technology. That is a second major factor. In contrast to the often tortuous progress affecting specialty recognition, progress in the clinical practice of anesthesia, and in education and research, was linear and steady. With some exceptions, new agents and techniques were incorporated into practice without too much delay, and knowledge and skills developed in progressive fashion. This occurred more obviously in the twentieth century. By then, chemistry and the pharmacological and physiological sciences had made great strides, while industry was manufacturing anesthetic agents and anesthetic equipment at a high level.

Science was a key factor because only through progress in science was it possible for the many inhalational, intravenous, local and regional anesthetic agents, as well as anesthetic techniques, to be researched and developed and made available to patient care. The fluorinated halogens, for example, were developed out of wartime research on fluorides in the atomic bomb; the many replacements for curare became available as the result of synthesis that was based on a knowledge of structure and activity relationships; and the same is true of the synthetic opioids and of local anesthetics. This new approach of "tailoring" by chemists—those who synthesized divinyl ether in 1930[33] and halothane in 1956,[34] for example—indicates how science continues to influence the development of anesthesia, as is apparent in the recent introduction of the new anti-neuromuscular blocking agent, sugammadex.[35] Such advances, incidentally, have contributed to our understanding of the mechanism of anesthesia.

Beginning in the mid-1950s, technology also made highly significant contributions. Technological advances had an impact on both anesthesia procedures and the nature of anesthetic practice in general. Some changes affected simple procedures such as intravenous injection, tracheal intubation, or placement of a laryngeal mask airway, in which the plastics industry fashioned equipment. Others affected more complex procedures such as monitoring and blood and gas analysis, which were facilitated by microprocessing and computerization. The planning and conduct of research too was affected by advances in technology, as also was teaching in the form of simulators, for example.

Along with science and technology, one must consider important auxiliaries such as the pharmaceutical industry and the contributions of chemists and engineers. They too made enormous contributions to progress in anesthesia.

Expansion of the Nature and Scope of Anesthesia

Expansion of the nature and scope of the practice is an obvious aspect of the evolution of anesthesia, and is the the third major factor to consider. Anesthesia changed in remarkable ways. Within the traditional role of anesthesia as a partner of surgery, the nature of anesthesia changed, as it adapted to the demands of highly complex surgery, such as that on the heart and brain. Anesthesia came to be recognized as a complex undertaking, and it would seem that the quest of early anesthetists for specialty recognition was fully justified.

But the expansion of anesthesia into areas outside the operating room also indicated a broadening of the scope of anesthesia. While pain relief in patients undergoing surgical operations remained a primary concern, the care of many other types of patients with pain became increasingly frequent. Anesthesiologists treated the pain of women in labor, of patients with cancer, and of patients with a variety of types of chronic pain. Anesthesiologists broadened the context of pain relief and developed a closer one-to-one relationship with patients and responsibility for a patient's overall health care than they had when confined to the operating room. They forged a new dimension of health care. Just one example of this is the work of Seattle anesthesiologist John Bonica. His seminal textbook on the management of pain[36] was but one of many manifestations of this new role in anesthesia—and of its participation in the management of what contributes a large part of disability in society.

But pain medicine was only one aspect of this new dimension. Critical care medicine and resuscitation medicine were two others. Anesthesiologists were closely involved with critical care from the start; indeed, critical care originated in part from the initiative of Danish anesthesiologist Bjorn Ibsen in 1952. He introduced a new concept of the management of respiratory involvement in acute poliomyelitis by using positive-pressure ventilation instead of negative-pressure ventilation.[37] That led to the recognition that the knowledge and skills of anesthesiologists should be applied in the care of patients with other respiratory disorders and with cardiac disorders. That is also true of the involvement of anesthesiologists with resuscitation medicine, such as the work of Peter Safar, of Baltimore and Pittsburgh.[38]

All these activities showed that the knowledge, techniques, and monitoring modalities that were routinely used in the operating room were applicable to the care of patients with a variety of medical and surgical problems. The role of anesthesiologists became larger than that of the administration of anesthesia. The anesthesiologist had become not simply a partner of the surgeon in the operating room, as a perioperative physician, but one whose special knowledge and skills were also valued in many areas of medicine and surgery beyond the operating room. Anesthesiologists were now specialists, but with many quivers in their bows. That aspect of the process of evolution leads to the second conclusion to be drawn from this history of anesthesia, concerning the way specialization in anesthesia came about.

The Relationship between Anesthesia and Society

A final evolutionary factor is the relationship between anesthesia and society. This relationship was a mutual one: anesthesia was influenced by society, and society was influenced by developments in anesthesia. A few points will illustrate this.

How has society influenced anesthesia? A starting point is the debate about the question as to whether it was right or wrong to use anesthesia to relieve the pain of childbirth.[39] Some obstetricians and clerics held that giving an anesthetic to a woman in labor was wrong, both medically (pain was natural and shouldn't be interfered with) and morally (according to the Bible, women should bear children "in sorrow"). These criticisms were successfully countered in the United Kingdom, both by obstetrician James Simpson and by women, including Queen Victoria. Early in the twentieth century, women also expressed themselves forcefully again on the matter of twilight sleep, having again to counter physicians' objections to this form of pain relief.[40] This suggests that society is prepared to enter into a debate whenever this seems called for.

The public was concerned again in the 1960s, when attitudes of some doctors toward health care, and even patient care, were discussed. Objections focused on several concerns, though anesthesia was affected only a little. In the liberal, even rebellious, decade of the 1960s, people were ready to question the doctor-oriented way medical care was organized and distributed; the public no longer accepted without questioning what doctors thought best as medical care for their patients. With respect to anesthesia, errors of omission or commission could no longer be dismissed, as they were initially when anesthesia-associated deaths were not uncommon and regarded as "acts of God." Anesthesiologists had to admit that they were sometimes at fault.[41] To their credit, anesthesiologists responded positively, and they recognized the need to instill guidelines concerning quality of care and of standards of anesthetic practice.[42] Indeed, anesthesiologists were in the forefront of the medical profession in this respect.

Anesthesiologists were more directly concerned, perhaps, by the economic constraints of the 1990s, which had their origin in the public's demand for the form of medical care that it would like to see delivered.[43] Anesthesiologists were made to feel conscious of the costs of anesthetics, and particularly hard hit were academic anesthesiologists, since costs for academic centers are, in general, greater than for nonacademic centers. Even in prestigious centers such as those of Harvard and Stanford universities,[44] academic productivity appeared to diminish as a result of financial constraints.[45] Progress in anesthesia is based on the growth of knowledge, and the possible effects of economics were not welcomed by those academic anesthesiologists who were affected; and eventually, their productivity in terms of research inevitably diminished.[46] The net result in the long term seemed to be that the growth of the knowledge base would become stunted.

The effects of societal changes on anesthesia, particularly in the last quarter of the twentieth century, can also be illustrated by examining the issue of professionalism in the context of the patient-physician relationship. In the 1970s, *knowledge* and its place and its transmission from authorities to others were what were emphasized,[47, 48] but thirty years later, the concept of professionalism was quite different. Professionalism was now viewed in terms of a *social contract* between medicine and society.[49] A new relationship had developed between medicine and society: knowledge had a part, but it did not predominate, and professionalism now stressed three principles: the primacy of patient welfare, of patient autonomy, and of social justice. Though anesthesiologists do not have them uppermost in their minds while giving an anesthetic, the new principles may begin shaping the niche that anesthesiologists occupy in society.

In contrast, how has anesthesia influenced society? In 1846, the introduction of anesthesia created a new form of health care. Initially, its role was related to the abolition of pain during surgery. This was a positive force in health care, and anesthesiologists have continued to relieve pain and to achieve excellence in anesthesia. As anesthesiologists expanded the scope of their activities, so society benefited, as newer dimensions of health care were developed.

By becoming a specialty, anesthesia has indeed benefited society. Physicians are trained in anesthesia, and their specialty organizations conduct their continuing education. Research in anesthesia is customarily closely related to the specialty organization; and the specialty, in formulating clinical guidelines, has continually upgraded the standard of anesthesia. In addition, anesthesia has responded to new concepts of professionalism. At one time, the term *professionalism* in medicine implied treatment of patients according to standards of care that were observed by most physicians, particularly with respect to knowledge and skills, and a certain type of conduct with respect to fellow physicians according to codes of ethics. Today, professionalism implies—in addition to commitment to scientific knowledge, to improvements in the quality of care, and to professional responsibilities as physicians—agreement to the clauses in a social contract between physicians and their patients.[50] That anesthesiologists have responded to such societal concerns is evident from the concern from 1978 onward with potentially adverse critical events[51] and, from 1986 onward, with the concern about standards of practice.[52] In such aspects of quality maintenance, anesthesia has been a leader within medicine.

*   *   *

In the century and a half since the advent of anesthesia, the growth of anesthesia has been a dynamic one. The growth was a process that was evolutionary and that resulted from the operation of factors both within and outside anesthesia itself. As it moved from being a craft to becoming a discipline and then a specialty, its practitioners proved adaptable and worthy of being regarded as specialists. Seen from a historical perspective, that augurs well for the future of anesthesia.

Appendix A

CHRONOLOGICAL OUTLINE OF HISTORY OF ANESTHESIA*

BCE

c.3500   Soothing applications for wound (Egypt)

c.2250   Henbane in cement: dental caries (Babylonia)
          Pressure on nerves, blood vessels: anesthesia (Saqquara)

c.1200   Nepenthe: potion for surgical patients (Greece)

c.1150   Opium: pain relief, amnesia (*Odyssey*)

c.1000   Wine: insensibility (India: Susruta, Charaka)

c.5th C   Hemp, henbane, opium: temple sleep (Hippocrates)

CE

60   Mandragora, wine: anesthesia (Dioscorides)

c.220   Wine, hemp: preoperative hypnosis (China: Hua T'o)

800   *Spongia somnifera* (Bavaria: Bamberg *Antidotarium*)

1200   "Sweet vitriol" discovery (Spain: Lullius)

1363   Opium: pain relief, narcosis (France: de Chauliac)

c.1536   Laudanum: pain relief (Switzerland: Paracelsus)
          "Sweet vitriol": hypnosis (Paracelsus)
          "Sweet oil of vitriol": (Germany: Cordus)

1564   Nerve compression: local anesthesia (France: Pare)

---

*Principal sources: C. Leake, *Letheon: The Cadenced Story of Anesthesia* (Austin: University of Texas Press, 1947). T. Keys, *The History of Surgical Anesthesia* (New York: Dover Publications, Inc., 1963)

1646	Snow, ice: local anesthesia (Italy: Severino)
1648	Carbon dioxide—"gas sylvestre": (Holland: van Helmont)
1660	Air necessary for life, combustion (England: Boyle)
1665	Intravenous opium in dog: anesthesia (Germany: Elsholtz)
1730	Ether: named as such (Switzerland: Frobenius)
1743	Ether: pain relief (England: Turner)
1754	Carbon dioxide: "fixed air" discovered (Scotland: Black)
1772	Nitrous oxide discovery (England: Priestley)
1775	Oxygen: co-discovery of oxygen (Priestley; Sweden: Scheele)
1784	Clamp on nerve trunks: local anesthesia (England: Moore)
1798	Pneumatic Medical Institution (England: Beddoes)
	Nitrous oxide: possible surgical use (England: Davy)
1806	Morphine: extraction (Germany: Serturner)
1824	Carbon dioxide: animal anesthesia (England: Hickman)
	Chloroform: co-discovery (USA: Guthrie; France: Soubeiran; Germany: von Liebig)
c.1840	Hypnosis: anesthesia (England: Elliotson; India: Esdaile)
	Ether: anesthesia (USA: Clarke, Long)
1844	Nitrous oxide: anesthesia (USA: Wells)
1846	Ether: anesthetic efficacy demonstrated (USA: Morton)
1847	Ether: pain relief in labor (Scotland: Simpson)
	Ether: anesthesia-specific inhaler (England: Snow)
	Chloroform: anesthesia (Simpson)
	Ether: first publication (England: Robinson)
1853	Chloroform *a la reine* (England [Victoria]: Snow)
	Hollow needle introduced (Scotland: Wood)
	Syringe introduced (France: Pravaz)
1860	Cocaine alkaloid isolated (Germany: Niemann)
1868	Nitrous oxide: resurgence of interest (France: Colton)
	Nitrous oxide: oxygen addition advocated (USA: Andrews)
1878	Tracheal intubation pre-induction (Scotland: Macewen)
1884	Cocaine: local anesthesia (Austria: Koller)
1885	Cocaine: nerve block (USA: Halsted)
	Cocaine: intravertebral anesthesia (USA: Corning)
	Two-cylinder anesthesia machine (USA: White Company)
1893	Society of Anaesthetists, London (England: Silk et al.)
1894	Ethyl chloride: anesthesia induction (Sweden: Carlson)
1898	Subarachnoid anesthesia (Germany: Bier)
1899	Fell-O'Dwyer device: artificial ventilation (USA: Matas)
1902	Anesthesia machine patented (USA: Teter)
1903	Barbital: synthesis as hypnotic (Germany: Fischer, v. Mering)
1904	Procaine: synthesis to replace cocaine (Germany: Eichorn)

1905	Long Island Society of Anesthetists (USA: Erdmann et al.)
1909	Insufflation anesthesia: established (USA: Meltzer, Auer)
1915	Anesthesia supplement to *Amer J Surg* (USA: McMechan)
1920	Endotracheal anesthesia (England: Magill, Rowbotham)
1922	*Current Researches in Anesthesia and Analgesia* (McMechan)
1923	Ethylene: codiscovery of anesthetic value (USA: Luckhardt, Herb; Canada: Brown)
1924	To-and-fro canister: CO_2 absorptionxide (USA: Waters)
1927	Tribromoethyl alcohol: rectal use (Germany: Butzengeiger)
	Pernoston: intravenous anesthesia (Germany: Bumm)
1928	Cuffed tracheal tube (USA: Guedel, Waters)
1929	Cyclopropane: anesthetic property (Canada: Lucas, Henderson)
	Sodium amytal: intravenous anesthesia (USA: Zerfas et al.)
1930	Divinyl ether: anesthetic property (USA: Leake, Chen)
1932	Hexobarbital: intravenous anesthesia (Germany: Weese)
1934	Thiopental sodium: improved iv induction (USA: Waters, Lundy)
1935	Trichloroethylene: inhalation agent (USA: Striker et al.)
1939	Meperidine: synthesis of opioid (Germany: Schaumann, Eisleb)
	Curare: muscle paralysis in anesthesia (Canada: Griffith)
1943	Lidocaine: synthesis of local anesthetic (Sweden: Lofgren)
1949	Succinylcholine: new class of relaxant (Italy: Bovet)
1952	Positive-pressure ventilation in polio (Denmark: Ibsen)
	Fluroxene: new class of fluorinated agent (USA: Krantz)
1959	Fentanyl: synthesis of potent opioid (Belgium: Jannsen)
1977	Propofol: intravenous induction agent (England: Kay, Rolly)

Appendix B

GLOSSARY OF TERMS

airway. The route for passage of air, gas, or vapor into and out of the lungs; may be natural (anatomical) or artificial in the form of a tubular device placed at certain pints in the respiratory tract.

analgesia. The absence of pain sensation. Note also **analgesic**.

anaesthesia (*UK*), **anesthesia** (*USA*). (1) Loss of feeling, sensation (2) In a general sense, the art and science of induction and maintenance of a state of loss of feeling of all or part of the body for surgical purposes, and aspects relating to that art and science.

anaesthetist (*UK*). A physician qualified to practice the specialty of anesthesia

anesthesia. See under **anaesthesia**.

anesthesiologist (*USA*). A physician qualified to practice the specialty of anesthesia

anesthesiology (*USA*). (1) The science, art, practice, and study of the state of anesthesia (2) The medical specialty of anesthesia

anesthetist (*USA*). (1) A general term indicative of a practitioner of anesthesia, especially before anesthesia became recognized as a specialty. (2) A nurse qualified to administer anesthesia (also nurse-anesthetist).

anodyne. A pain-relieving substance

anoxemia. Abnormally low oxygen concentration in the blood

anoxia. Abnormally low oxygen concentration in body tissues

Apgar score. Numerical assessment of the condition of a newborn infant based on heart rate, respiratory rate and effort, muscle tone, reflex irritability, and color.

apnea. Absence or cessation of breathing

arrhythmia. Any abnormal heart rhythm

arterial gases. Oxygen and carbon dioxide, us. their concentration and analysis

arterial line. Tubing inserted into an artery for recording of pressure

asphyxia. Deficient oxygenation of the blood; suffocation.

balanced anesthesia. The triad of hypnosis, analgesia, and muscle relaxation whereby small amounts of specific drugs are given so that light rather than deep anesthesia is required.

Blalock-Taussig shunt. An operation for the correction of congenital pulmonary stenosis by anastomosing the subclavian artery to the pulmonary artery.

brachial block, plexus. Injection of local anesthetic into the bundle of radial, ulnar, and median nerves as they pass below the clavicle into the axilla before separating the their distribution in the upper limb.

bronchoscopy. Visual examination by instrumentation of the bronchi

bronchus. The tubular part of the airway between the trachea and the lungs, anatomically divided into right and left bronchi and then into the smaller bronchioles.

cardiac arrest. Cessation of the action of the heart

cardiac massage. Manipulation of the heart so as to start its action after it has ceased; either closed, with chest closed, or open, with chest surgically opened.

capnograph. Graphic representation of the concentration of inspired and expired carbon dioxide Note also **capnometer**. Measuring device

caudal block, space. Injection of local anesthetic into the space within the sacrum, or tailbone.

cervical block, plexus. Injection of local anesthetic into the cervical nerves between the neck muscles

coarctation of aorta. Localized narrowing of the aorta

craft. Art requiring special knowledge and skill, usually based on experience and manual dexterity.

critical care. Intensive care of patients who are critically ill. (See also **intensive care**.)

cyanosis. Bluish tinge of the skin and mucous membranes resulting from an excess of reduced (deoxygenated) hemoglobin in the blood .

dead space. Space in which respiratory exchange of oxygen and carbon dioxide does, or can, not take place; usually anatomical or mechanical.

defibrillation. Correction of the abnormal heart rhythm of ventricular fibrillation by electrical means

discipline. A branch of learning or instruction; in anesthesia, objective application of formal knowledge to clinical practice.

dissociation, dissociative. Separation of mental or emotional processes from consciousness

echocardiography. Technique of examining the heart and its function by radiographic and sonic means to obtain moving images

electrocardio-graph,—gram. Electrical recording of rate and rhythm of the heart

electroencephalograph. Electrical recording of brain activity

epidural block, space. Injection of local anesthetic into the anatomical, negative-pressure space surrounding the dura mater of the spinal cord and through which spinal nerves pass; sometimes, injection of an opioid for this purpose. May also be referred to as extradural or peridural block.

fiberoscopy, fiberscope. Visualization based on illumination provided by the passage of light along a myriad of glass fibers or other light-transmitting solids

gate theory of pain. A theory to explain the occurrence of pain based on the concept that pain perception is not mediated only by impulses from pain receptors but can be inhibited by other, nonociceptive nerve cells, thus closing a gate to the transmission of pain perception.

general anesthesia. Absence of feeling and sensation resulting from a reversible state of unconsciousness induced by chemical agents (general anesthetics).

geriatric. Pertaining to the elderly. Also **geriatrics**, the specialty of medicine relating to the elderly.

glottis. The vocal apparatus of the larynx (*q.v.*), including the aperture between the vocal cords.

halogen. In anesthesia, a member of group of gaseous or liquid, non-metallic electronegative chemical elements characterized by volatility and anesthetic properties, especially bromine, chlorine, and fluorine.

hemoglobin. The oxygen-carrying pigment of the red blood cells

homoeostasis. A tendency to normality of the internal environment of the body, especially with respect to the blood.

hypercapnia. (1) An abnormally high concentration of carbon dioxide in the blood (cf. hypercarbia) (2) An abnormally high concentration of carbon dioxide in expired gas

hypercarbia. An abnormally high concentration of carbon dioxide in the blood

hyperthermia. High body temperature

hypnosis, hypnotic. In anesthesia, the state of sleep induced by anesthetic agents, especially as a member of the anesthesia triad of unconsciousness, analgesia, and muscle relaxation.

hypothermia. Low body temperature

hypoxemia. Low oxygen content of the blood

hyper-, hypo-ventilation. Over- or under-activity of respiration

hypoxia. The state of low concentration of oxygen in the tissues or in inhaled air

induction of anesthesia. The process whereby the state of anesthesia is produced by means of chemical agents or drugs

infiltration anesthesia. Anesthesia of a limited area of the body produced by infiltration, or subcutaneous injection, of tissues with a local anesthetic drug.

inhaler. An apparatus for administering a volatilized liquid or vapor into the respiratory tract

inhalation (-al) anesthesia. Anesthesia induced or maintained by the administration of a gaseous or volatile agent

insufflation anesthesia. Anesthesia by means of a continuous flow of anesthetic gas or vapor in and out of the trachea

intensive care. Specialized medical care of the critically ill. (See also **critical care**.)

intravenous. Occurring in or pertaining to veins; in anesthesia, with reference to administration of drugs or other chemical substances.

intubation. Placement of a tube, especially through the larynx into the trachea.

ischemia. Inadequate blood supply to body tissue

larynx. The musculocartilaginous anatomical structure situated at, and guarding, the proximal end of the trachea and containing the glottis (*q.v.*).

minimum alveolar concentration. Concentration of an anesthetic vapor that is needed to prevent movement in response to a painful, surgical stimulus in 50 percent of individuals.

local anesthesia. Anesthesia restricted to a small area of the body

monitor. A device that records changes in physiological conditions and is equipped with a warning device that alerts an individual to the occurrence of a potentially critical abnormality.

morbidity. Prevalence of disease; in relation to surgery and anesthesia, especially of postoperative complications.

mortality. Ratio of deaths to expected deaths; death rate.

narcotic. In anesthesia, a drug inducing drowsiness or unconsciousness.

neonate. An infant under four weeks of age

nerve block. Injection of a local anesthetic drug in the vicinity of a nerve in order to produce anesthesia in the distribution of that nerve

neuraxial block. Regional anesthesia induced by injection of a local anesthetic and/or an opioid into the subarachnoid or epidural space

neuroleptanalgesia. A dissociative state characterized by diminished initiative, emotional response, and interest in the surroundings as well as by analgesia.

neuromuscular block. Prevention of transmission of nerve impulse from nerve to muscle resulting from the administration of a particular class of muscle relaxant drug

opiate. A drug derived from opium; a drug that induces sleep or drowsiness.

opioid. A synthetic drug with morphine-like neurochemical, especially analgesic, properties.

oximeter. An instrument for measuring the oxygen saturation of the blood

paracervical block. Anesthesia in the distribution of the paravertebral nerves achieved by the injection of a local anesthetic drug.

patent ductus arteriosus. Abnormal persistence after birth of an opening in the connection between the pulmonary artery and the descending aorta

patient-controlled analgesia. Technique enabling a patient to self-administer analgesic drugs under controlled safety conditions; may be intravenous or epidural.

pneumothorax. Presence of air or gas in the pleural cavity of the thorax

premedication. Drug administration shortly before operation in order to calm a surgical patient

pulse oximeter. A monitoring device that records the saturation level of oxygen in the arterial blood, usually at a finger, and the pulse rate.

regional anesthesia. Anesthesia of a specific region of the body related to a particular nerve distribution produced by injection of a local anesthetic drug close to that nerve

resuscitation. Restoration of the vital functions in a parson who has suddenly and unexpectedly collapsed and is apparently dead

sedation. A state of drug-induced calmness of mind

specialty. A special or particular branch of a profession, the practice of which mandates special training, certification, and general oversight by a specialist's peers and often adherence to the specific guidelines relating to practice and professional conduct.

sphygmomanometer. An instrument to determine blood pressure

spinal anesthesia. Subarachnoid or epidural anesthesia.

stellate block. Injection of local anesthetic close to the stellate ganglion in the neck to produce anesthesia in the neck and arm

subarachnoid block, space. Anesthesia induced by injection of a local anesthetic into the subdural space surrounding the spinal cord; sometimes, injection of an opioid for this purpose.

subspecialty. In anesthesia, a subdivision of the specialty that is dedicated to care of a particular group of patients.

tamponade. Pathological compression of a part of the body by a fluid

thoracotomy. Surgical opening of the thorax

topical anesthesia. Anesthesia restricted to a particular surface

trachea. The windpipe

tracheostomy. Incision of the trachea for the purpose of inserting an artificial airway

trepanotomy. Perforation of the skull with a trephine

vaporizer. A device for the administration of a vapor; sometimes, converting a liquid into a vapor.

venous line. Tubing inserted into a vein in order to administer liquids or drugs, or to measure pressure.

ventricular fibrillation. Potentially lethal arrhythmia characterized by rapid, uncoordinated fibrillary and non-productive contraction of the ventricles.

Select Bibliography

Most of the sources listed in this Bibliography are given in the chapter footnotes, but texts that are of primary significance and aids to further reading on the history of anesthesia are included here. They are in two categories: those pertaining specifically to the history of anesthesia, and those relating to the history of medicine (excepting standard texts) and the history of science.

History of Anesthesia

W. H. Archer. Chronological history of Horace Wells, discoverer of anesthesia. *Bull Hist Med* 1939; 7:1140-68.

Anaesthesia Centenary Issue. *Brit Med Bull* 1946; 4:81-155.

R. Atkinson, T. Boulton (eds.).*A History of Anaesthesia* (London: Royal Society of Medicine, 1989).

D. Bacon. "Regional Anesthesia and Chronic Pain Therapy: A History," in D. Brown, *Regional Anesthesia and Analgesia* (Philadelphia: W. B. Saunders Company, 1996).

D. Bacon, K. McGoldrick, M. Lema (eds.). *The American Society of Anesthesiologists: A Century of Challenges and Progress* (Park Ridge: Wood Library-Museum of Anesthesiology, 2005).

A. Barr, T. Boulton, D. Wilkinson (eds.). *Essays on the History of Anaesthesia* (London: Royal Society of Medicine Press, 1996).

P. Baskett, T. Baskett (eds.). *Resuscitation Greats* (Bristol: Clinical Press, Ltd., 2007).

N. Bergman. *The Genesis of Surgical Anesthesia* (Park Ridge: Wood Library-Museum of Anesthesiology, 1998.

C. Bernard. *Lectures on Anaesthetics and on Asphyxia* [Transl. B. R. Fink] (Park Ridge: Wood Library-Museum of Anesthesiology, 1989).

A. Betcher, B. Ciliberti, p. Wood, L. Wright. The Jubilee Year of Organized Anesthesia. *Anesthesiology* 1955; 17:226-64.

T. Boulton, D. Wilkinson. "The Origins of Modern Anaesthesia," in T. Healy, P. Cohen (eds.), *Wylie and Churchill-Davidson's A Practice of Anaesthesia* [6th ed.] (London: Edward Arnold, 1995).

H. Braun. *Local Anesthesia: Its Scientific Basis and Practice* (Philadelphia: Lea & Febiger, 1914).

D. Brown, B. R. Fink. "The History of Neural Blockade and Pain Management," in M. Cousins, P. Bridenbaugh (eds.), *Neural Blockade in Clinical Anesthesia and Management of Pain* (Philadelphia: Lippincott-Raven Publishers, 1998 [3rd edition]).

J. Bunker. *The Anesthesiologist and the Surgeon: Partners in the Operating Room* (Boston: Little, Brown and Company, 1972).

D. Buxton. *Anaesthetics: Their Uses and Administration* (London: H. K. Lewis, 1888).

R. Calverley, M. Scheller. "Anesthesia as a Specialty: Past, Present, and Future," in P. Barash, B. Cullen, R. Stoelting (eds.), *Clinical Anesthesia* [2nd ed.] (Philadelphia: J. B. Lippincott and Company, 1989, pp. 3-33.

F. Cartwright. *The English Pioneers of Anaesthesia (Beddoes, Davy, Hickman)* (Bristol: John Wright & Sons, Ltd., 1952).

D. Caton. Obstetric anesthesia: The first ten years. *Anesthesiology* 1970; 33:102-09.

D. Caton. Obstetric anesthesia and concepts of placental transport: A historical review of the nineteenth century. *Anesthesiology* 1977; 46:132-37.

D. Caton. The secularization of pain. *Anesthesiology* 1985; 62:493-501.

D. Caton. *What a Blessing She Had Chloroform: The Medical and Social Response to the Pain of Childbirth From 1800 to the Present* (New Haven: Yale University Press, 1999).

M. Armstrong Davison. *The Evolution of Anaesthesia* (Altrincham: John Sherratt, 1965).

D. Davis. *Historical Vignettes of Modern Anesthesia.* In J. F. Artusio [ed.], *Clinical Anesthesia*, vol.2 (Oxford: Blackwell, 1968).

H. Davy. *Researches, Chemical and Philosophical; Chiefly Concerning Nitrous Oxide, or Dephlogisticated Nitrous Air and Its Respiration* [1800] (London: Butterworths, 1972).

J. Diaz, A. Franco, D. Bacon et al. (eds.). *The History of Anesthesia* [Fifth International Symposium on the History of Anesthesia] (Amsterdam: Elsevier Science, 2003).

P. Drury. Published anaesthesia history. *Curr Anaesth Crit Care* 2000; 11:338-43.

B. Duncum. *The Development of Inhalation Anaesthesia With Special Reference to the Years 1846-1946* (London: Wellcome Historical Medical Museum and Oxford University Press, 1947). Reprinted by Royal Society of Medicine Press, Ltd., 1994.

J. Dundee. Fifty years of thiopentone. *Brit J Anaesth* 1984; 56:211-13.

J. Eckenhoff. A wide-angle view of anesthesiology. *Anesthesiology* 1978; 48:472-79.

E. S. Ellis. *Ancient Anodynes* (London: Heinemann, 1946).

R. Ellis (ed.). W. S. Sykes: *Essays on the First Hundred Years of Anaesthesia*, vol.3 (London and Edinburgh: Churchill Livingstone, 1982).

R. Ellis (ed.). *On Narcotism by the Inhalation of Vapours by John Snow, MD* (London: Royal Society of Medicine Services, Ltd., 1991 [facsimile edition]).

R. Ellis (ed.). *The Case Books of Dr. John Snow* (London: Wellcome Institute, 1994).

J. Esch, M. Goerig (eds.). *Proceedings of the Fourth International Symposium on the History of Anaesthesia* (Lubeck: Drager-Druck, 1997).

A. Faulconer, T. Keys. *Foundations of Anesthesiology* (Springfield: Charles C Thomas, 1965). Reprinted 1993 by Wood Library-Museum of Anesthesiology, Park Ridge, IL.

B. R. Fink. Leaves and needles: The introduction of surgical anesthesia. *Anesthesiology* 1985; 63:77-83.

B. R. Fink, L. Morris, C. R. Stephen (eds.). *The History of Anaesthesia: Proceedings of the Third International Symposium* (Park Ridge: Wood Library-Museum of Anesthesiology, 1992).

B. R. Fink, K. McGoldrick (eds.). *Careers in Anesthesiology* [ongoing series of autobiographical memoirs by anesthesiologists]. (Park Ridge: Wood Library-Museum of Anesthesiology).

P. Flagg. *The Art of Anesthesia* (Philadelphia: J. B. Lippincott Company, 1916).

G. Foy. *Anaesthetics Ancient and Modern* (London: Bailliere Tindall and Cox, 1889).

R. Fulop-Miller. *Triumph Over Pain* (London: Hamish Hamilton, 1938).

J. Fulton. The vision and daring of youth: The story of the introduction of surgical anesthesia. *Anesthesiology* 1947; 8:464-70.

N. Gillespie. *Endotracheal Anaesthesia* (Madison: University of Wisconsin Press, 1941).

R. Gill. *White Water and Black Magic* (New York: Doubleday, 1940).

N. Greene. A consideration of factors in the discovery of anesthesia and their effects on its development. *Anesthesiology* 1971; 35:515-22.

N. Greene. *Anesthesia and the University* (New Haven: Yale University Press, 1975).

N. Greene. Anesthesia and the development of surgery (1846-1896). *Anesth Analg* 1979; 58:5-12.

J. T. Gwathmey. *Anesthesia* (New York: D. Appleton Company, 1914).

A. Guedel. *Inhalation Anesthesia: A Fundamental Guide* (New York: Macmillan and Company, 1937).

W. Hammonds, J. Steinhaus. Crawford Long: Pioneer physician in anesthesia. *J Clin Anesth* 1993; 5:163-67.

F. Hewitt. *Anaesthetics and Their Administration* (London: Griffin, 1893).

F. Hewitt. *Administration of Nitrous Oxide and Oxygen for Dental Operations* (London: C. Ash, 1897).

H. Hickman. *Centenary Exhibition 1830-1930*, Souvenir Catalogue (London: Wellcome Historical Medical Museum, 1930).

T. Keys. *The History of Surgical Anesthesia* (New York: H. Schuman, 1945). Revised and enlarged edition by Dover Publications, Inc., 1963; reprinted by Wood Library-Museum of Anesthesiology, 1996.

T. Keys. The early pneumatic chemists and physicians: Their influence on the development of surgical anesthesia. *Anesthesiology* 1969; 30:447-62.

C. Koller. On the use of cocaine for producing anaesthesia on the eye. *Lancet* 1884; 2:990-92.

M. Larson. "History of Anesthetic Practice," in R. Miller (ed.), *Millers Anesthesia* (New York: Elsevier Churchill Livingstone, 6th edition, 2005), pp. 3-52.

C. Leake. *The Cadenced Story of Anesthesia* (Austin: University of Texas Press, 1947).

J. Lundy. *Clinical Anesthesia: A Manual of Clinical Anesthesiology* (Philadelphia: W. B. Saunders Company, 1942.

H. Lyman. *Artificial Anaesthesia and Anaesthetics* (New York: William Wood & Company, 1881).

R. Maltby (ed.). *Notable Names in Anaesthesia* (London: Royal Society of Medicine Press, Ltd., 2003).

R. Macintosh, F. B. Pratt. *Essentials of General Anaesthesia, With Special Reference to Dentistry* (Oxford: Blackwell Scientific Publications, 1940).

R. Matas. Local and regional anesthesia: A retrospect and prospect. *Amer J Surg* 1934; 25:189-96.

A. McIntyre. *Curare: Its History, Nature and Clinical Use* (Chicago: University of Chicago Press, 1947).

A. McIntyre. Historical background, early use and development of muscle relaxants. *Anesthesiology* 1959; 20:409-16.

W. Mushin, L. Rendell-Baker, p. Thompson et al. *Automatic Ventilation of the Lungs* (Oxford: Blackwell Scientific Publications [3rd ed.], 1980).

S. Nuland. *The Origins of Anesthesia* (Birmingham: The Classics of Medicine Library, 1983).

E. Papper. The influence of Romantic literature on the understanding of pain and suffering—the stimulus to the discovery of anesthesia. *Persp Biol Med* 1992; 35:401-15.

M. Pernick. *A Calculus of Suffering: Pain, Professionalism and Anesthesia in Nineteenth-century America* (New York: Columbia University Press, 1985).

C.B. Pittinger. *James Tayloe Gwathmey, M.D.: American Pioneer Anesthesiologist* (Nashville: Vanderbilt University School of Medicine, 1989).

P. Raj. "Historical Aspects of Regional Anesthesia," in P. Raj, *Textbook of Regional Anesthesia* (New York: Churchill Livingstone, 2002), pp. 3-21.

H. Raper. *Man Against Pain: The Epic of Anesthesia* (New York: Prentice Hall, 1945).

K. Rehder, A. Southorn, A. Sessler. *Art to Science* (Rochester, MN: Mayo Clinic, 2000).

B. Robbins. *Cyclopropane Anesthesia* (Baltimore: Williams and Wilkins, 1940).

J. Robinson. *A Treatise on the Inhalation of the Vapour of Ether* [1847]. With preface to facsimile edition by R. Ellis. (Eastbourne: Bailliere Tindall, 1983).

V. Robinson. *Victory Over Pain* (New York: H. Schuman, 1945).

J. Rupreht, M. Van Leiburg, J. A. Lee, N. Erdmann. *Anaesthesia: Essays on Its History* (Berlin: Springer-Verlag, 1985).

G. Rushman, N. Davies, R. Atkinson. *A Short History of Anaesthesia: The First 150 Years* (Oxford: Butterworth-Heinemann, 1996).

A. Sansom. *Chloroform: Its Action and Administration* (London: John Churchill, 1865.

David Shephard

O. Secher. *Bibliography on the History of Anaesthesia* (Copenhagen: Rigshospitalet, 1984).

D. Shephard. John Snow and research. *Can J Anaesth* 1989; 36:224-41.

D. Shephard. *John Snow, Anaesthetist to a Queen and Epidemiologist to a Nation* (Cornwall, Prince Edward Island: York Point Publishing, 1985).

D. Shephard. The evolution of anaesthesia as a specialty in Canada. *Can J Anaesth* 1990; 37:134-42.

D. Shephard. *Watching Closely Those Who Sleep: A History of the Canadian Anaesthetists' Society 1943-1993* (Toronto: Canadian Anaesthetists'Society, 1993).

J. Y. Simpson. *Account of a New Anaesthetic Agent as a Substitute for Sulphuric Ether in Surgery and Midwifery* (Edinburgh: Sutherland and Knox, 1848).

W. G. Simpson (ed.). *The Collected Works of James Young Simpson* (Edinburgh: Adam and Charles Black, 1874).

H. Smith, D. Bacon. "The History of Anesthesia," in P. Barash, B. Cullen, R. Stoelting (eds.), *Clinical Anesthesia* (Philadelphia: Lippincott, Williams & Wilkins [5th ed.], 2006), pp. 3-26.

G. Smith, N. Hirsch. Gardner Quincy Colton: Pioneer of nitrous oxide anesthesia. *Anesth Analg* 1991; 72:382-91.

P. Smith. *Arrows of Mercy* (New York: Doubleday, 1969).

W. D. A. Smith. *Under the Influence—A History of Nitrous Oxide and Oxygen Anaesthesia* (Park Ridge: Wood Library-Museum of Anesthesiology, 1982).

W. D. Smith. Surgery without pain—Part I: Background. *Anaesth Int Care* 1986; 14:70-78.

W. D. Smith. Surgery without pain—Part II:1800-1847. *Anaesth Int Care* 1986; 14:186-92.

J. Snow. *On the Inhalation of the Vapour of Ether in Surgical Operations* (London: John Churchill, 1847).

J. Snow. *On Chloroform and Other Anaesthetics* (London: John Churchill, 1858).

J. Snow. [1991] See Ellis, 1991.

S. Snow. *Operations Without Pain: The Practice and Science of Anaesthesia in Victorian Britain* (Basingstoke: Palgrave Macmillan, 2006).

K. Sykes, J. Bunker. *Anaesthesia and the Practice of Medicine: Historical Perspectives* (London: Royal Society of Medicine Press, Ltd., 2007).

W. S. Sykes. *Essays on the First Hundred Years of Anaesthesia*, vols.1 and 2 (Edinburgh: E. and S. Livingstone, 1961, 1962). [For details of Volume3, see Ellis, 1982.).

K. B. Thomas. *Curare—Its History and Usage* (London: Pitman, 1964).

K. B. Thomas. *The Development of Anaesthetic Apparatus: A History Based on the Charles King Collection of the Association of Anaesthetists of Great Britain and Ireland* (Oxford: Blackwell Scientific Publications, 1975).

P. Thompson, D. Wilkinson. Development of anaesthetic machines. *Brit J Anaesth* 1985; 57:640-48.

L. Turnbull. *The Advantages and Accidents of Artificial Anaesthesia* (Philadelphia: Lindsay and Blakiston, 1875).

L. D. Vandam. Early American anesthetists: The origins of professionalism in anesthesia. *Anesthesiology* 1973; 38:264-74.

L. D. Vandam. On the origin of intrathecal anesthesia. *Int Anesth Clin* 1989; 27:2-7.

P. Vinten-Johansen, H. Brody, N. Paneth et al. *Cholera, Chloroform, and the Science of Medicine: A Life of John Snow* (Oxford: Oxford University Press, 2003).

P. Volpitto, L.D. Vandam. *The Genesis of Contemporary Anesthesiology* (Springfield: Charles C Thomas, 1982).

R. Waters. Endotracheal anesthesia and its historical development. *Anesth Analg* 1933; 12:196-203.

R. Waters. The evolution of anesthesia. *Proc Staff Meet Mayo Clin* 1942; 17:186-92.

R. Waters. The development of anesthesiology in the United States: Personal observations, 1913-1946. *J Hist Med All Sci* 1946; 1:595-606.

R. Waters. *Chloroform: A Study After 100 Years* (Madison: University of Wisconsin, 1951).

C. Wells. Horace Wells. *Anesth Analg* 1935; 14:176-89, 216-24.

H. Wells. *Dentist. Proceedings of the Centenary Commemorations of Wells' Discovery in 1844* (American Dental Association, 1948).

R. Wolfe, L. Meczer (eds.). *I Awaken to Glory: Essays Celebrating Horace Wells and the Sesquicentennial of His Discovery of Anesthesia* (Boston: Boston Medical Library, 1994).

R. Wolfe. *Tarnished Idol: William T.G. Morton and the Introduction of Surgical Anesthesia* (San Anselmo: Norman Publishing, 2001).

History of Medicine and History of Science

R. G. Frank. *Harvey and the Oxford Physiologists: Scientific Ideas and Social Interaction* (Berkeley: University of California Press, 1980).

J. Fulton (ed.). *Selected Readings in the History of Physiology* (Springfield: Charles C Thomas, 2nd edition, 1966).

L. King. *The Medical World of the Eighteenth Century* (Chicago: University of Chicago Press, 1958).

L. King. Medicine in the USA. Historical vignettes: XXI. Medical practice: Specialization. *JAMA* 1984; 251:1333-38.

T. Kuhn. *The Structure of Scientific Revolutions* (Chicago: University of Chicago Press, 2nd edition, 1970).

J. Liebenau. *Medical Science and Medical Industry* (Baltimore: Johns Hopkins University Press, 1987).

J. Luce, R. Byyny. The evolution of medical specialization. *Persp Biol Med* 1979; 22:377-88.

R. Melzack, P. Wall. Pain mechanisms: A new theory. *Science* 1965; 150:971-79.

J. M. Peterson. *The Medical Profession in Mid-Victorian London* (Berkeley: University of California Press, 1978).

R. Porter. *The Greatest Benefit to Mankind: A Medical History of Humanity* (New York: Norton, 1997).

G. Rosen. *The Specialization of Medicine with Particular Reference to Ophthalmology* (New York: Froben Press, 1944).

R. Shryock. *The Development of Modern Medicine: An Interpretation of the Social and Scientific Factors Involved* (Madison: University of Wisconsin Press, 1979).

R. Stevens. *Medical Practice in Modern England: The Impact of State Medicine* (New Haven: Yale University Press, 1960).

R. Stevens. *American Medicine and the Public Interest* (New Haven: Yale University Press, 1971). [2nd edition published with additional subtitle *A History of Specialization* (Berkeley: University of California Press, 1998).]

M. Vogel, C. Rosenberg (eds.). *The Therapeutic Revolution: Essays in the History of American Medicine* (Philadelphia: University of Pennsylvania Press, 1979).

J. H. Warner. *The Therapeutic Perspective: Medical Practice, Knowledge and Identity in America, 1820-1885* (Cambridge: Harvard University Press, 1986).

G. Weisz. *Divide and Conquer: A Comparative History of Medical Specialization* (Oxford: Oxford University Press, 2006).

G. Whitteridge. *William Harvey and the Circulation of the Blood* (London: Macdonald, 1971).

Endnotes

Introduction

[1]   C. Singer, E. Underwood. *A Short History of Medicine* (Oxford: Clarendon Press, 1968), p. 349.

[2]   J. C. Warren. Inhalation of ethereal vapor for the prevention of pain in surgical operations. *Boston Med Surg J* 1846; 35:375-39.

[3]   See, for example: D. Shephard, *John Snow: Anaesthetist to a Queen and Epidemiologist to a Nation—A Biography* (Chapel Hill: Professional Press, 1995); P. Vinten-Johansen, N. Brody, N. Paneth et al, *Cholera, Chloroform, and the Science of Medicine: A Life of John Snow* (Oxford: Oxford University Press, 2003).

[4]   O. P. Dinnick. "The First Anaesthesia Society," in *Progress in Anaesthesiology*, Proceedings of the Fourth World Congress of Anaesthesiology, London, Sept. 9-13 (Amsterdam: Excerpta Medica Foundation, International Congress Series, no. 200, 1970), pp. 181-86.

[5]   J. Erickson, "In the Beginning: Adolph Frederick Erdmann and the Long Island Society of Anesthetists," in D. Bacon, K. McGoldrick, M. Lema (eds.), *The American Society of Anesthesiologists: A Century of Challenges and Progress* (Park Ridge: Wood Library-Museum of Anesthesiology, 2005), pp. 1-9.

[6]   L. D. Vandam. Early American anesthetists: The origins of professionalism in anesthesia. *Anesthesiology* 1973; 38:264-74.

[7]   K. Rehder, P. Southorn, A. Sessler. *Art to Science* (Rochester, MN: Dept. of Anesthesiology, Mayo Clinic and Foundation, nd.), pp. 14-16.

[8]   D. Caton. *What a Blessing She Had Chloroform: The Medical and Social Response to the Pain of Childbirth From 1800 to the Present* (New Haven: Yale University Press, 1998), pp. 106-07.

[9]   J. Cooper, R. Newblower, C. Long, B. McPeek. Preventable anesthesia mishaps: A study of human factors. *Anesthesiology* 1978; 49:399-406.

[10] K. Sykes, J. Bunker. *Anaesthesia and the Practice of Medicine: Historical Perspectives* (London: Royal Society of Medicine Press, Ltd., 2007), p. 77.

11 S. Smith, H. Brown, J. Toman, L. Goodman. The lack of cerebral effects of d-tubocurarine *Anesthesiology* 1947; 8:1-14.

12 B. Ibsen. The anaesthetist's viewpoint on the treatment of respiratory complications in poliomyelitis in Copenhagen, 1952. *Proc Roy Soc Med* 1954; 47:72-75.

13 R. Ellis (ed.). *On Narcotism by the Inhalation of Vapours by John Snow MD* (London: Royal Society of Medicine Services, Ltd., 1991).

14 G. Edwards. Frederic William Hewitt (1857-1916) *Ann Roy Coll Engl* 1951; 8:233-45.

15 W. Boothby. Determination of anaesthetic tension of ether vapor in man, with some theoretical determinations therefrom, as to mode of action of common volatile anaesthetics. *J Lab & Exper Therap* 1914; 5:379-92.

16 W. Boothby. Nitrous oxide-oxygen anesthesia with description of new apparatus. *Boston Med Surg J* 1912; 166:86-90.

17 J. Snow. On the administration of chloroform in the public hospitals. *Med Times Gaz* 1852; 4:349-50.

18 F. Hewitt. The past, present and future of anaesthesia. *Practitioner* 1896; 57:347-56.

19 S. O. Goldan. Anesthetization as a specialty: Its present and future. *American Medicine* 1901; 2:101-04.

20 S. Snow. *Operations Without Pain: The Practice and Science of Anaesthesia in Victorian Britain* (Basingstoke: Palgrave Macmillan, 2006).

21 B. Bamforth, K. Siebecker. "Ralph M. Waters," in P. Volpitto, L. D. Vandam (eds.), *The Genesis of Contemporary American Anesthesiology* (Springfield: Charles C Thomas, 1982), pp. 51-68.

22 J. Bunker. *The Anesthesiologist and the Surgeon* (Boston: Little, Brown and Company, 1972), p. 17.

23 T. Keys. *The History of Surgical Anesthesia* (New York: H. Schuman, 1945). [Reprinted by Wood Library-Museum of Anesthesiology, Park Ridge, IL, 1996.]

24 B. Duncum. *The Development of Inhalation Anaesthesia With Special reference to the Years 1896-1900* (Oxford: Wellcome Historical Medical Museum and Oxford University Press, 1947).

25 K. B. Thomas. *The Development of Anaesthetic Apparatus: A History Based on the Charles King Collection of the Association of Anaesthetists of Great Britain and Ireland* (Oxford: Blackwell Scientific Publications, 1975).

26 N. Bergman. *The Genesis of Surgical Anesthesia* (Park Ridge: Wood Library-Museum of Anesthesiology, 1998).

27 G. Rushman, N. Davies, R. Atkinson. *A Short History of Anaesthesia: The First 150 Years* (London: Butterworth-Heinemann, 1996).

28 Sykes, Bunker, 2007.

29 J. Burnham. *What Is Medical History?* (Malden, MA: Polity Press, 2005), p. 9.

30 R. Fulop-Miller. *Triumph Over Pain* (New York: Literary Guild of America, Inc., 1938) [transl. E&C. Paul], p. vii.

Chapter 1

1. M. H. Armstrong Davison. *The Evolution of Anaesthesia* (Baltimore: Williams & Wilkins, 1965), p. 208.
2. V. Cordus. *De Artificionis Extractionibus*, 1561. Reprinted in part in A. Faulconer, T. Keys, *Foundations of Anesthesiology* (Park Ridge: Wood Library-Museum of Anesthesiology, 1993), vol. I, pp. 267-75.
3. Paracelsus. *Opera Medico-chemica Sive Paradoxa . . .* (Frankfurt, 1605), p. 125.
4. M. Morris. *A Letter from Michael Morris M.D. to the Medical Society Describing the Process for Making Aether, with Some Observations on its Medical Use.* Article XII, read Dec. 18, 1758. *Medical Observations and Inquiries by a Society of Physicians in London*, 1764; 2:176-86 (London: W. Johnson, 1764).
5. R. Pearson. *A Short Account of the Nature and Properties of Different Kinds of Airs, so far as Related to Their Medicinal Use, etc.* (Birmingham: R. Baldwin, 1795).
6. W. Harvey. *An Anatomical Disputation Concerning the Movement of the Heart and Blood in Living Creatures* [1628]. Translated with Introduction and Notes by G. Whitteridge (Oxford: Blackwell Scientific Publications, 1976).
7. R. Frank. *Harvey and the Oxford Physiologists* (Berkeley: University of California Press, 1980).
8. J. Priestley. Observations on different kinds of air. *Phil Trans Roy Soc Lond* 1772; 62:210-22. See also A. Faulconer, T. Keys, *Foundations of Anesthesiology* (Park Ridge: Wood Library-Museum of Anesthesiology, 1993), p. 396.
9. J. Priestley. *Experiments and Observations on Different Kinds of Air.* Vol II, Sections III-V (London, 1775), pp. 29-103. See also Faulconer, Keys, 1993, pp. 39-70.
10. Davison, 1965, p. 16.
11. Ibid., pp. 16-17.
12. R. Wolfe. *Tarnished Idol: William T. G. Morton and the Introduction of Surgical Anesthesia* (San Anselmo: Norman Publishing, 2001), p. 85.
13. Accounts of ancient anodynes are legion. See, among many, the following: E. H. Ackernecht, Aspects of the history of therapeutics, *Bull Hist Med* 1962; 36:389-419; C. Benedetti, L. Premuda, The history of opium and its derivatives, *Adv Pain Research Therap* 1990; 14:1-35; Bergman, 1998, pp. 1-28; A. Castigloni, *A History of Medicine* (New York: James Aronson, 1969); Davison, 1965; E. Ellis, *Ancient Anodynes: Primitive Anaesthesia and Allied Conditions* (London: William Heinemann, 1946); L. Freeman, Surgery of the ancient inhabitants of the Americas, *Art and Archeology* 1924; 18:21-35; T. Keys, *The History of Surgical Anesthesia* (New York: Henry Schuman, 1945), pp. 3-11; C. Leake, The historical development of surgical anesthesia, *Sci Monthly* 1925; 20:304-28; H. Lyman, *Artificial Anaesthesia and Anaesthetics* (New York: William Wood and Co., 1888); C. Mettler, *A History of Medicine* (Philadelphia: Blakiston Company, 1947); S. Nuland, "The anodynes of antiquity," in S. Nuland (ed.), *The Origins of Anesthesia* (Birmingham: Classics of Medicine Library, 1983), pp. 3-9; C. Randolph, The mandragora of the ancients in folk-lore and medicine,

Daedalus 1905; 40:487-537; J. Snow, "Historical Introduction," in *Chloroform and Other Anaesthetics: Their Action and Administration* (London: John Churchill, 1858), pp. 3-24; G. Tallmadge, Some anesthetics of antiquity, *J Hist Med All Sci* 1946; 1:515-20.

[14] Saint Hilary, *The Trinity* (New York: Fathers of the Church, Inc., 1954. Cited by Bergman, 1998, p. 1.

[15] R. Fulop-Miller. *Triumph Over Pain* (London: Hamish Hamilton, 1938 [transl. E. and C. Paul]), p. 16.

[16] P. Raj. *Textbook of Regional Anesthesia* (New York: Churchill Livingstone, 2002), p. 8.

[17] J. Duns. *Memoir of Sir James Y. Simpson, Bart.* (Edinburgh: Edmonston and Douglas, 1873).

[18] Homer. *The Odyssey* (Cambridge: Houghton Mifflin, 1929 [transl. G. Palmer]), p. 42.

[19] Celsus. *De Re Medicina.* Cited by Nuland, 1983, p. 4.

[20] W. Archer. The history of anesthesia. *Proc Dental Centenary Celebration*, 1940, pp. 333-63.

[21] Davison, 1965, p. 42.

[22] Randolph, 1905.

[23] Shakespeare. *Romeo and Juliet*, act I, sc. v, ll. 13-16.

[24] Dioscorides. *Dioscorides Opera*, Liber iv, Cap. 76.

[25] R. von Steinbuchel. Die Scopolamine-Morphium-Halbnarkose in der Gerburtshulfe. *Gerburtst* 1903; 1:294-326.

[26] Snow, 1858, p. 5.

[27] Ibid., p. 4.

[28] N. Saliternatus. *Antidotarium* (Venice: Nicolas Jenson, 1471), f. 33b.

[29] Boccaccio. *Il Decameron* (Firenze: Adriano Salani, 1928), vol. I, Giornata Quarta, Novella Decima, pp. 438-37.

[30] Bergman, 1998, p. 25.

[31] H. Raper. *Man Against Pain—The Epic of Anesthesia* (New York: Prentice Hall, 1945), p. 7.

[32] Cordus, 1561, pp. 265-75

[33] Paracelsus, 1605, p. 125.

[34] J. Frobenius. An account of a spiritus vini aethereus. *Phil Trans Roy Soc Lond* 1730; 36:283-89.

[35] H. Davy, 1800. *Researches, Chemical and Philosophical; Chiefly Concerning Nitrous Oxide or Dephlogisticated Nitrous Oxide and Its Respiration* (London: J. Johnson, 1800), p. 556.

[36] W. Bullein. *Bulwarke of Defence Against All Sickness* (London: John Kyngston, 1652), f. 44, recto.

[37] R. Pitcairn. *Ancient Criminal Trials in Scotland, Compiled from the Original Records and Manuscripts* (Edinburgh: Ballantyne Club, 1833), vol. I, part III.

[38] J. Fernel. *De Naturali Parte Medicinae . . .* (Paris, 1544).

[39] Vesalius. *De Humani Corporis Fabrica* (Basel, 1543).

[40] W. Harvey. *Exercitatio Anatomica de Motu Cordis et Sanguinis in Animalibus*, 1628. Transl. K. Franklin (Oxford: Blackwell Scientific Publications, 1957).

[41] Harvey, 1957, pp. 9-10.

[42] L. Wilson. The transformation of ancient concepts of respiration in the seventeenth century. *Isis* 1960; 51 (Part 2), no. 2:161-72.

[43] T. Keys. The early pneumatic chemists and physicians: Their influence on the development of surgical anesthesia. *Anesthesiology* 1969; 30:447-62.

[44] F. Cartwright. *The English Pioneers of Anaesthesia (Beddoes, Davy, Hickman)*. (Bristol: John Wright & Sons, Ltd., 1952), p. 27.

[45] Frank, 1980.

[46] R. Boyle. *The Sceptical Chymist* [1661] (London: J. M. Dent and Sons Everyman's Library, 1911).

[47] L. King. *The Medical World of the Eighteenth Century* (Chicago: University of Chicago Press, 1958).

[48] Boyle, 1661.

[49] R. Major. *A History of Medicine* (Springfield: Charles C Thomas, 1954), p. 515.

[50] Wolf. *A History of Science, Technology, and Philosophy in the 16th and 17th Centuries* (New York: Macmillan, 1939), p. 339.

[51] T. Sprat. *The History of the Royal Society of London for the Improving of Natural Knowledge* (London: J. Martin and J. Allestry, 1667), p. 232.

[52] Bergman, 1998, p. 49.

[53] M. Malpighi. *Opera Omnia* (Leyden, 1687), pp. 328-29.

[54] R. Lower. *Tractatus de Corde, Item de Motu, et Coloris Sanguinis et Chyli in eum Transitu* (London, 1669).

[55] Wilson, 1960.

[56] Ibid.

[57] Bergman, 1998, p. 43.

[58] Ibid., pp. 53-63.

[59] Davy, 1800, p. 556.

[60] S. Hales. *Statical Essays* (London, 1731-1733), vol. II: *Haemastatics*.

[61] M. Kerker. Herman Boerhaave and the development of pneumatic chemistry. *Isis* 1955; 46:36-49.

[62] Cournand. "Air and Blood," in A. Fishman, D. Richards (eds.), *Circulation of the Blood: Men and Ideas* (New York, Oxford University Press, 1964).

[63] Kerker, 1955.

[64] Bergman, 1998, p. 56.

[65] C. Mettler. *History of Medicine: A Correlative Text, Arranged According to Subjects* (Philadelphia: The Blakiston Company, 1947), p. 124.

[66] J. Black. *Experiments Upon Magnesia Alba, Quicklime, and Some Other Alcaline Substances* (Edinburgh: Alembic Club, 1944).

[67] H. Guerlac. Joseph Black and fixed air. A bicentenary perspective, with some new or little known material. *Isis* 1957; 48:124-51.

[68] H. Cavendish. Three papers, containing experiments on factitious air. *Phil Trans Roy Soc* 1766; 56:141-84.

[69] Bergman, 1998, p. 63.

[70] Idem.

[71] J. Priestley. Observations on different kinds of air. *Phil Trans Roy Soc* 1772; 62:210-22. Reprinted in Faulconer and Keys, 1993, vol. I, p. 396.

[72] Davison, 1965, p. 72.

[73] Priestley, 1772.

[74] Idem.

[75] P. Hartog. Date and place of Priestley's discovery of oxygen. *Nature* 1933; 132:25-26.

[76] R. Schofield (ed.) *A Scientific Biography of Joseph Priestley (1733-1804)* (Cambridge: MIT Press, 1966), Letters 53, 54.

[77] J. Priestley. *Experiments and Observations on Different Kinds of Air*, vol. II, 1775, p. 34.

[78] Hartog, 1933.

[79] Keys, 1996, note, p. 14.

[80] F. Holmes. *Lavoisier and the Chemistry of Life: An Exploration of Scientific Creativity* (Madison: University of Wisconsin Press, 1985), p. 146.

[81] Wolf, 1939, p. 370.

[82] Lavoisier. *Traite Elementaire de Chimie* (Paris: Cuchet, 1789).

[83] Bergman, 1998, p. 175.

[84] Ibid., pp. 91-92.

[85] Ibid., p. 93.

[86] R. Pearson. *A Short Account of the Nature and Properties of Different Kinds of Airs* (Birmingham: R. Baldwin, 1795).

[87] J. Barzun. Thomas Beddoes or medicine and social conscience. *JAMA* 1992; 220:50-53.

[88] Cartwright, 1952, p. 49.

[89] J. Cottle. *Early Recollections: Chiefly relating to the Late Samuel Taylor Coleridge, During His Long Residence in Bristol* (London: Longman Rees, 1837). Cited by Cartwright, 1952, p. 123.

[90] Cartwright, 1952, p. 86.

[91] Ibid., p. 88.

[92] Ibid., p. 86.

Chapter 2

[1] H. Davy. *Researches, Chemical and Philosophical; Chiefly Concerning Nitrous Oxide or Dephlogisticated Nitrous Air and Its Respiration* (London: J. Johnson, 1800), p. 556. (Reprinted by Butterworth, London, 1972.)

[2] Davy, 1800, p. 465.

[3] Davy, 1800, p. 464.

[4] H. Wells. *A History of the Discovery of the Application of Nitrous Oxide Gas, Ether, and Other Vapors, to Surgical Operations* (Hartford: J. G. Wells, 1847).

5   As indicated in Chapter 1, endnotes 2 and 3, ether was certainly known to Valerius
    Cordus and Paracelsus in the sixteenth century, Paracelsus observing its ability to
    induce sleep in chickens.

6   R. Pearson. *A Short Account of the nature and Properties of Different Kinds of Airs, so
    far as related to the Medicinal Use . . .* (Birmingham: R. Baldwin, 1795).

7   T. Beddoes. *Considerations on the Medicinal Use . . . of Factitious Airs* (Bristol: Bulgin
    and Rosser, for J. Johnson, London, 1796), p. 3.

8   T. Mitchell. *Elements of Chemical Philosophy* (Cincinnati: Corey and Fairbank, 1832),
    pp. 167-74.

9   W. D. A. Smith. *Under the Influence: Nitrous Oxide and Oxygen Anaesthesia* (Park
    Ridge: Wood Library-Museum of Anesthesiology, 1982), pp. 31-35, 37-39.

10 H. Lyman. *Artificial Anaesthesia and Anaesthetics* (New York: William Wood and
    Co., 1881), p. 6.

11 C. W. Long. An account of the first use of sulphuric ether by inhalation as an
    anesthetic in surgical operations. *South Med J* 1849; 5:705-13.

12 H. Hickman. *A Letter on Suspended Animation, Containing Experiments Showing That
    It May Safely be Employed During Operations on Animals, with the View of Ascertaining
    Its Probable Utility in Surgical Operations on the Human Subject . . . .* (Ironbridge,
    1824).

13 N. P. Rice. *Trials of A Public Benefactor, as Illustrated in the Discovery of Etherization*
    (New York: Pudney and Russell, 1859).

14 Hickman, 1824.

15 Davy, 1800.

16 N. Bergman. *The Genesis of Surgical Anesthesia* (Park Ridge: Wood Library-Museum
    of Anesthesiology, 1998), p. 278.

17 M. Jacob, M. Sauter. Why did Humphry Davy and associates not pursue the pain-
    alleviating effects of nitrous oxide? *J Hist Med All Sci* 2002; 57:161-76.

18 J. H. van den Berg. *Leven in Meervoud* (Nijkerk: G. F. Callenbach, 1963), pp. 248-
    53. Cited by D. de Moulin, A historical-phenomenological study of bodily pain in
    western man, *Bull Hist Med* 1974; 48:540-570.

19 D. Beales. *From Castlereagh to Gladstone:1815-1885* (New York: W. W. Norton &
    Company, 1969), p. 74.

20 J. Cottle. *Early Recollections; Chiefly Relating to the Late Samuel Taylor Coleridge,
    During His Long Residence in Bristol* (London: Longman Rees, 1837).

21 H. Davy, Nov. 21, 1800. Cited by Jacob, Sauter, 2002.

22 Davy, 1800, p. 471.

23 S. Snow. *Operations Without Pain: The Practice and Science of Anaesthesia in Victorian
    Britain* (Basingstoke: Palgrave Macmillan, 2006), p. 19.

24 E. Ackerknecht. *A Short History of Medicine* (Baltimore: Johns Hopkins University
    Press [revised edition], 1982), p. 129.

25 Bergman, 1998, p. 280.

26 Jacob, Sauter, 2002.

27 S. L. Mitchill. *Remarks on the Gaseous Oxyd of Azote or of Nitrogene qnd on the Effects it Produces When Generated in the Stomach, Inhaled into the Lungs, and Applied to the Skin: Being an Attempt to Ascertain the True Nature of Contagion, and to Explain thereupon the Phenomenon of Fever* (New York: T. and J. Swords, 1795).

28 Annotation. *Lancet* 1827-28; 13:455.

29 B. Brodie. *Lecture Notes on Poisonous Gases*—Vol. 1 (London: Royal College of Surgeons, 1812).

30 B. Brodie. *Physiological Researches* (London: Longman, Brown, Green, and Longmans, 1851), p. 143.

31 J. Bell. *The Principles of Surgery in Two Volumes* (Edinburgh: Cadell, 1801). Cited by W. D. A. Smith, Surgery without pain—Part II:1800-1847, *Anaesth Int Care* 1986; 14:186-92.

32 Smith, 1986.

33 M. Pernick. *A Calculus of Suffering: Pain, Professionalism and Anesthesia in Nineteenth-Century America* (New York: Columbia University Press, 1985), p. 45.

34 L. Velpeau. *Nouveau Elements de Medecine Operatoirs* (Paris, 1839).

35 J. Cosnett. Surgery without anesthesia: A historical perspective. *Sem Anesth* 1988; 7:315-22.

36 R. Hunt. "Biographical Sketch of Tiberius Cavallo," in L. Stephen (ed.), *Dictionary of National Biography* (London: Oxford Publishing Co., 1975), vol. 1, p. 334.

37 J. Stock. *Memoirs on the Life of Thomas Beddoes, MD, With an Analytical Account of His Writings* (London: John Murray, 1811).

38 F. Cartwright. *The English Pioneers of Anaesthesia (Beddoes, Davy, Hickman)* (Bristol: John Wright and Sons, 1952), pp. 86-89.

39 Hickman, 1824.

40 Ibid.

41 J. Berzelius. Hydrogen gas. *Amer J Sci Arts* 1824; 8:375.

42 Hickman, 1824.

43 Ibid.

44 S. Snow, 2006, p. 26.

45 Bergman, p. 370.

46 R. French. *Antivivisection and Medical Science in Victorian Society* (Princeton: Princeton University Press, 1975).

47 "Antiquack." Surgical humbug. *Lancet* 1846; 2:646-47.

48 Wellcome Foundation. *Souvenir of the Henry Hill Hickman Centenary Exhibition, 1830-1930.* Wellcome Medical Museum, London, 1930, pp. 37-45.

49 E. M. Papper. The influence of Romantic literature on the understanding of pain and suffering—The stimulus to the discovery of anesthesia. *Persp Biol Med* 1992; 35:401-15.

50 J. Bentham. *An Introduction to the Principles of Morals and Legislation* (J. H. Burons, H. L. A. Hart, eds.) (New York: Methuen, 1982), p. 34.

51 J. S. Mill. *Nature, The Philosophy of John Stuart Mill* (M. Cohen, ed.) (New York: Modern Library, 1961), pp. 463-67.

52 N. Greene. A consideration of factors in the discovery of anesthesia and their effects on its development. *Anesthesiology* 1971; 35; 515-22.

53 D. Caton. The secularization of pain. *Anesthesiology* 1985; 62:493-501.

54 R. Descartes. Cited by P. Gay, *The Enlightenment: An Interpretation. The Rise of Modern Paganism* (New York: W. W. Norton, 1977), p. 6.

55 B. R. Fink. Background of scientific law to the discovery of surgical anesthesia, in R. S. Atkinson, T. B. Boulton (eds.), *The History of Anesthesia* (Carnforth: Royal Society of Medicine Publishing Services, 1989), pp. 52-56.

56 N. Greene. Eli Ives and the medical use of ether prior to 1846. *J Hist Med All Sci* 1960; 15:297.

57 Hickman, 1824.

58 W. Wright. *The Aurist or Medical Guide for the Deaf.* 1825:3 (May):76-80.

59 J. Curtis. Nitrous oxide as a remedy in chronic diseases of the chest. *Lancet* 1829; 2:376.

60 J. Hudson. Nitrous oxide in cholera. *Lancet* 1832; 2:629.

61 Back and Morgan. Hydrophobia. Inhalation of nitrous oxide gas. *Lancet* 1834; 2:703.

62 R. M. Waters. The evolution of anesthesia. I. *Staff Proc Mayo Clin* 1942; 17:428-445.

63 Fink, 1989.

64 W. D. A. Smith. Surgery without pain—Part II:1800-1847. *Anaesth Intens Care* 1986; 14:186-92.

65 S. Morison. *The Oxford History of the American People* (New York: Oxford University Press, 1965), p. 535.

66 Ibid., p. 470.

67 Fink, 1989.

68 Cartwright, 1952, p. 328.

69 H. R. Raper. *Man Against Pain: The Epic of Anesthesia* (New York: Prentice-Hall, Inc., 1945), p. 141.

70 Cartwright, 1952, p. 282.

71 H. Hickman. Memorial to Charles X of France, 1828. In Wellcome Foundation *Souvenir of the Henry Hill Hickman Centenary Exhibition, 1830-1930* (London: Wellcome Foundation, 1930), pp. 37-45.

72 Cartwright, 1952, p. 309.

73 Bergman, 1998, p. 135.

74 W. Wright. *On the Varieties of Deafness and Diseases of the Ear, With Proposed Methods of Relieving Them* (London: Hurst, Chance and Co., 1829).

75 Smith, 1982, pp. 39-40, 54.

76 G. Smith, N. Hirsch. Gardner Quincy Colton: Pioneer of nitrous oxide anesthesia. *Brit J Anaesth* 1991; 72:382-91.

77 C. Wells. Horace Wells. *Anesth Analg* 1935; 14:176-89, 216-24.

78 H. Wells. *An Essay on Teeth, Comprising a Brief Description of Their Formation, Diseases and Proper Treatment* (Hartford: Case, Tiffany and Co., 1838).

[79] W. H. Archer. Chronological history of Horace Wells, discoverer of anesthesia. *Bull Hist Med* 1939; 7:1140-69.

[80] Smith, 1982, p. 54.

[81] Ibid., p. 55.

[82] H. Wells. To the European and American public. *Lancet* 1847; 1:471-73. (1847b.)

[83] C. Wells, 1935.

[84] Smith, 1982, p. 55.

[85] Ibid., p. 57.

[86] H. Wells. Letter to Hartford *Courant*, Dec. 9, 1846.

[87] Archer, 1939.

[88] Wells, Letter to *Courant*, Dec. 9, 1846.

[89] R. J. Wolfe. *Tarnished Idol: William Thomas Green Morton and the Introduction of Surgical Anesthesia—A Chronicle of the Ether Controversy* (San Anselmo, CA: Norman Publishing, 2001), p. 507.

[90] E. E. Marcy. Removal of a large scirrhous testicle from a man while under the influence of nitrous oxide. *Boston Med Surg J* 1847; 37:97-99.

[91] P. W. Ellsworth. Amputation of the thigh under the influence of the nitrous oxide gas. *Boston Med Surg J* 1848; 37:498-99.

[92] Though Wells' use of ether is well documented, it appears to have been downplayed in accounts of the introduction of ether. *Vide infra* and also, for example: P. Ellsworth, The discoverer of the effects of sulphuric ether, *Boston Med Surg J* 1846; 35:397-98; E. Marcy, Inhalation of ether to prevent pain, Ibid., 495-97; C. Wells, Horace Wells, *Anesth Analg* 1935; 14:176-89.

[93] R. J. Wolfe. Who was the discoverer of surgical anesthesia? A brief for Horace Wells, in R. J. Wolfe, L. F. Menczer (eds.), *I Awaken to Glory* . . . . (Boston: Boston Medical Library, 1994), p. 26.

[94] Lyman, 1881, p. 6.

[95] R. Stone. *Biography of Eminent American Physicians and Surgeons* (Indianopolis: Carlon and Hollenbeck, 1894), p. 89.

[96] Stetson, 1992

[97] W. Hammonds, J. Steinhaus. Crawford W. Long: Pioneer physician in anesthesia. *J Clin Anesth* 1993; 5:163-67.

[98] J. Ball. The ether tragedies. *Ann Med Hist* 1925; 7:264-66.

[99] W. Channing. Notes of difficult labors, in the second of which etherization by sulphuric ether was successfully employed nineteen years ago. *Boston Med Surg J* 1853; 46:113-16.

[100] R. Collyer. Patent for inhalation. *Lancet* 1847; 1:163.

[101] E. Smilie. Insensibility produced by the inhalation of the vapor of the ethereal solution of opium. *Boston Med Surg J* 1846; 35:263-64.

[102] Wolfe, 2001, p. 59, citing J. C. Warren III, Warren Family Papers, Massachusetts Historical Society 23:11.

[103] E. W. Emerson. *A History of the Gift of Painless Surgery* (Boston: Houghton Mifflin and Company, 1896), p. 2.

[104] Ibid., pp. 2-3.

[105] Ibid., p. 3.

[106] Wolfe, 2001, p. 520.

[107] Idem.

[108] Idem.

[109] Wolfe, 2001, p. 509.

[110] W. T. G. Morton. Memoir. *Littell's Living Age*, 1848; 16 (no. 16, 18 March), pp. 566-67.

[111] Wolfe, 2001, p. 509.

[112] *Littell's Living Age*, p. 535.

[113] Morton, 1848, p. 568.

[114] J. Stetson. William E. Clarke and his 1842 use of ether, in B. R. Fink, L. Morris (eds.), *The History of Anesthesia* (Park Ridge: Wood Library-Museum of Anesthesiology, 1992), pp. 406-07.

[115] Lyman, 1881, p. 6.

[116] Stone, 1894.

[117] Stetson, 1992, pp. 400-07.

[118] Hammonds, Steinhaus, 1993

[119] Ibid.

[120] Long, 1849.

[121] Wolfe, 2001, p. 502 and p. 630, n. 17.

[122] Cited by W. S. Sykes, "The Jump-up-behinder." *Essays on the First Hundred Years of Anaesthesia*, vol. III (R. H. Ellis [ed.]), (Park Ridge, IL: Wood Library-Museum of Anesthesiology, 1982), p. 46.

[123] Sykes, 1982, p. 52.

[124] Wolfe, 2001, p. 59.

[125] H. Wells. The discovery of ethereal inhalation. *Boston Med Surg J* 1847:36:297-301.

[126] Ellsworth, 1847.

[127] Marcy, 1847.

[128] C. Wells, 1935.

[129] Wolfe, 2001.

[130] B. P. Poore. *Historical Materials for a Biography of W. T. G. Morton, MD, Discoverer of Etherization, with an Account of Anaesthesia* (Washington: G. S. Gideon, 1856).

[131] N. P. Rice. *Trials of a Public Benefactor, as Illustrated in the Discovery of Etherization* (New York: Pudney & Russell, 1859).

[132] L. D. Vandam. Benjamin Perley Poore and his historical materials for a biography of W. T. G. Morton, MD. *J Hist Med All Sci* 1994; 49:5-23.

[133] H. J. Bigelow. Insensibility during surgical operations produced by inhalation. *Boston Med Surg J* 1846; 35:310-17.

[134] Rice, 1859.

[135] Wolfe, 2001, p. 543.

[136] Wolfe, 2001.

[137] H. Wells, 1847b.

[138] Wolfe, 2001, p. 3.

[139] Idem.

[140] Archer, 1939.

[141] H. Wells, 1846.

[142] *Littell's Living Age*, p. 534.

[143] Wolfe, 2001, p. 62.

[144] *Littell's Living Age*, p. 535.

[145] Wolfe, 2001, pp. 64-65.

[146] Ibid., p. 534.

[147] Rice, 1859, pp. 61-62.

[148] *Littell's Living Age*, p. 535.

[149] Idem.

[150] Morton, Memoir, 1848, p. 568.

[151] C. Eddy. *Littell's Living Age*, p. 541.

[152] Wolfe, 2001, p. 72, citing *Boston Daily Journal*, Oct. 1, 1846.

[153] Wolfe, 2001, p. 72.

[154] Ibid., p. 86.

[155] *Littell's Living Age*, pp. 535-56.

[156] W. J. Morton. In Discussion of W. W. Babcock, The uses and limitations of general anesthesia as produced by subcutaneous and intravascular injections. *JAMA* 1911; 22:1677.

[157] *Littell's Living Age*, p. 536.

[158] Wolfe, 2001, p. 70.

[159] J. C. Warren, cited by S. B. Nuland, *The Origins of Anesthesia* (Birmingham: Classics of Medicine Library, 1983), p. 70.

[160] D. D. Slade. Historic moments: The first capital operation under the influence of ether. *Scribner's Magazine* 1892; 12:518-24.

[161] R. H. Ellis. Early ether anesthesia: The news of anaesthesia spreads to the United Kingdom. In R. S. Atkinson, T. B. Boulton (eds.), *The History of Anaesthesia* (Carnforth: RSM Services and Parthenon Publishing Group, 1989), pp. 69-76.

[162] Ibid.

[163] H. J. Bigelow. Insensibility during surgical operations produced by inhalation. *Boston Med Surg J* 1846; 35:309-17.

[164] *Boston Daily Advertiser* 1846, Nov. 19, p. 2, cols. 2-4.

[165] T. Baillie. *From Boston to Dumfries* (Dumfries: Robert Dinwiddie & Co., 1969).

[166] Cited by Wolfe, 2001, p. 84.

[167] J. Robinson. *A Treatise on the Inhalation of the Vapour of Ether for the Prevention of Pain in Surgical Operations* (London: Webster & Co., 1847).

[168] Baillie, 1969.

[169] J. Ruprecht. The knowledge spreads through Europe, in Atkinson, Boulton, 1989, pp. 82-86.

[170] J. R. Maltby. Early anaesthesia in North America, in Atkinson, Boulton, 1989, pp. 112-19.

[171] Ruprecht, 1989.

[172] Ibid.

[173] G. Wilson. The news spreads along the trade routes of the British Empire, in Atkinson, Boulton, 1989, pp. 134-46.

[174] R. Nunn. Operation for stone in the bladder. *Lancet* 1847; 1:343.

[175] Genesis 3:16.

[176] J. Y. Simpson. "Answers to the Religious Objections Advanced Against the Employment of Anaesthetic Agents in Surgery and Obstetrics in Anaesthesia, Hospitalism, Hermaphrodites and a proposal to Stamp Out Small-Pox and other Contagious Diseases," in W. G. Simpson (ed.), *The Collected Works of James Young Simpson* (Edinburgh: Adam and Charles Black, 1874), pp. 42-64.

[177] Wolfe, 2001.

[178] G. Hayward. Some account of the first use of sulphuric ether by inhalation, in surgical practice. Extract cited by S. Nuland, 1983, Chapter XI, p. 48.

[179] Morton, 1848, p. 537.

[180] Wolfe, 2001, p. 123.

[181] *Littell's Living Age*, p. 545.

[182] Wolfe, 2001, p. 120.

[183] Wolfe, 2001, pp. 120-21.

[184] C. T. Jackson. Antidote to physical suffering. *Boston Daily Advertiser*, March 1, 1847, p. 2.

[185] W. T. G. Morton, *Boston Daily Advertiser* 1847, March 5, p. 2.

[186] Idem.

[187] Wolfe, 2001, p. 217.

[188] *Littell's Living Age*, p. 569.

[189] M. Gay. *A Statement of the Claims of Charles T. Jackson, MD, to the Discovery of the Applicability of Sulphuric Ether to the Prevention of Pain in Surgical Operations* (Boston: D. Clapp, 1847).

[190] Wolfe, 2001, pp. 143-44.

[191] H. Wells, 1847a.

[192] Wolfe, 2001, pp. 127-28, citing letter from C. T. Jackson to C. S. Brewer, 30 March 1847.

[193] Wolfe, 2001, p. 340.

[194] American Medical Association, June 24, 1864, cited by Nuland, 1983, p. 99.

[195] W. Osler. The first printed documents relating to modern surgical anesthesia. *Proc Roy Soc Med* 1918; 11:65-69.

[196] Wolfe, 2001, p. 542.

[197] "A." Discovery of the effects of ether. *Boston Med Surg J* 1847; 36:297-98.

[198] J. Fulton. The vision and daring of youth: The story of the introduction of surgical anesthesia. *Anesthesiology* 1947; 8:464-70.

[199] "A," 1847.

Chapter 3

1   O. W. Holmes. Letter to W. T. G. Morton, 21 Nov. 1846. Cited by N. P. Rice, *Trials of a Public Benefactor* (New York, 1859), p. 137.

2   J. Snow. *On Chloroform and Other Anaesthetics: Their Administration* (London: John Churchill, 1858), pp. 329-44.

3   M. Pernick. *A Calculus of Suffering* (New York: Columbia University Press, 1985), p. 249, Table 1.

4   Ibid., 196-205.

5   Ibid., pp. 42-58

6   Anonymous. Insensibility during surgical operations. *Phil Med Exam* 1847; n. s. 3:229-30.

7   J. Lister. On the antiseptic principle in the practice of surgery. *Lancet* 1867; 2:353-56, 668-69.

8   B. Duncum. *The Development of Inhalation Anaesthesia With Special Reference to the Years 1846-1900* (London: Wellcome Historical Medical Museum, 1947), p. 29.

9   N. Greene. Anesthesia and the development of surgery (1846-1896). *Anesth Analg* 1979; 58:5-12.

10 The literature on Snow is vast. See, in the present context, the following especially: J. Snow. *On the Inhalation of the Vapour of Ether in Surgical Operations . . .* (London: John Churchill, 1847); R. Ellis (ed.), *On Narcotism by the Inhalation of Vapours by John Snow MD* (London: Royal Society of Medicine Services, Ltd., 1991; J. Snow, *On Chloroform and Other Anaesthetics: Their Action and Administration* (London: John Churchill, 1858; D. Shephard. *John Snow: Anaesthetist to a Queen and Epidemiologist to a Nation—A Biography* (Chapel Hill: Professional Press, 1995), pp. 279-94; and P. Vinten-Johansen, H. Brody, N. Panath et al. *Cholera, Chloroform, and the Science of Medicine: A Life of John Snow* (Oxford: Oxford University Press, 2003), p. 143.

11 J. A. Lee. Joseph Clover and the contributions of surgery to anaesthesia. *Ann Roy Coll Surg Engl* 1960; 26:280-99.

12 G. Edwards. Frederic William Hewitt (1857-1916). *Ann Roy Coll Surg Engl* 1951; 8:233-45.

13 F. Hewitt. The past, present, and future of anaesthesia. *Practitioner* 1896; 57:347-56.

14 R. Ellis (ed.). *The Case Books of Dr. John Snow* (London: Wellcome Institute for the History of Medicine, 1994), p. xxxi.

15 S. Snow. *Operations Without Pain: The Practice and Science of Anaesthesia in Victorian Britain* (Basingstoke: Palgrave Macmillan, 2006), p. 154.

16 J. Robinson. *A Treatise on the Inhalation of the Vapour of Ether* (London: Webster, 1847). Facsimile edition, with introductory essay by R. H. Ellis (Eastbourne: Bailliere Tindall, 1983).

17 Snow, 1847 J. Snow. *On the Inhalation of the Vapour of Ether in Surgical Operations . . .* (London: John Churchill, 1847).

18 J. Snow, 1858.

19 D. Buxton. *Anaesthetics: Their Uses and Administration* (London:1888).

20 F. Hewitt. *Anaesthetics and Their Administration: A Textbook for Medical and Dental Practitioners and Students* (London: Griffin, 1893).

21 J. Snow, 1847, pp. 15-23.

22 G. Smith. Gardner Quincy Colton: Pioneer of nitrous oxide anesthesia. *Anesth Analg* 1991; 72:382-91.

23 Duncum, 1947, pp. 274-75

24 Duncum, 1947, pp. 289-91.

25 J. Y. Simpson. On a new anaesthetic agent, more efficient than sulphuric ether. *Lond Med Gaz* 1847; 5 (n. s.):934-37.

26 S. Guthrie. New mode of preparing a spirituous colution of chloric ether. *American Journal of Science and Arts* 1831; 21:64-65.

27 E. Soubeiran. Recherches sur quelques combinaisons du chlore. *Ann Chim Phys* 1831; 48:113-57.

28 J. von Liebig. Ueber der Verbindungen, welche durch die Einwirkung des Chlors auf Alkohol, Aether, olbildendes Gas und Essiggeist entstehen. *Ann Phamacie* 1832; 1:182-230.

29 J. Simpson. On the inhalation of sulphuric ether in the practice of midwifery. *Edin Month J Med Sci* 1846-47; 1 (n. s.):721-32.

30 H. Gordon. *Sir James Young Simpson and Chloroform (1811-1870)* (London: T. Fisher Unwin, 1897).

31 J. Simpson. On a new anaesthetic agent, more efficient than sulphuric ether. *Lancet* 1847; 2:549-50.

32 J. Bell. Note. *Pharm J* 1846-1847; 6; 357.

33 H. Coote. Surgical operations performed on patients rendered insensible to pain by the inhalation of chloroform. *Lancet* 1847; 2:571-72.

34 F. Sertuerner. *J der. Pharmacie* (Trommsdorff's), 1805. Cited by A. Faulconer, T. Keys, *Foundations of Anesthesiology* (Park Ridge: Wood Library-Museum of Anesthesiology, 1993), vol. 2, p. 1078.

35 C. Bernard. *Lecons sur les Anesthesiques et sur l'Asphyxie.* (Paris, 1875), p. 234.

36 E. Lowenstein. The birth of opioid anesthesia. *Anesthesiology* 2004; 100:1013-15.

37 Duncum, 1947, p. 133, ftn.

38 Duncum, 1947), p. 133.

39 Duncum, 1947, p. 131.

40 Ellis, 1991, pp. xix-xxi.

41 Snow, 1847, p. 15.

42 J. Snow. On the inhalation of the vapour of ether. *Lond Med Gaz* 1847; 4:156-57.

43 Snow, 1847, p. 15.

44 Snow, 1847, p. 26.

45 Snow, 1847, p. 20.

46 Snow, 1847, pp. 5-6.

47 Snow, 1847, pp. 35-36.

[48] Snow, 1858, p. 89.

[49] J. Snow. Death from chloroform in a case of fatty degeneration of the heart. *Med Times Gaz* 1852; 5:361-62.

[50] J. Snow. Further remarks on amylene. *Med Times Gaz* 1857; 14:379-82.

[51] J. Snow. Case of death from amylene. *Med Times Gaz* 1857; 15:133-34.

[52] D. Caton. *What a Blessing She Had Chloroform: The Medical and Social Response to the Pain of Childbirth from 1800 to the Present* (New Haven: Yale University Press, 1999), p. 68.

[53] J. Snow. On the inhalation of chloroform and ether. With description of an apparatus. *Lancet* 1848; 1:177-80.

[54] Ellis, 1994, p. 271.

[55] Ibid., p. 471.

[56] Vinten-Johansen et al, 2003), p. 143.

[57] B. Richardson, "The Life of John Snow, MD," in Snow, 1858, p. xxxv.

[58] J. Snow. Remarks on the fatal case of chloroform. *Lond Med Gaz* 1848; 6 n. s.:277-78.

[59] Ellis, 1991, pp. xvi-xvii.

[60] J. Snow. *On the Mode of Communication of Cholera* (Pamphlet, 31 pp., 1849). This is rare. Another reference is Snow's article in the *London Medical Gazette* (1849; 44:745-52, 923-29) titled "On the pathology and mode of communication of cholera."

[61] J. Snow. *On the Mode of Communication of Cholera* (London: John Churchill, 1854, 2nd edition).

[62] Snow, 1858, pp. 120-99.

[63] Ellis, 1991, pp. xix-xxi.

[64] Duncum, 1947, p. 463.

[65] Ellis, 1991, pp. xvi-xvii.

[66] Shephard, 1995, pp. 279-94.

[67] J.-L. Gay-Lussac. "The Expansion of Gases by Heat," reprinted in W. Magie (ed.), *A Source Book in Physics* (New York: McGraw-Hill, 1935).

[68] J. Dalton. "Experimental Enquiry Into the Proportion of the Several Gases or Elastic Fluids, Constituting the Atmosphere, Read Nov. 12, 1802," in *Memoirs of the Literary and Philosophical Society of Manchester* 1805; 1:244-58.

[69] A. Ure. New experimental researches on some of the leading doctrines of caloric . . . . *Phil Trans Roy Soc Lond* 1818; 108:388-94.

[70] Caton, 1999), pp. 68-69.

[71] Ellis, 1991, p. xxi.

[72] Lee, 1960.

[73] Anon. *Med Times Lond* 1862; 2; 149.

[74] J. Clover. Apparatus for administering nitrous oxide gas and ether, singly or combined. *Brit Med J* 1876; 2:74.

[75] J. Clover. Portable regulating ether inhaler. *Brit Med J* 1877; 1:69-70.

[76] K. B. Thomas. *The Development of Anaesthetic Apparatus: A History Based on the Charles King Collection of the Association of Anaesthetists of Great Britain and Ireland* (Oxford: Blackwell Scientific Publications, 1975), p. 121.

[77] Edwards, 1951.

[78] E. Andrews. The oxygen mixture, a new anaesthetic combination. *Chicago Med Exam* 1868; 9:656-61.

[79] P. Bert. Anesthesie par le protoxyde d'azote employe sous tension. *Compt Rend Soc Biol* 1880; 152.

[80] Edwards, 1951.

[81] F. Hewitt. *Anaesthetics* . . . (London: Griffin, 2nd ed., 1901), p. 277.

[82] F. Hewitt. An artificial airway for use during anaesthetisation. *Lancet* 1908; 1:490.

[83] Edwards, 1951.

[84] F. Hewitt. *Select Methods in the Administration of Nitrous Oxide and Ether* (London, 1888).

[85] Edwards, 1951.

[86] Duncum, 1947

[87] Buxton, 1888.

[88] D. Caton. Obstetric anesthesia: The first ten years. *Anesthesiology* 1970; 33:102-09.

[89] J. Snow, citing J. Miller in *Surgical Experience of Chloroform* (Edinburgh, 1848), pp. 16-17, in *On Chloroform*, 1858, p. 79.

[90] Odontological Society of Great Britain; J. Parkinson. Dental Notes and Critical Reports (March 2). *Brit J Dent Sci* 1868; 11:123-41.

[91] J. Snow. On the administration of chloroform during parturition. *Assoc Med J* 1853; 1:500-02.

[92] Duncum, 1947, pp. 135, 136, 204.

[93] *Med Times Lond* 1868; 2:9. Cited by Duncum, 1947, pp. 16-17.

[94] M. J.-P. Flourens. Note touchant les effets de l'inhalation de l'ether sur la moelle allongee. *Compte Rendu des Sceances de l'Academie des Sciences* 1847; 24:253-58.

[95] C. Bernard. *An Introduction to the Study of Experimental Medicine* (New York: Macmillan Company, 1927, transl. H. Greene).

[96] Bernard, 1875, p. 149.

[97] C. Bernard. *Lecon sur les Effets des Substances Toxiques et Medicamenteuses* (Paris: Bailliere, 1851).

[98] J. Snow. On narcotism by the inhalation of vapours, part 16. *Med Gaz* 1851; 12 (ns):1053-57.

[99] Bernard, 1875, p. 234.

[100] P. Bert. The feasibility of producing lasting anesthesia with nitrous oxide, with a note on the innocuous nature of this agent. *Compt Rend* 1878; 87:728-30.

[101] Duncum, 1947, pp. 56-63.

[102] T. Keys. *The History of Surgical Anesthesia* (New York: Dover Publications, Inc., 1945), p. 107

[103] L. Turnbull. *The Advantages and Accidents of Artificial Anaesthesia* (Philadelphia: Lindsay and Blakiston, 1870).

[104] H. Lyman. *Artificial Anaesthesia and Anaesthetics* (New York: William Wood and Co., 1881).

[105] G. Smith, N. Hirsch. Garner Quincy Colton: Pioneer of Nitrous Oxide Anesthesia. *Anesth Analg* 1991; 72:382-91.

[106] Duncum, 1947, p. 274.

[107] E. Andrews. *Brit J Dent Sci* 1869; 12:22-26. Cited by Duncum, 1947, pp. 305-07.

[108] Clover, 1876.

[109] Hewitt, 1893.

[110] Duncum, 1947, p. 253.

[111] Report of the Nitrous Oxide Committee [Odontological Society]. *Lancet* 1872; 2:687.

[112] Duncum, 1947, p. 279.

[113] Ibid., pp. 285-87.

[114] Ibid., p. 287.

[115] Duncum, 1947, pp. 235-36.

[116] Ibid., pp. 489-91.

[117] Thomas, 1975, p. 133.

[118] Ibid.

[119] E. von Bibra, E. Harless. *Die Wirkung des Schwefelathers in chemischr und physiologischer Beziehung* (Erlangen, 1847), p. 183.

[120] F. Heyfelder. *Experiments with Ethyl Chloride* (Erlangen: Carl Heyder, 1848), pp. 83-85.

[121] *ibid.*

[122] B. Richardson. On a new and ready mode of producing local anesthesia. *Med Times Gaz* 1866; 1:115-17.

[123] C. Redard. Ethyl chloride as a local anesthetic. *Verhandlungen des X Internationalen Medicinischen Congresses*, Berlin, Aug. 4-9, 1890 (Berlin: August Hirschwald, 1891), vol. 5, pp. 71-73.

[124] Duncum, 1947, p. 499.

[125] Ibid., p. 500.

[126] K. B. Thomas. Ferdinand Ethelbert Junker. *Anaesthesia* 1073; 28:531-34.

[127] Thomas, 1975, pp. 68-77.

[128] K. Rehder, P. Southorn, A. Sessler. *Art to Science* (Rochester, MN: Mayo Clinic, 2000), pp. 14-17.

[129] I. Herb. Ethylene. Notes taken from the clinical records. *Anesth Analg* 1923; 2:230-32.

[130] Duncum, 1947, p. 413.

[131] Ibid., p. 253.

[132] Ibid., p. 258.

[133] *Brit Med J* 1868; 2:622.

[134] Report of the Nitrous Oxide Committee. *Lancet* 1872; 2; 687.

[135] *Brit Med J* 1875; 2:781.

[136] Ibid., p. 214.

[137] Duncum, 1947, pp. 429-439.

[138] E. Lawrie: The Hyderabad Chloroform Commission. *Lancet* 1889; 1:394.

[139] Ibid., p. 438.

[140] *Lancet* 1889; 2:606.

[141] Ibid., p. 1183.

[142] *Lancet* 1893; 1:629, 693, 761, 899, 971, 1111, 1236, 1479.

[143] F. Hewitt. *Anaesthetics and Their Administration: A Textbook for Medical and Dental Practitioners and Students* (London: Macmillan and Company, Ltd., 1912), pp. 137-39.

[144] J. McWilliam. Cardiac failure and sudden death. *Brit Med J* 1889; 1:6-8.

[145] Levy, 1911.

[146] Duncum, 1947, p. 469.

[147] Duncum, 1947, pp. 460-64.

[148] Ibid.

[149] Buxton, 1888.

[150] C. Singer. Medical progress from 1850 to 1900. *Brit Med J* 1950; 1:57-60.

[151] Hewitt, 1896.

Chapter 4

[1] C. Koller. On the use of cocaine for producing anaesthesia on the eye. *Lancet* 1884; 2:990-92.

[2] J. Moore. *A Method of Preventing or Diminishing Pain in Several Operations of Surgery* (London: J. Cadell, 1784).

[3] D. Wilkinson. "The History of Trauma Anesthesia," in C. Grande, *Textbook of Trauma Anesthesia and Critical Care* (St. Louis: C. V. Mosby, 1993), p. 15.

[4] Physiological Society of London. Snow "On the Production of Local Anaesthesia." *Lancet* 1854; 1:448.

[5] B. W. Richardson. On a new and ready mode of producing local anesthesia. *Med Times Gaz* 1866; 1:115-17.

[6] C. Redard. X International Medical Congress, 1890; 5:14, abstract 71.

[7] H. Braun. *Local Anesthesia: Its Scientific Basis and Practice* (Philadelphia: Lea & Febiger, 1914), p. 51.

[8] Ibid., p. 52.

[9] S. O. Goldan. Anesthetization as a specialty: Its present and future. *Amer Med* 1901; 2:101-04.

[10] S. O. Goldan. Intraspinal cocainization for surgical anesthesia. *Phil Med J* 1900; 6:850-57.

[11] S. O. Goldan. Intraspinal cocainization from the anaesthetist's standpoint. *New York Med J* 1900; 72; 1089-91.

[12] *idem.*

[13] C. Van Dyke, R. Byck. Cocaine. *Sci Amer* 1982; 246:128-41.

[14] R. C. Petersen. "History of Cocaine," in National Institute on Drug Abuse Research Monograph Series No. 13 (Rockville, MD: Dept Health, Education and Welfare, Public Health Service, May 1977), p. 17.

[15] C. Singer, E. A. Underwood. *A Short History of Medicine* (Oxford: Clarendon Press, 1962), p. 349.

[16] J. Catalayud, A. Gonzalez. History of the development and evolution of local anesthesia since the coca leaf. *Anesthesiology* 2003; 98:1503-08.

[17] C. Van Dyke, P. Jatlow, J. Ungerer et al. Oral cocaine: Plasma concentrations and central effects. *Science* 1978; 200:211-13.

[18] A. Niemann. Ueber eine neue organische Base in den Cocablatten. *Arch Pharm* 1860; 153:129-55, 291-308.

[19] K. Courtney, G. Strichartz. "Structural Elements Which Determine Local Anesthetic Activity," in G. Strichartz (ed.), Local Anesthetics, in *Handbook of Experimental Pharmacology*, 1987, vol. 81, pp. 53-94. The activity of local anesthetic agents, like many other anesthetic agents, is influenced by their chemical structure. Those, including procaine, that replaced cocaine contains an ester linkage. Others, from lidocaine onward, contain an amide linkage and are stable since they are not readily metabolized and are safer.

[20] W. Lossen. Ueber das Cocain. *Ann Chem Pharm* 1865; 133:351-71.

[21] B. von Anrep. Ueber die physiologische Wirkung des Cocain. *E Pfluger Arch Ges Physiol* 1880; 21:38-77.

[22] T. Moreno y Maiz. Recherches chimiques et physiologiques sur l'erythroxylum coca de Perou at la cocaine. Ph. D. Thesis. (Paris: Louis Leclerc Libraire-Editeur, 1868), pp. 76-79.

[23] H. Davy. *Researches, Chemical and Philosophical; Chiefly Concerning Nitrous Oxide . . . .* (London: J. Johnson, 1800), p. 556.

[24] E. R. Palmer. Erythroxylon coca as an antidote to the opium habit. *Therap Gaz* 1880; 1:163-64.

[25] C. Koller. Historical notes on the beginnings of local anesthesia. *JAMA* 1928; 90:1742-43.

[26] Von Anrep, 1880.

[27] T. Aschenbrandt. Die physiologische Wirkung und Bedeutung des Cocain auf den Menschlichen organismus. *Dtsch Medizin Wchschr* 1883; 50:730-32. (Reprinted in R. Byck [ed.], *Cocaine Papers: Sigmund Freud* [New York: Stonehill Publishing Co., 1974]).

[28] S. Freud. Ueber Coca. *Zentrabl Gesamte Ther* 1884; 2:289-314.

[29] Koller, 1928.

[30] idem.

[31] Fink, 1985.

[32] C. Koller. *Bericht ueber die sechszehnte Versammlung der ophthalmologischen Gesellschaft* (Heidelberg, 1884).

[33] H. Noyes. The ophthalmological congress in Heidelberg. *New York Med J* 1884; 26:417-18.

[34] C. Koller. Ueber die Verwendung des Cocain zur Anasthesirung am Auge. *Wien Med Wschr* 1884; 34:1309-11.

[35] Fink, 1985.

36 *idem.*

37 J. S. Spillane. *Cocaine: From Medical Marvel to Modern Menace in the United States, 1884-1920* (Baltimore: Johns Hopkins University Press, 2000), title page and p. 7.

38 R. Ashley. *Cocaine: Its History, Uses and Effects* (New York: St Martin's Press, 1975), p. 18.

39 B. R. Fink. Leaves and needles: The introduction of surgical anesthesia. *Anesthesiology* 1985; 63:77-83.

40 R. Matas. Local and regional anesthesia: A retrospect and prospect. *Amer J Surg* 1934; 25:189-96.

41 Anon. Cocaine. *Brit Med J* 1979; 1:971-72.

42 J. Y. Simpson. Local anaesthesia, notes on its production by chloroform etc in the lower animals, and in man. *Lancet* 1848; 2:39-42.

43 H. Cushing. On the avoidance of shock in major amputations by cocainization of large nerve-trunks preliminary to their division. With observations on blood-pressure changes in surgical cases. *Ann Surg* 1902; 36:321.

44 W. Burke. Hydrochlorate of cocaine in minor surgery. *New York Med J* 1884; 40:616-17.

45 R. Hall. Hydrochlorate of cocaine. *New York Med J* 1884; 40:643-44.

46 W. Halsted. Practical comments on the use and abuse of cocaine; suggested by its invariably successful employment in more than a thousand minor surgical operations. *New York Med J* 1885; 42:294-95.

47 A. Winnie. "The Early History of Regional Anesthesia in the United States," in D. B. Scott, J. Wildsmith (eds.), *Regional Anesthesia 1884-1994* (Sodertalje, Sweden: Information Consulting Service, 1994), pp. 35-38.

48 J. L. Corning. Spinal anaesthesia and local medication of the cord. *New York Med J* 1885; 42:483-85.

49 D. Cotugno. *De Ischiade Nervosa Commentarius* (Neapoli: apud Fratres Simomios, 1764).

50 H. Quincke. Die Lumbalpuncture des Hydrocephalus. *Berl Klin Wchschr* 1891; 28:929-33.

51 W. E. Wynter. Four cases of tuberculous meningitis in which paracentesis of the theca vertebralis was performed. *Lancet* 1891; 1:981-82.

52 C. L. Schleich. A new method of local anaesthesia (infiltration anaesthesia). *Internat Clinics* (series 5) 1895; 2:177-92.

53 Bier, 1899.

54 L. D. Vandam. On the origins of intrathecal anesthesia. *Int Anesth Clin* 1989; 27:2-7.

55 M. Larson. Tait and Caglieri: The first spinal anesthetic in America. *Anesthesiology* 1996; 85; 915-99.

56 D. Tait, G. Caglieri. Experimental and clinical notes on the subarachnoid space. *JAMA* 1900; 35:6-10.

57 R. Matas. Intraspinal cocainization. *JAMA* 1899; 33:1659.

58 R. Matas. Local and regional anesthesia with cocain and other analgesic drugs, including the subarachnoid method, as applied in general surgical practice. *Phil Med J* 1900; 6:820-43.

59 T. Tuffier. Anesthesie medullaire chirurgicale par infection sous-arachnoidienne. *Sem Med* 1900; 20:167-68.

60 H. Cushing. Letter to W. Osler, August 23, 1918. In J. Fulton, *Harvey Cushing: A Biography* (Springfield: Charles C. Thomas, 1946), p. 142.

61 P. Reclus. Analgesie locale par la cocaine. *Rev Chir* 1889; 9:913.

62 G. de Takats. *Local Anesthesia: A Short Course for Students and Surgeons* (Philadelphia: W. B. Saunders Company, 1928). Cited by T. Keys, *The History of Surgical Anesthesia* (New York: Dover Publications, Inc., 1945), p. 42.

63 C. L. Schleich. Zur Infiltrationsanasthesie. *Therapeutisch Monathefte* 1884; 8:429.

64 Brown, Fink, 1998, p. 9.

65 J.-A. Sicard. Les injections medicamenteuses extradurales par voie sacroccygienne. *Compt Rend* 1901; 53:396-98.

66 F. Cathelin. Une nouvelle voie d'injection rachidienne. Methode des injections epidurals par le procede du canal sacre. Applications a l'homme. *Compt Rend* 1901; 53:452-53.

67 A. Bier. Ueber einen neuen Weg Localanasthesie an den Gliedmassen zu erzeugen. *Arch Klin Chir* 1908; 86:1007.

68 H. Braun. *Local Anesthesia: Its Scientific Basis and Practical Use* (Philadelphia: Lea& Febiger, 3rd edition, 1914).

69 Cushing, 1902.

70 H. T. Gray, L. Parsons. Blood pressure variations associated with lumbar puncture and the induction of spinal anaesthesia. *Quart J Med* 1912; 5:339.

71 G. S. Smith, W. T. Porter. Spinal anesthesia in the cat. *Am J Physiol* 1915; 38:108.

72 G. Labat. Circulatory disturbances associated with subarachnoid nerve block. *Long Island Med J* 1927; 21:573.

73 A. Barker. Clinical experiences with spinal analgesia in 100 cases and some reflections on the procedure. *Brit Med J* 1907; 1:665-74.

74 Vandam, 1989.

75 W. Babcock. Spinal anesthesia; with report of surgical clinics. *Surg Gynecol Obstet* 1912; 15:606-22.

76 Matas, 1934.

77 T. Jonnesco. Remarks on general spinal analgesia. *Brit Med J* 1909; 2:1396-1401.

78 H. Koster. Spinal anesthesia, with special reference to its use in surgery of the head, neck, and thorax. *Am J Surg* 1928; 5:554.

79 O. Kreis. Ueber Medullnarkose bei Gebarenden. *Zentrabl Gynakol* 1900; 24:724-29.

80 S. Marx. Analgesia in obstetrics produced by medullary injections of cocain. *Phil Med J* 1900; 6:857, 915.

81 Bier, 1898.

82 Tait, Caglieri, 1900.

83 J. V. Menendez, T. Burns, D. Bacon. Lincoln Fleetwood Sise: Regional anesthesia's forgotten man? *Reg Anesth Pain Med* 1999; 24:364-68.

[84] C. Burkle, R. Sands, D. Bacon. "Beyond Blocks: The History of the Development of Techniques in Regional Anesthesia," in P. Raj, *Textbook of Regional Anesthesia* (New York: Churchill Livingstone, 2002, p. 25.

[85] Menendez et al, 1999.

[86] W. T. Lemmon. A method for continuous spinal anesthesia: A preliminary report. *Ann Surg* 1940; 111:141-44.

[87] G. Labat. *Regional Anesthesia: Its Technic and Clinical Application* (Philadelphia: W. B. Saunders Company, 1922).

[88] A. Cote, C. Vachon, T. Horlocker et al. From Victor Pauchet to Gaston Labat: The transformation of regional anesthesia from a surgeon's practice to the physician anesthesiologist. *Anesth Analg* 2003; 96:1193-1200.

[89] B. Deschner, C. Robards, L. Somasundaram, W. Harrop-Griffiths. "The History of Local Anesthetics," in A. Hadzic (ed.), *Textbook of Regional Anesthesia and Acute Pain Management* (New York: McGraw Hill Medical, 2007), p. 15.

[90] B. Bamforth, K. Siebecker. "Ralph M. Waters," in P. P. Volpitto, L. D. Vandam (eds.), *The Genesis of Contemporary Anesthesiology* (Springfield: Charles C Thomas, 1982, pp. 51-68.

[91] J. Lundy. Balanced anesthesia. *Minn Med* 1926; 9:399-404.

[92] Brown, Fink, 1998, Appendix D.

[93] Ibid.

[94] Ibid.

[95] Ibid.

[96] Cathelin, 1901.

[97] Sicard, 1901.

[98] W. Stoeckel. Ueber sakrale Anasthesie. *Zentrabl Gynaekol* 1909; 33:1.

[99] W. Edwards, R. Hingson. Continuous caudal anesthesia in obstetrics. *Am J Surg* 1942; 57:549-64.

[100] W. Edwards, R. Hingson. Continuous caudal anesthesia: An analysis of the first ten thousand confinements thus managed with the report of authors' first thousand cases. *JAMA* 1943; 123:538-46.

[101] S. A. Manalan. Caudal block anesthesia in obstetrics. *J Indiana State Med Assoc* 1942; 35:564.

[102] A. Lawen. Ueber die Verwertung der Sakralanasthesie fur chirurgisch Operationen. *Zentrabl Chir* 1910; 37:708.

[103] F. Pages. Anestesia metamerica. *Rev San Milit Argen* 1921; 11:351-56.

[104] A. M. Dogliotti. Eine neue Methode der regionaren Anasthesie. *Zentrabl Chir* 1931; 58:3141-45.

[105] E. Aburel. L'anesthesie locale continue (prolongee) en obstetrique. *Bull Soc Obstet Gynecol* 1931; 20:35.

[106] P. C. Lund. *Peridural Analgesia and Anesthesia* (Springfield: Charles C Thomas, 1966), pp. 3-10.

[107] R. de Jong. *Local Anesthetics* (St Louis: Mosby, 1994), p. 7.

[108] Brown, Fink, 1998.

[109] T. Gordh. Anesthesiology Topics/January-February 1986. Karolinska Hospital, Stockholm.

[110] N. Lofgren. *Studies on Local Anaesthetics. Xylocaine: A New Synthetic Drug* (Stockholm: Hoeggstroms, 1948).

[111] Vandam, 1989.

Chapter 5

[1] G. Edwards. Frederic William Hewitt (1857-1916). *Ann Roy Coll Surg Engl* 1951; 8:233-45.

[2] S. Meltzer, J. Auer. Continuous respiration without respiratory movements. *J Exp Med* 1909; 11:622-25.

[3] A. G. Levy. Sudden death under light chloroform anaesthesia. *J Physiol* 1911; 42: iii-iv.

[4] H. Cushing. On routine determination of arterial tensions in operating-room and clinic. *Boston Med Surg J* 1903; 148:250-56.

[5] I. Magill. Endotracheal anaesthesia. *Proc Roy Soc Med* 1928; 22:83-88.

[6] J. Liebenau. *Medical Science and Medical Industry: The Formation of the American Pharmaceutical Industry* (Baltimore: Johns Hopkins University Press, 1987)

[7] E. Pellegrino. "The Sociocultural Impact of Twentieth-century Therapeutics," in M. Vogel, C. Rosenberg (eds.), *The Therapeutic Revolution: Essays in the Social History of American Medicine* (Philadelphia: University of Pennsylvania Press, 1979), p. 248.

[8] T. Nunneley. On anesthesia and anaesthetic substances generally; being an experimental inquiry into their nature, properties, and action, their comparative value and danger, and the best means of counteracting the effects of an over dose. *Trans Prov Med Surg Ass Lond* 1849; 16:228-30, 330-31.

[9] T. Keys. *The History of Surgical Anesthesia* (New York: Dover Publications, Inc., 1963), p. 49.

[10] W. Crocker, L. Knight. Effect of illuminating gas and ethylene on flowering carnations. *Bot Gaz* 1908; 46; 259-76.

[11] A. Luckhardt, R. Thompson. "Ethylene Anesthesia," in J. T. Gwathmey, *Anesthesia* (New York: Macmillan Company, 2nd ed., 1924), pp. 711-31.

[12] A. Luckhardt, J. Carter. Ethylene as a gas anesthetic: Preliminary communication. *JAMA* 1923; 80; 1440-42.

[13] I. Herb. Ethylene: Notes taken from the clinical records. *Anesth Analg* 1923; 2:230-32.

[14] J. Cotton. Anesthesia from commercial ether-administration and what it is due to. *Can Med Ass J* 1917; 7; 769-77.

[15] W. E. Brown. Preliminary report: Experiments with ethylene as a general anesthetic. *Can Med Ass J* 1923; 13:210.

[16] A. Luckhardt. An adventure in research. *Bull Conn State Dent Ass* 1944 (May); 46-56.

[17] J. Snow. *On Chloroform and Other Anaesthetics: Their Action and Administration* (London: John Churchill, 1958), pp. 408-16.

[18] J. Lundy. *Clinical Anesthesia* (Philadelphia: W. B. Saunders Company, 1942), p 714.

[19] L. Hewer. Trichlorethylene as a general analgesic and anaesthetic. *Brit J Anaesth* 1923; 1:27-29.

[20] A. Freund. Ueber trimetylen. *Monatshafte f. Chimie* 1882; 3:625-35.

[21] W. E. Brown. Experiments with anesthetic gases, propylene, methane, dimethyl ether. *J Pharmacol Expet Ther* 1924; 23:485-96.

[22] G. Lucas, V. Henderson. A new anesthetic gas: Cyclopropane; A preliminary report. *Can Med Ass J* 1929; 21:173-75.

[23] V. Henderson, G. Lucas. Cyclopropane: A new anesthetic. *Anesth Analg* 1930; 9:1-6.

[24] G. Lucas. The discovery and pharmacology of cyclopropane. *Can Anaesth Soc J* 1960; 7:237-56.

[25] R. Waters. Letter to V. Henderson, Aug. 20, 1930. Cited by Lucas, 1960.

[26] M. Seevers, W. Meek, E. Rovenstine, J. Stiles. A study of cyclopropane anesthesia with especial reference to gas concentrations, respiratory and electrocardiographic changes. *J Pharmacol Exper Ther* 1934; 51:1-17.

[27] J. Stiles, W. Neff, E. Rovenstine, R. Waters. Cyclopropane as an anesthetic agent: A preliminary report. *Anesth Analg* 1934; 13:56-60.

[28] B. Sword. The closed circle method of administration of gas anesthesia. *Anesth Analg* 1930; 9:198-202.

[29] R. Waters, E. Schmidt. Cyclopropane anesthesia. *JAMA* 1934; 103:975-83.

[30] C. Leake. "Introductory Essay," in T. Keys, *The History of Surgical Anesthesia* (New York: Dover Publications, Inc., 1963), pp. xxv-xxvi.

[31] A. Faulconer, T. Keys. *Foundations of Anesthesiology* (Park Ridge: Wood Library-Museum of Anesthesiology, 1993), vol. 1, p. 573. (German source: F. Semmler, *Ann Chimie [Liebig's]*, 1867; 241:90-116.)

[32] R. Major, R. Ruigh. The preparation and properties of pure divinyl ether. *J Amer Chem Soc* 1931; 53:2662-71.

[33] C. Leake, M. Y. Chen. The anesthetic properties of certain unsaturated ethers. *Proc Soc Exper Med Biol* 1930; 28:151-54.

[34] S. Gelfan, I. Bell. The anesthetic action of divinyl oxide in humans. *J Pharmacol Exper Ther* 1933; 47:1-3.

[35] C. Leake, P. Knoefel, A. Guedel. The anesthetic action of divinyl oxide in animals. *J Pharmacol Exper Ther* 1933; 47:5-16.

[36] Faulconer, Keys, 1993. p. 582. (German source: E. Fischer. *Jena Z. Med Naturw* 1864; 1:123.)

[37] W. Plessner. Diseases of the trigeminal nerve following poisoning with trichloroethylene. *Berliner Klin Wchschr* 1916; 53:25.

[38] H. Gerbis. Irreparable facial paralysis in industrial poisoning. *Zentralblatt f. Gewerbehyg* 1928; 16:97-101.

[39] K. Roholm. Trichlorethylene intoxication in industry. *Ugeskrift for Laeger* (Copenhagen) 1933; 95:1185. Abstract: *JAMA* 1933, Dec.23.

[40] K. Stuber. Injuries to health in industrial use of trichloroethylene and possibility of their prevention. *Arch f. Gewerbepath u. Gewerbehyg* 1931:2:398.

[41] T. Christiansen. Clinical contributions to trichloroethylene intoxication. *Ugeskrift for Laeger* (Copenhagen) 1933; 95:1187. Abstract: *JAMA* 1933, Dec.23.

[42] Oppenheim, cited by D. Jackson. Tic douloureux—its etiology and character. *Arch Int Pharmacodynamie et Therapie* 1934; 48, fasc.2:129.

[43] Oppenheim, cited by D. Jackson. Observations concerning the etiology and nature of trigeminal neuralgia(tic doulereux).*J Med* 1934; 15:127-29.

[44] I. Olenjeck. Trichlorethylene treatment of trigeminal neuralgia. *JAMA* 1928; 91:1085-87.

[45] M. Glaser. Treatment of trigeminal neuralgia with trichloroethylene. *JAMA* 1931; 96:916-20.

[46] K. Lehmann. Experimentelle Studien ueber den Einfluss technisch und hygienisch wichtiger Gase und Dampfe auf den Organismus . . . . *Arch Hyg Munch Berlin* 1911; 74:1-60.

[47] C. Striker, S. Goldblatt, I. Warm, D. Jackson. Clinical experiences with the of trichloroethylene in the production of over 300 analgesias and anesthesias. *Anesth Analg* 1935; 14:68-71.

[48] C.L. Hewer, C. Hadfield. Trichloroethylene as an inhalation anesthetic. *Brit Med J* 1941; 1:924-27.

[49] J. Lundy. Balanced anesthesia. *Minn Med* 1936; 9:399-404.

[50] W. Harvey. *An Anatomical Disputation Concerning the Movement of the Heart and Blood in Living Creatures* [1628]. Translated with an introduction and notes by G. Whitteridge (Oxford: Blackwell Scientific Publications, 1976).

[51] C. Wren. An account of the rise and attempts, of a way to coneigh liquors into the mass of blood. *Phil Trans Roy Soc Lond* 1665; 1:129-30.

[52] E. Lowenstein. The birth of opioid anesthesia. *Anesthesiology* 2004; 100:1013-15.

[53] J. S. Elsholtz. *Clysmatica Nova* (Berlin: D. Reichel, 1665).

[54] J. Major. *Chirurgia Infusoria* (Kiel:1667).

[55] T. Boulton. "The Development of the Syringe," in A. Barr, T. Boulton, D. Wilkinson (eds.), *Essays on the History of Anaesthesia* (London: Royal Society of Medicine Press, 1996), pp. 79-84.

[56] L. Pasteur. Memoires sur les corpuscles organisees qui existent dans l'atmosphere. Examen de la doctrine des generations spontanees. *Ann Chim Phys* 1862; 64:5-110.

[57] J. Lister. On the antiseptic principle in the practice of surgery. *Lancet* 1867; 2:353-56, 668-69.

[58] N. Pirogoff. *Recherches Pratiques et physiologiques sur l'etherisation* (St Petersbourg: F. Bellizard & Cie, 1847).

[59] N. Pirogoff. Nouveau procede pour produire, au moyen de la vapeur d'ether, l'insensibilite chez les soumis a des operations chirurgicals. *Compt rend hebdom Acad*

Sci 1847; 24:789. See also A. Faulconer, T. Keys, *Foundations of Anesthesiology* (Park Ridge: Wood Library-Museum of Anesthesiology, 1993), vol. 2, p. 726.

[60] J. Gwathmey. The story of oil-ether colonic anesthesia. anesthesia. *Anesthesiology* 1942; 3:171-75.

[61] P.-C. Ore. Des injections intra-veineuses de chloral. *Bull Soc Chir* (Paris) 1872; 1:400-12.

[62] Ore, 1872.

[63] P.-C. Ore. De l'anesthesie produite chez l'homme par les injections de chloral dans les veines. *Compt Rend Hebdom Acad Sci* 1874; 78:515-17.

[64] W. Babcock. A new method of surgical anesthesia. *Proc Phila County Med Soc* 1905; 26:347-57.

[65] O. Schmiedeberg. Ueber die pharmakologischem Wirkungen und die therapeutische Anwendung einiger Carbaminsaure-Ester. *Arch Exp Pathol Pharmakol* 1885-1886; 20:203-16.

[66] R. C. Adams. *Intravenous Anesthesia* (New York: Paul B. Hoeber, 1944), p. 2.

[67] N. Krakow. On hedonal-chloroform anesthesia. *Russ Vrach* 1903; 2:1697-1703.

[68] S. Fedoroff. *Russ Med Rund* 1911; 8:457-61.

[69] A. Jeremitsch. Die intravenose Hedonalnarkose. *Deutsche Zeitschr Chirurg* 1911; 108:551-63.

[70] Kissin, Wright, 1988.

[71] C. Page. Hedonal as a general anaesthetic administered by intravenous infusion: A report on 75 cases. *Brit Med J* 1912; 1:1258-64.

[72] H. Noel, H. Souttar. The anaesthetic effects of the intravenous injection of paraldehyde. *Ann Surg* 1913; 57:64-67.

[73] C. Peck, S. Meltzer. Anesthesia in human beings by intravenous injection of magnesium sulphate. *JAMA* 1916; 67:1131-33.

[74] K. Naragawa. Experimentelle studien ueber die intraveose infusionsnarkose mittels alcohols. *J Exp Med* 1921; 2:81-126.

[75] M. Kirschner. Eine psycheschonende und steuerbaure Form der Allgemeinbetaubung. *Der Chirurg* 1929; 1:673-82.

[76] D. Davis. "The Collapse and Resuscitation of Intravenous Anesthesia," in J. Artusio (ed.), *Clinical Anesthesia* (Philadelphia: F. A. Davis, 1968), p. 78.

[77] E. Pellegrino. "The Sociocultural Impact of Twentieth-Century Therapeutics," in M. Vogel, C. Rosenberg (eds.), *The Therapeutic Revolution: Essays in the Social History of American Medicine* (Philadelphia: University of Pennsylvania Press, 1979), p. 248.

[78] E. Fischer, J. von Mering. Ueber eine neue Klasse von Schlafmitteln. *Die Therapie der Gegenwert* 1903; 44:97-107.

[79] D. Bardet. Sur l'utilisation, comme anesthesique general, d'un produit nouveau, le diethyl-diallyl-barbiturate de diethylamine. *Bull Gen Ther Med Chir Obstet Pharm* 1921; 172:27-33.

[80] R. Bumm. Intravenose narkosen mit barbitursaure-derivaten. *Klin Wchschr* 1927; 6:725-26.

[81] L. Zerfas, J. McCallum, H. Shonle et al. Induction of anesthesia in man by intravenous injection of sodium iso-amyl-ethyl barbiturate. *Proc Soc Exper Biol Med* 1929; 26:399-403.

[82] R. Fitch, R. Waters, A. Tatum. Barbituric acid hypnotics in surgery. *Amer J Surg* 1930; 9:110-14.

[83] J. Lundy. Experience with sodium ethyl (1-methylbutyl) barbiturate (Nembutal) in more than 2, 300 cases. *Surg Clin N Amer* 1931; 11; 905-15.

[84] Fitch et al., 1930.

[85] H. Weese, W. Scharpff. Evipan, ein neuartiges einschlaffmittel. *Deutsch Med Wchschr* 1932; 58:1205-07.

[86] D. Tabern, E. Volweiler. The development of the thiobarbiturates. *J Am Chem Soc* 1935; 57:1961-63.

[87] T. Pratt, A. Tatum, H. Hathaway, R. Waters. Sodium ethyl (1-methyl butyl) thiobarbiturate. *Am J Surg* 1936; 31:464-66.

[88] J. Lundy, R. Tovell. Some of the newer local and general anesthetic agents. Methods of their administration. *Northwest Med* (Seattle) 1934; 33:308-11.

[89] J. Lundy, R. Tovell. Annual report for 1934 of the Section of Anesthesia: Including data on blood transfusion. *Proc Staff Meet Mayo Clin* 1935 (April 24):257-71.

[90] J. Lundy. Intravenous anesthesia: preliminary report of the use of two new thiobarbiturates. *Proc Staff Meet Mayo Clin* 1935; 10:536-43.

[91] J. Dundee. Fifty years of thiopentone. *Brit J Anaesth* 1984; 56:211-13.

[92] R. C. Adams, H. Gray. Intravenous anesthesia with pentothal sodium in the case of gunshot wound associated with accompanying severe traumatic shock and loss of blood: report of a case. *Anesthesiology* 1943; 4:70-71.

[93] F. Halford. A critique of intravenous anesthesia in war surgery. *Anesthesiology* 1943; 4:67-69.

[94] Editorial. The question of intravenous anesthesia in war surgery. *Anesthesiology* 1943; 4:71-77.

[95] T. de Quincey. The Confessions of an English opium-eater. *London Magazine* 1821, Oct.-Nov.

[96] The year in which Serturner isolated morphine has been given as 1803, 1804, and 1806. 1804 is the date given by A. Faulconer and T. Keys in *Foundations of Anesthesiology* (Springfield: Charles C Thomas, 1993), vol. 2, p. 1078.

[97] G. Wedel. *Opiologia, ad Mentem Academiae Naturae Curiosum* (Jena, 1682), pp. 129-30.

[98] J. Douglas. *Cheselden's Method of Performing the Lateral Operation for Stone* (London, 1731), p. 35.

[99] J. Clover. Remarks on the production of sleep during surgical operations. *Brit Med J* 1874; 2:74-75.

[100] A. Dogliotti. *Anesthesia: Narcosis, Local, Regional, Spinal* (Chicago: S. B. Debour, 1939), p. 20.

[101] C. Bernard. Des effets physiologiques de la morphine et de leur combinaison avec ceux du chloroform. *Bull Gen de Therapeutique Med et Chirurg* 1869; 77:241-56. Cited by Faulconer, Keys, 1993, p. 1089.

102 Anon. Hypodermic injections supplementary to chloroformising [on J. von Nussbaum's technique]. *Med Times Lond* 1864; 1:259.

103 C. Uterhart. Mittheilungen aus der chirurgischen Klinik der Rostocker Krankenhauses (Communication from the surgical clinic of the Rostock Hospital). *Berliner Klin Wchschr* 1868; 5:329-30.

104 L. Labbe, E. Guyon. Sur l'action combine de la morphine et du chloroforme (Note). *Compt Rendus Acad Sci Paris* 1872; 74:627-29.

105 Pitha, 1861. Cited by B. Duncum, *The Development of Inhalation Anaesthesia: With Special Reference to the Years 1846-1900* (London: Wellcome Historical Medical Museum and Oxford University Press, 1947), p. 377.

106 B. Bell. The therapeutic relations of opium and belladonna. *Edin Med J* 1858-1859 (n. s.); 4:1-7.

107 C. Brown-Sequard. Sur l'importance de l'emploi simultane de la morphine et de l'atropine . . . . *Compt Rend Acad Sci Biol* Paris 1883; 5:289.

108 W. Munro. On watching the pulse during the administration of chloroform. *Brit Med J* 1880; 2:240, 761.

109 A. Dastre. Sur un procede d'anesthesie. *Compt Rend Soc Biol* 1883; 7. s., v, 259-63.

110 Duncum, 1947, pp. 397-98.

111 P. Aubert. Anesthesies mixtes par la morphine; l'atropine et le chloroforme. *Compt Rend Soc Biol Paris* 1883; 5:626-32.

112 Liverpool Medical Institution, Report of Society Meeting, Nov. 11, 1906 [citing W. Fingland]. *Lancet* 1906; 2:1514.

113 D. Buxton. Treatment of shock during anesthesia. *Proc Roy Soc Med* 1908-09; ii, Sect. Anaesth., 55-70.

114 B. Gardner, 1912. Cited by Duncum, 1947, p. 401.

115 J. Schneiderlin. Eine neue narkose. *Aertz Mitth a Baden* 1900; 54:104. Cited by B. Duncum, 1947, p. 402.

116 Cited by Duncum, 1947, p. 402.

117 Hocheisen. Geburten mit Skopolamin-Morphium. *Munch med Wchschr* 1906; 53:1801, 1872.

118 O. Bass. Hundertundsieben Geburten in Skopolamin-Morphin-Halbnarkose. *Munch med Wchschr* 1907; 54:519-24.

119 R. Smith. Scopolamine-morphine anesthesia. *Surg Gynecol Obst* 1908; 7:424-20.

120 Beckett, Wright, 1875.

121 O. Eisleb, O. Schaumann. Dolantin, ein neuartiges Spasmolyticum und Analgetikum . . . . *Deutsch Med Wchschr* 1939; 65:967-68.

122 R. Waters. The evolution of anesthesia. I, *Proc Staff Meet Mayo Clin* 1942; 17:428-40.

123 H. Beecher, D. Todd. A study of the deaths associated with anesthesia and surgery, *Ann Surg* 1954; 140:2-34.

124 A fine account of the work of those individuals, and, indeed of the history of the transmission of impulses at the neuromuscular junction is that of W. Maxwell Cowan and Eric Kandel ("A Brief History of Synapses and Synaptic Transmission") in the

text edited by W. M. Cowan, T. Sudhof, C. Stevens, and K. Davies titled *Synapses* (Baltimore: Johns Hopkins University Press, 2001), pp. 1-87.

[125] The literature on curare is extensive. Useful texts are the following: R. Gill, *White Water and Black Magic* (New York: Doubleday, 1940); A. McIntyre, *Curare. Its History, Nature and Clinical Use* (Chicago: University of Chicago Press, 1947); L. Stevenson, *The Meaning of Poison* (Lawrence: University of Kansas Press, 1959); K. B. Thomas, *Curare. Its History and Usage* (London: Pitman, 1964); and P. Smith, *Arrows of Mercy* (New York: Doubleday, 1969).

[126] B. Brodie. Letter to P. Flourens, 1811. Cited by Armstrong Davison, *The Evolution of Anaesthesia* (Baltimore: Williams and Wilkins Company, 1965), p. 156.

[127] H. Griffith, E. Johnson. The use of curare in general anesthesia. *Anesthesiology* 1942; 3:418-20.

[128] E.-F.-A. Vulpian. De l'emploi du curare comme antidote de la strychnine, et comme traitement du tetanus. *L'Union Medicale* 1857; 11:25-26.

[129] L. Sayres, F. Burrall. Two cases of traumatic tetanus. *New York J Med* 1858; 4:250-53.

[130] A. Bennett. Preventing traumatic complications in convulsive shock therapy by curare. *JAMA* 1940; 114:322-24.

[131] P. M. d'Anghiera. *De Rebus Oceanicis et Novo Orbo* (New York: G. P. Putnam's Sons, 1912 [transl. P. MacNutt]). See also Faulconer and Keys, 1993, pp. 1135-36.

[132] J. Carman. History of curare. *Anaesthesia* 1968; 23:706-07.

[133] C. M. de la Condamine. Relation abregee d'un voyage fait dans l'interieur de l'Amerique Meridionale. *Memoires de l'Academie des Sciences* 1745; 62:391.

[134] F. Fontana. Traite sur le venin de la vipere sue les poisons americains. *Philos Trans* 1780-1781; 70:34.

[135] R. Schomburgk. On the Urari, the arrow poison of the Indians of Guiana. *Ann & Mag Nat Hist* 1841; 7:407-27.

[136] A. von Humboldt. *Voyage de Humboldt et Bonpland, Premiere Partie. Relation Historique* (Paris: N. Maze, 1819), tome II, p. 554.

[137] E. Bancroft. *Essay on the Natural History of Guiana and South America*, 1769, p. 281.

[138] B. Brodie. Experiments on the different modes in which death is produced by certain vegetable poisons. *Philos Trans* 1811; 101:194-205.

[139] B. Brodie. Further experiments and observations on the actions of poisons on the animal system. *Philos Trans* 1812; 102:205-27.

[140] R. Maltby. Charles Waterton (1782-1865): Curare and a Canadian national park. *Can Anaesth Soc J* 1982; 29:195-202.

[141] W. Smith. Waterton and Wourali. *Brit J Anaesth* 1983; 55:221-25.

[142] R. Irwin (ed.). *Letters of Charles Waterton* (London: Rockcliffe, 1955).

[143] Smith, 1983.

[144] Maltby, 1982.

[145] C. Bernard. *An Introduction to the Study of Experimental Medicine* (New York: Dover Publications, 1957 (transl. H. Greene]). Cited by J. Olmsted, E. Olmsted, *Claude*

Bernard and the Experimental Method in Medicine (New York: Collier Books, 1953), p. 77.

[146] A. McIntyre. Historical background, early use and development of muscle relaxants. *Anesthesiology* 1959; 20:409-16.

[147] C. Bernard. *Lecons sur les Effets des Substances Toxiques et Medicamenteuses* (Paris: J. B. Bailliere et Fils, 1857), pp. 311-25.

[148] C. Bernard. Etudes physiologiques sue quelques poisons americains. *Revue des deux mondes* 1864; 53:164-90.

[149] Bernard, 1857.

[150] Ibid.

[151] Bernard, 1864.

[152] Vulpian, 1857.

[153] M. Rouget. Note sur la termination des nerfs moteurs dans les muscles chez les reptiles, les oiseaux et les mammiferes. *J de la Physiol de l'Homme* (Paris) 1862; 11:25-26.

[154] Cited by A. Heeter, *Handbuch der Experimentellen Pharmakologie* (Berlin: Julius Springer, 1920).

[155] A. Lawen. Ueber die Verbindung der Lokalanesthesie mit der Narkose, ueber hohe Extraduralanesthesie und epidurale Injektionen anesthesierender Losungen bei tabischen Magenkrisen. *Beit z Klin Chir* 1912; 80:168-69.

[156] D. Wilkinson. Dr F. P. de Caux—the first user of curare for anaesthesia in England. *Anaesthesia* 1991; 46:49-51.

[157] Dale, 1914.

[158] Cowan, Kandel, 2001, p. 24.

[159] H. Dale. Clinical transmission of the effects of nerve impulses. *Brit Med J* 1934; 1:835-41.

[160] J. Aeschlimann, M. Reinert. The pharmacological action of some analogues of physostigmine. *J Pharmacol* 1931; 43:413-444.

[161] R. West. Curare in man. *Proc Roy Soc Med* 1932; 25:1107-16.

[162] L. Cole. Tetanus treated with curare. *Lancet* 1934; 2:475-77.

[163] H. King. Curare alkaloids. Part I. *J Chem Soc Lond* 1935; part 2:1381-89.

[164] M. Burman. Therapeutic use of curare and erythroidine hydrochloride for spastic and dystonic states. *Arch Neurol Psychiat* 1939; 41:307-27.

[165] A. Bennett. Preventing traumatic complications in convulsive shock therapy by curare. *JAMA* 1940; 114:332-24.

[166] A. Bennett. How Indian arrow poison curare became a useful drug. *Anesthesiology* 1967; 28:446-52.

[167] McIntyre, 1947.

[168] O. Wintersteiner, J. Dutcher. Curare alkaloids from *Chondrodendron tomentosum*. *Science* 1943; 97:467-79.

[169] R. Hughes. "Neuromuscular Blocking Agents," in R. Atkinson, T. Boulton (eds.), *The History of Anaesthesia* (London: Royal Society of Medicine Services, 1989), p. 264.

[170] Ibid.

[171] A. Bennett. The history of the introduction of curare into medicine. *Anesth Analg* 1968; 47:484-92.

[172] Ibid.

[173] A. Betcher. The civilizing of curare: A history of its development and introduction into anesthesiology. *Anesth Analg* 1977; 56:305-19.

[174] Griffith, Johnson, 1942.

[175] Ibsen, 1954.

[176] Meltzer, Auer, 1909.

[177] C. Jackson. The technique of insertion of intratracheal insufflation tubes. *Surg Gynecol Obst* 1913; 17:507-09.

[178] Y. Henderson. A lecture on respiration in anesthesia: Control by carbon dioxide. *Brit Med J* 1925; 2:1170-75.

[179] W. Einthoven. Die galvanometrische registrirung des menschlichen capillary-elektrometers in der physiologie. *Arch Ges Physiol* 1903; 99:472-80.

[180] Levy, 1911.

Chapter 6

[1] J. Lister. On a new method of treating compound fracture, abscess, etc., with observations on the condition of suppuration. *Lancet* 1867; 1:326-29, 357-59, 507-09; 2:95-96.

[2] F. Sibson. On the treatment of facial neuralgia by the inhalation of ether, and on a new inhaler. *Lond Med Gaz* 1847; 39:358-64.

[3] J. Snow. *On Chloroform and Other Anaesthetics: Their Action and Administration* (London: John Churchill, 1858), p. 280.

[4] J. Snow. *On the Inhalation of the Vapour of Ether . . .* (London: John Churchill, 1847), p. 21.

[5] J. Heiberg. A new expedient in administering chloroform. *Med Times Gaz* 1874; 36.

[6] B. Howard. Observations on the upper air passages in the anaesthetic state. *Lancet* 1880; 1:796-8.

[7] Cited by B. Duncum, *The Development of Inhalation Anaesthesia With Special Reference to the Years 1846-1900* (London: Wellcome Historical Medical Museum, Oxford University Press, 1947), p. 285.

[8] Duncum, 1947, p. 285.

[9] Ibid., p. 287.

[10] J. Snow. On narcotism by the inhalation of vapours. XV, XVI, *Lond Med Gaz* 1850; 11 (n. s.); 749-54, and 1851; 12 (n. s.):622-27.

[11] Duncum, 1947, p. 491.

[12] J. O'Dwyer. Intubation of larynx. *New York Med J* 1885; 42:145-47.

[13] G. Fell. Forced respiration in opium poisoning—its possibilities, and the apparatus best adapted to produce it. *Buffalo Med Surg J* 1887; 28:146-57.

[14] R. Matas. On the management of acute traumatic pneumothorax. *New York Med J* 1899; 29:409-34.

[15] F. Hewitt. An artificial 'air-way' for use during anaesthetization. *Lancet* 1908; 1:490-91.

[16] F. Hewitt. Clinical observations upon respiration during anaesthesia. *Proc Roy Med Chir Soc* 1891; 3:31-38.

[17] C. Ball, R. Westhorpe. Clearing the airway—the development of the pharyngeal airway. *Anaesth Intens Care* 1997; 25:451.

[18] A. Guedel. A non traumatic pharyngeal airway. *JAMA* 1933; 100:1862.

[19] L. Brandt. The first reported oral intubation in the human trachea. *Anesth* Analg 1987; 66:1198-99.

[20] Andreas Vesalius. *De Humani Corporis Fabrica* (Libri Septem) (Basel [1543], 1555), pp. 255, 708.

[21] C. Kite. *An Essay on the Recovery of the Apparently Dead* (London: Dilly, 1788).

[22] J. Herholdt, C. Rafn. *An Attempt at an Historical Survey of Life-saving Measures for Drowning Persons and Information of the Best Means by Which They Can Again be Brought Back to Life* (Copenhagen: Tikioby, 1796), 1-88.

[23] W. Macewen. Clinical observations on the introduction of tracheal tubes by the mouth instead of performing tracheotomy or laryngotomy. *Brit Med J* 1880; 1:163-65.

[24] R. Waters. Endotracheal anesthesia and its historical development. *Anesth Analg* 1933; 12:196-203.

[25] J. Snow, 1858, p. 117.

[26] F. Trendelenburg. Tamponade de Trachea. *Arch Klin Chir* 1871; 12; 121.

[27] Macewen, 1880, pp. 122-24.

[28] R. Matas. On the management of acute traumatic pneumothorax. *Ann Surg* 1899; 29:409-34.

[29] P. J. Koltai, R. E. Nixon. The story of the laryngoscope. *Ear, Nose and Throat J* 1989; 68:494-502.

[30] M. Mackenzie. *The Use of the Laryngoscope in Diseases of the Throat: With an Appendix on Rhinoscopy* (London: Robert Hardwicke, 1866), p. 3.

[31] Ibid., p. 6.

[32] Ibid., p. 9.

[33] B. G. Babington. The glottiscope. *Lond Med Gaz* 1829; 3:555.

[34] Mackenzie, 1866, p. 13.

[35] M. Garcia. *Physiological Observations of the Human Voice.* (London: Royal Society of London, 1855).

[36] Mackenzie, 1866, p. 28.

[37] Ibid., p. 28.

[38] W. S. Sykes. *Essays on the First Hundred Years of Anaesthesia* (Edinburgh: E. & S. Livingstone, 1961), vol. II, p. 97.

[39] N. P. Hirsch, G. Smith, P. Hirsch. Alfred Kirstein: Pioneer of direct laryngoscopy. *Anaesthesia* 1986; 41:42-45.

[40] A. Kirstein. Direct laryngoscopy. *Lancet* 1895; 1:1132.

[41] S. Zeitels. Chevalier Jackson's contributions to direct laryngoscopy. *Journal of Voice* 1998; 12:1-6.

[42] Ibid.

[43] Koltai, Nixon, 1989.

[44] C. Jackson. The technique of insertion of intratracheal insufflation tubes. *Surg Gynecol Obstet* 1913; 17:507-09.

[45] H. Janeway. Intra-tracheal anesthesia from the standpoint of the nose, throat and oral surgeon with a description of a new instrument for catheterizing the trachea. *Laryngoscope* 1913; 23:1082-90.

[46] N. Gillespie. *Endotracheal Anaesthesia* (Madison: University of Wisconsin Press, 1941), p. 20.

[47] S. Meltzer, J. Auer. Continuous respiration without respiratory movements. *J Exper Med* 1909; 11:622-25.

[48] Gillespie, 1941, p. 21.

[49] R. Waters. Clinical scope and utility of carbon dioxide filtration in inhalation anesthesia. *Anesth Analg* 1924; 3; 20-2.

[50] D. Jackson. A new method for the production of general analgesia and anaesthesia with a description of the apparatus used. *J Lab Clin Med* 1915; 1:1-12.

[51] A. Guedel, R. Waters. A new intra-tracheal catheter. *Anesth Analg* 1928; 7:238-39.

[52] V. Eisenmenger. *Wien Med Wschr* 1893; 43:199. (Duncum, 1947, p. 611.)

[53] B. Sword. The closed circle method of administration of gas anesthesia. *Anes Analg* 1930; 9:198-202.

[54] C. Burkle, F. Zepeda, D. Bacon. A historical perspective on the use of the laryngoscope as a tool in anesthesiology. *Anesthesiology* 2004; 100:1003-06.

[55] R. Waters, E. Schmidt. Cyclopropane anesthesia. *JAMA* 1934; 103:975-83.

[56] W. Mushin, L. Rendell-Baker, P. Thompson et al. *Automatic Ventilation of the Lungs* (Oxford: Blackwell Scientific Publications, 3rd edition, 1980), p. 16.

[57] Ibid., p. 16.

[58] H. Griffith, E. Johnson. The use of curare in general anesthesia. *Anesthesiology* 1942; 3:418-20.

[59] S. Thesleff, O. van Dardel, F. Holmberg. Succinylcholine iodide: New muscle relaxant. *Brit J Anaesth* 1952; 24:238-44.

[60] S. Cooper. "The Evolution of Upper-Airway Retraction: New and Old Laryngoscopy Blades," in J. Benumof (ed.). *Airway Management: Principles and Practice* (St Louis: Mosby, 1996), p. 377.

[61] Ibid.

[62] J. Lundy. *Clinical Anesthesia: A Manual of Clinical Anesthesiology* (Philadelphia: W. B. Saunders Company, 1942), p 287.

[63] R. Miller. A new laryngoscope. *Anesthesiology* 1941; 2:317-20.

[64] W. Cassels. Advantages of a curved laryngoscope. *Anesthesiology* 1942; 3:580.

[65] R. Macintosh. A new laryngoscope. *Lancet* 1943; 1:205.

[66] R. Macintosh. A new laryngoscope. *Lancet* 1943; 1:205.

[67] E. Siker. A mirror laryngoscope. *Anesthesiology* 1956; 17:38-42.

[68] J. Huffman, J. Elam. Prisms and fiber optics for laryngoscopy. *Anesth Analg* 1971; 50:64-67.

[69] C. Bellhouse. An angulated laryngoscope for routine and difficult tracheal intubation. *Anesthesiology* 1988; 69:126-29.

[70] M. Gorback. Management of the challenging airway with the Bullard laryngoscope. *J Clin Anesth* 1991; 3:473-77.

[71] R. Carr, K. Belani. Clinical assessment of the Augustine guide for endotracheal intubation. *Anesth Analg* 1994; 78:983-87.

[72] J. Tyndall. On some phenomena connected with the motion of liquids. *Proc Roy Inst Great Britain 1*, 1854:446-48.

[73] H. Hopkins, N. Karpany. A flexible fiberscope using static scanning. *Nature* 1954; 173:39-41.

[74] B. Hirschowitz, L. Curtiss, C. Peters et al. Demonstration of a new gastroscope, the fiberscope. *Gastroenterology* 1958; 35:50-53.

[75] P. Murphy. A fibre-optic endoscope used for nasal intubation. *Anaesthesia* 1967; 22:489-91.

[76] A. Ovassapian, S. Yelich, M. Dykes et al. Fiberoptic nasotracheal intubation—incidence and causes of failure. *Anesth Analg* 1983; 62:692-95.

[77] J. Brimacombe. *Laryngeal Mask Anesthesia: Principles and Practice* (Philadelphia: W. B. Saunders Company, 2005 [2nd edition]), p. 10.

[78] O'Dwyer, 1885.

[79] B. Leech. The pharyngeal gasway: A new aid in cyclopropane anesthesia. *Anesth Analg* 1934; 13:22-27.

[80] A. Brain. The laryngeal mask—a new concept in airway management. *Brit J Anaesth* 1983; 55:801-05.

[81] Brimacombe, 2005, p. 14.

[82] Ibid., p. 20.

[83] A. Ovassapian. *Fiberoptic Endoscopy and the Difficult Airway* (Philadelphia: Lippincott-Raven Publishers, 1996, 2nd ed., p. 244.

[84] Brimacombe, 2005, p 22.

Chapter 7

[1] Editorial. Fifty years of medicine. *Brit Med J* 1950; 1:61-63.

[2] C. Singer. Medical progress from 1850 to 1900. *Brit Med J* 1950; 1:57-60.

[3] F. Hewitt. A new method of administering and economizing nitrous oxide gas. *Lancet* 1885; 1:840.

[4] S. S. White Dental Manufacturing Company. *Seventy Five Years of Service 1844-1919. A History of the House of White* (Philadelphia: S. S. White Dental Manufacturing Company, 1920. (Collection of Wood Library-Museum of Anesthesiology.)

[5] B. Duncum. *The Development of Inhalation Anaesthesia With Special Reference to the Years 1846-1900* (London: Wellcome Historical Medical Museum and Oxford University Press), 1947, p. 106.

[6] K. B. Thomas. *The Development of Anaesthetic Apparatus: A History Based on the Charles King Collection of the Association of Anesthetists of Great Britain and Ireland* (Oxford: Blackwell Scientific Publications, 1975), pp. 168-71.

[7] Duncum, 1947.

[8] Thomas, 1975.

[9] D. Wilkinson. "Anaesthetic Equipment—A Historical Perspective," in H. C. Churchill-Davidson (ed.), *A Practice of Anaesthesia* (London: Lloyd Luke, 1984, 5th edition), pp. 1157-1187.

[10] Thomas, p. 5.

[11] Duncum, 1947, p. 106.

[12] Duncum, p. 133.

[13] J. Snow. *On Chloroform and Other Anaesthetics: Their Action and Administration* (London: John Churchill, 1858), p. 79.

[14] T. Skinner. Anaesthesia in midwifery: With new apparatus for its safer induction with chloroform. *Brit Med J* 1862; 2:108. Also see Duncum, 1947, pp. 247-48, and Thomas, 1975, p. 252.

[15] Ibid., p. 252.

[16] J. Snow. *On the Inhalation of the Vapour of Ether . . . .* (London: John Churchill, 1847), pp. 15-30.

[17] J. Snow. *On Chloroform and Other Anaesthetics* (London: John Churchill, 1858), pp. 81-85.

[18] R. Ellis (ed.). *On Narcotism by the Inhalation of Vapours by John Snow MD* (London: Royal Society of Medicine Services Ltd., 1991), pp. 11-12.

[19] Duncum, 1947, pp. 225-27.

[20] Duncum, 1947, pp. 241-44.

[21] F. Junker. Description of a new apparatus for administering narcotic vapours. *Med Times & Gaz London* 1867; 1:171.

[22] Thomas, 1975, p. 72.

[23] Duncum, 1947, p. 289, infers that nitrous oxide was first made available in cylinders in 1868. W. D. A. Smith, however, stated that Armstrong Davison (The first cylinder of gas, *Brit J Anaesth* 1954; 26:40) had found evidence for the iron-bottling of "oxygen and other gases" as early as 1856 (W. D. A. Smith, *Under the Influence: A History of Nitrous Oxide and Oxygen Anaesthesia* [Park Ridge: Wood Library-Museum of Anesthesiology, 1982], p. 129).

[24] Duncum, 1947, p. 286.

[25] J. Clover. On an apparatus for administering nitrous oxide gas and ether singly or combined. *Brit Med J* 1876; 2:74-75.

[26] J. Clover. Portable regulating ether inhaler. *Brit Med J* 1877; 1:69-70.

[27] Thomas, 1975, p. 25.

[28] F. Hewitt. *Anaesthetics and Their Administration* (London: C. Griffin, 1893), pp. 122-24.

[29] F. Hewitt. The past, present, and future of anaesthesia. *Practitioner* 1896; 57:347-56.

[30] G. Edwards. Frederic William Hewitt (1857-1916). *Ann Roy Coll Surg Engl* 1951; 8:233-45.

[31] F. Hewitt. The past, present, and future of anaesthesia. *Practitioner* 1896; 57:347-56.

[32] P. Thompson, D. Wilkinson. Development of anaesthetic machines. *Brit J Anaesth* 1985; 57:640-48.

[33] O. P. Dinnick. "The First Anaesthesia Society," in *Progress in Anaesthesiology*, Proceedings of 4th World Congress of Anaesthesiology, London, Sept. 9-13, 1968 (Amsterdam: Excerpta Medica Foundation, International Congress Series, no. 200), pp. 181-86.

[34] J. Erickson. "In the Beginning: Adolph Frederick Erdmann and the Long Island Society of Anesthetists," in D. Bacon, K. McGoldrick, M. Lema (eds.), *The American Society of Anesthesiologists: A Century of Challenges and Progress* (Park Ridge: Wood Library-Museum of Anesthesiology, 2005), pp. 1-8.

[35] L. D. Vandam. Early American anesthetists: The origins of professionalism in anesthesia. *Anesthesiology* 1973; 38:264-74.

[36] A. V. Harcourt. Special Chloroform Committee. 1903; 2 (Suppl.); 142.

[37] A. Waller, V. Geets. The rapid estimation of the quantity of chloroform vapour present in mixtures of chloroform vapour and air. *Brit Med J* 1903; 1:1421.

[38] E. Andrews. The oxygen mixture, a new anaesthetic combination. *Chicago Med Examiner* 1868; 19:656-61. (See also *Survey Anesthesiol* 1963; 7:74)

[39] P. Bert. *Barometric Pressure: Researches in Experimental Physiology* (1878). Trans. M. and F. Hitchcock (Columbus, OH: College Book Company, 1943).

[40] S. S. White Company History, 1920.

[41] Thomas, 1975, p. 133.

[42] Duncum, 1947, pp. 289-90.

[43] W. Boothby. Nitrous oxide and oxygen anaesthesia and a new apparatus. *Surg Gynec Obstet* 1912; 14:198-201.

[44] L. D. Vandam. Walter M. Boothby, M. D.—The wellsprings of anesthesiology. *New Engl J Med* 1967; 276:258-63.

[45] Duncum, 1947, pp. 516-18.

[46] Gwathmey, 1914, pp. 317-20.

[47] Ibid., p. 318.

[48] Thomas, 1975, p. 134.

[49] S. S. White, 1920.

[50] J. Heidbrink. Memoirs. *Newsmonthly of the American Dental Society of Anesthesiology*, 1957, pp. 1-12.

[51] Thomas, 1975, pp. 137-39.

[52] Gwathmey, 1914, p. 159.

[53] K. Connell. A new ether-vaporizer: A preliminary report on the technic of intrapharyngeal insufflations anesthesia. *JAMA* 1913; 60:892-94.

[54] Thomas, 1975, p. 169.

[55] K. Connell. An apparatus—Anaesthetometer—for measuring and mixing anaesthetic and other vapors and gases. *Surg Gynecol Obst* 1913; 16:245-55. (Hereinafter, Connell 1913b.)

[56] Connell, 1913a.

[57] Connell, 1913b.

[58] W. Boothby. Ether percentages. *JAMA* 1913; 61:830-34.

[59] F. Mann. Some bodily changes during anesthesia; an experimental study. *JAMA* 1916; 67:172-75.

[60] F. Mann. Vascular reflexes with various tensions of ether vapor. *Amer J Surg: Anesth Suppl* 1917; 31:107-12.

[61] W. Boothby. Nitrous oxide-oxygen-ether anaesthesia, with a description of a new apparatus. *Boston Med Surg J* 1912; 15:281-89.

[62] F. Cotton, W. Boothby. Nitrous oxide-oxygen-ether anaesthesia: Notes on administration; a perfected apparatus. *Surg Gynecol Obstet* 1912; 15:281-89.

[63] W. Boothby. Nitrous oxide-oxygen anesthesia, with a description of a new apparatus. *Comm Mass Med Soc* 1911; 22:3-15.

[64] J. Gwathmey, W. Woolsey. The Gwathmey-Woolsey nitrous oxide-oxygen apparatus. *New York Med J* 1912; 96:943-46.

[65] H. Boyle. Nitrous oxide-oxygen-ether outfit. *Proc Roy Soc Med* 1917-18; 11 (Anaesth Sect.):30.

[66] G. Marshall. Two types of portable gas-oxygen apparatus. Ibid. 1919-20; 13 (Anaesth Sect.):16-19.

[67] Y. Henderson. Respiration in anesthesia: control by carbon dioxide. *Brit Med J* 1925; 2:1170-75.

[68] Vandam, 1967.

[69] Thomas, 1975, p. 169.

[70] G. Rushman, N. Davies, R. Atkinson. *A Short History of Anaesthesia: The First 150 Years* (Oxford: Butterworth-Heinemann, 1996), p. 56.

[71] M. Neu. Ein Verfahren zur Stickoxydulsauerstoffnarkose. *Munch Med Wchschr* 1910; 57:1873-75.

[72] Thomas, 1975, p. 169.

[73] Ibid.

[74] S. Meltzer, J. Auer. Continuous respiration without respiratory movements. *J Exper Med* 1909; 11:622-25.

[75] An account of an experiment made by M. Hook [sic], of preserving animals alive by blowing through their lungs with bellows. *Phil Trans Roy Soc* 1667; 2:539-40.

[76] Thomas, 1975, p. 179.

[77] C. Elsberg. Anaesthesia by the intratracheal insufflation of air and ether. *Ann Surg* 1911; 53:161-68.

[78] R. Kelly. Intratracheal anaesthesia. *Brit J Surg* 1911; 1:90-95.

[79] D. Buxton. *Anaesthesia* (London: H. K. Lewis, 6th edition, 1924), p. 197.

80 E. McKesson. Fractional rebreathing in anesthesia—Its physiologic basis. Technic and conclusions. *Amer J Surg* 1915; 29 (xxix):51-57.

81 W. Gatch. Nitrous-oxid-oxygen anesthesia by the method of rebreathing: With especial reference to the prevention of surgical shock. *JAMA* 1910; 54:775-80.

82 E. McKesson. Nitrous oxide-oxygen anaesthesia, with a description of a new apparatus *Surg Gynecol Obst* 1911; 13:456-62.

83 E. McKesson. Some physical factors in the administration of gaseous anaesthetics. *Brit Med J* 1926; 2:1113-17.

84 Thomas, pp. 160-61.

85 Z. Mennell. Second Embley Lecture. *Brit J Anaesth* 1935; 13:18-23.

86 Thomas, pp. 162-68.

87 R. Minnitt. Self-administered analgesia for the midwifery of general practice. 1934; 27:1313-18.

88 Ellis, 1991, p. 80.

89 A. Coleman. Modern anaesthetics: Reinhalation of nitrous oxide. *Brit Med J* 1868; 2:114-15.

90 Andrews, 1868.

91 D. Jackson. New method for the production of general analgesia and anaesthesia. *J Lab Clin Med* 1915; 1:1-12.

92 D. Jackson. Anesthesia equipment from 1914 to 1954 and experiments leading to its development. *Anesthesiology* 1955; 16; 953-69.

93 R. Waters. Clinical scope and utility of carbon dioxid filtration in inhalation anesthesia. *Anesth Analg* 1924; 3:20-26.

94 B. Sword. The closed circle method of administration of gas anesthesia. *Anesth Analg* 1930; 9:198-202.

95 P. Flagg. *The Art of Anaesthesia* (Philadelphia: J. B. Lippincott Company, 1916), pp. 123-24.

96 H. Epstein, R. Macintosh, K. Mendelsohn. The Oxford vaporizer no. 1. *Lancet* 1941; 2:62-64.

97 H. Epstein, R. Macintosh. An anaesthetic inhaler with automatic thermo-compensation. *Anaesthesia* 1956; 11:83-88.

98 H.-G. Schaefer, J. Farman. Anaesthetic vapour concentration in the EMO system. *Anaesthesia* 1984; 39:171-80.

Chapter 8

1 B. Duncum. *The Development of Inhalation Anaesthesia With Special Reference to the Years 1846-1900* (Oxford: Wellcome Historical Medical Museum and Oxford University Press, 1947), pp. 412-14, 428-39, 448-56, 46-64.

2 F. Hewitt. The past, present, and future of anaesthesia. *Practitioner* 1896; 57:347-56.

3 Editorial. A plea for public anaesthetizers. *Medical Record* (New York) 1894; 46:239-40.

4 Hewitt, 1896.

5   O. P. Dinnick. "The First Anaesthesia Society," in *Progress in Anaesthesiology*, Proceedings of the Fourth World Congress of Anaesthesiology, London, Sept. 9-13, 1968 (Amsterdam: Excerpta Medica Foundation, International Congress Series, no. 200, 1970, pp. 181-86).

6   J. Erickson. "In the Beginning: Adolph Frederick Erdmann and the Long Island Society of Anesthetists," in D. Bacon, K. McGoldrick, M. Lema (eds.), *The American Society of Anesthesiologists: A Century of Challenges and Progress* (Park Ridge: Wood Library-Museum of Anesthesiology, 2005), pp. 1-8.

7   R. Ellis (ed.). *On Narcotism by the Inhalation of Vapours by John Snow MD* (London: Royal Society of Medicine Services, Ltd., 1991).

8   F. Hewitt. *Anaesthetics and Their Administration* (London: Macmillan and Co., Ltd., 1912 [4th ed.]), pp. 304, 315-318.

9   J. Snow. *On the Inhalation of the Vapour of Ether in Surgical Operations* (London: John Churchill, 1847).

10 J. Robinson. *A Treatise on the Inhalation of the Vapour of Ether* [1847]. With preface to facsimile edition by R. Ellis. (Eastbourne: Bailliere Tindall, 1993.)

11 J. Snow. *On Chloroform and Other Anaesthetics: Their Action and Administration* (London: John Churchill, 1858).

12 J. Flagg, 1851, cited by T. Keys, *The History of Surgical Anesthesia* (New York: Dover Publications, Inc., 2nd edition, 1963), p. 107.

13 H. Lyman. *Artificial Anaesthesia and Anaesthetics* (New York: William Wood and Co., 1881).

14 G. Foy. *Anaesthetics Ancient and Modern* (London: Bailliere Tindall, & Cox, 1889).

15 L. Turnbull. *The Advantages and Accidents of Artificial Anaesthesia* (Philadelphia: Lindsay and Blakiston, 1875).

16 D. Buxton. *Anaesthetics: Their Uses and Administration* (London: H. K. Lewis, 1888).

17 F. Hewitt. *Select Methods in the Administration of Nitrous Oxide and Ether, a Handbook for Practitioners and Students* (London, 1888).

18 F. Hewitt. *Anaesthetics and Their Administration, a Manual for Medical and Dental Practitioners and Students* (London: C. Griffin, 1893).

19 F. Hewitt. *The Administration of Nitrous Oxide and Oxygen for Dental Operations* (London: C. Ash, 1897).

20 J. T. Gwathmey. *Anesthesia* (New York: D. Appleton and Company, 1914).

21 P. Flagg. *The Art of Anesthesia* (Philadelphia: J. B. Lippincott Company, 1916).

22 A. McKenzie. Early books and pamphlets on anaesthesia. *Anaesthesia* 2003; 58:499-500.

23 Hewitt, 1896.

24 S. O. Goldan. Anesthetization as a specialty: Its present and future. *Amer Med* 1901; 2:101-04.

25 F. Hewitt. *Anaesthetics and Their Administration: A Text-Book for Medical and Dental Practitioners and Students* (London: Macmillan and Co., 4th edition, 1912), p. 138.

[26] N. Buck, H. Devlin, J. Lunn. Nuffield Provincial Hospitals Trust: *Report of a Confidential Enquiry into Perioperative Deaths* (London: The King's Fund Publishing House, 1987). Cited in R. D. Miller (ed.), *Miller's Anesthesia* (New York: Elsevier Churchill Livingstone, 6th edition, 2005), p. 901.

[27] Miller, 2005, pp. 897-903.

[28] W. S. Sykes. *Essays on the First Hundred Years of Anaesthesia* (Edinburgh: E. &S. Livingstone, 1961), Chart I, facing p. 32.

[29] Hewitt, 1896.

[30] Goldan, 1901.

[31] F. McMechan. Address to AMA Council on Medical Education and Hospitals, 1935. Cited by R. Waters, The development of anesthesiology in the United States: Personal observations 1913-946. *J Hist Med All Sci* 1946; 1:595-606.

[32] J. Eckenhoff. A wide-angle view of anesthesiology. *Anesthesiology* 1978; 48: 272-79.

[33] M. Shield. The need for better instructions in the administration of anaesthetics. *Practitioner* 1896; 57:387-93.

[34] H. Beecher. The first anesthesia records (Codman, Cushing). *Surg Gynecol Obstet* 1940; 71:689-93.

[35] H. Cushing. On routine determinations of arterial tension in operating room and clinic. *Boston Med Surg J* 1903; 148:250-56.

[36] F. Hewitt. On the effects produced in the human subject by the administration of nitrous oxide and air an of nitrous oxide and oxygen. *Med. Chir Trans* 1899; 82:163.

[37] Duncum, 1947, pp. 436-39, 460-64, 469.

[38] R. Waters. *Chloroform, A Study After 100 Years* (Madison: University of Wisconsin, 1951).

[39] L. Vandam. Early American anesthetists: The origins of professionalism in anesthesia. *Anesthesiology* 1973; 38:264-74.

[40] See, for example, J. Fulton, *Selected Readings in the History of Physiology* (Springfield: Charles C Thomas, 2nd edition, 1966).

[41] L. D. Vandam. Walter M. Boothby, M. D.—The wellsprings of anesthesiology. *New Engl J Med* 1967; 276:558-63.

[42] W. Boothby. The determination of the anaesthetic tension of ether vapor in man, with some theoretical deductions therefrom, as to the mode of action of the common volatile anaesthetics. *J Pharmacol & Exper Ther* 1914; 5:379-92.

[43] W. Boothby. Nitrous oxide-oxygen anesthesia, with a description of a new apparatus. *Boston Med Surg J* 1912; 146:86-90.

[44] D. Bacon. "The New York Society of Anesthetists: Building the Foundation," in Bacon, McGoldrick, Lema, 2005, p. 9.

[45] K. B. Thomas. *The Development of Anaesthetic Apparatus: A History Based on the Charles King Collection of the Association of Anaesthetists of Great Britain and Ireland* (Oxford: Blackwell Scientific Publications, 1975), pp. 140-42.

[46] C. Pittinger. *James Tayloe Gwathmey, M. D.: Pioneer American Anesthesiologist* (Nashville: Vanderbilt University School of Medicine, 1989).

[47] F. Clement. "Elmer I. McKesson," in P. Volpitto, L. D. Vandam (eds.), *The Genesis of Contemporary American Anesthesiology* (Springfield: Charles C Thomas, 1982), pp. 21-27.

[48] D. Jackson. A new method for the production of general analgesia and anaesthesia with a description of the apparatus used. *J Lab Clin Med* 1915; 1:1-12.

[49] H. Thomason, D. Jackson. Carbon dioxide filtration method for general analgesia and anaesthesia. *Anesth Analg* 1927; 6:181-83.

[50] Thomas, 1975), pp. 137-39.

[51] B. Bamforth, K. Siebecker. "Ralph. M. Waters," in Volpitto, Vandam, 1982, pp. 51-68.

[52] J. Eckman. "John Silas Lundy," in Volpitto, Vandam, 1982, pp. 35-48.

[53] R. Waters. Pioneering in anesthesiology. *Postgrad Med* 1948; 4:265-70.

[54] R. Waters. Clinical scope and utility of carbon dioxide filtration in inhalation anesthesia. *Anesth Analg* 1924; 3:20-22.

[55] R. Waters, E. Schmidt. Cyclopropane anesthesia. *JAMA* 1934; 103:975-83.

[56] T. Pratt, A. Tatum, H. Hathaway, R. Waters. Sodium ethyl (1-methyl butyl) thiobarbiturate. *Amer J Surg* 1936; 31:464-46.

[57] C. Leake, R. Waters. The anesthetic properties of carbon dioxide. *Anesth Analg* 1929; 8:17.

[58] W. Meek, H. Hathaway, O. Orth. The effects of ether, chloroform and cyclopropane on cardiac automaticity. *J Pharm Exper Therap* 1937; 61:240-52.

[59] M. Seevers, W. Meek, E. Rovenstine, J. Stiles. A study of cyclopropane anesthesia with especial reference to gas concentrations, respiratory and electrocardiographic changes. *J Pharmacol Exp Ther* 1934; 51:1-17.

[60] B. Sword. The closed circle method of administration of gas anesthesia. *Anesth Analg* 1930; 9:198-202.

[61] A. Guedel, R. Waters. A new intratracheal catheter. *Anesth Analg* 1928; 7:238-39.

[62] A. Guedel. Third stage ether anesthesia: a subclassification regarding the significance of the position and movements of the eyeball. *Nat Anesth Res Soc Bull* 1920; no. 3 (May), 4 pp.

[63] A. Guedel. *Inhalational Anesthesia: A Fundamental Guide* (New York: Macmillan Company, 1937).

[64] J. Lundy. The barbiturates as anesthetics, hypnotics and antispasmodics: Their use in more than 1000 surgical and non-surgical clinical cases and in operations on animals. *Curr Res Anesth Analg* 1929; 8:360-65.

[65] J. Lundy. Intravenous anesthesia: preliminary report of the use of two new thiobarbiturates. *Proc Staff Meet Mayo Clin* 1935; 10:536-43.

[66] J. Lundy. *Clinical Anesthesia* (Philadelphia: W. B. Saunders Company, 1942).

[67] J. Lundy. A cart for use in the postanesthesia room or for general hospital use. *Proc Staff Meet Mayo Clin* 1952; 27:234-35.

68 J. Lundy. The blood bank. *Minn Med* 1940; 22:870.

69 J. Lundy. Plastic stylet for plastic needle. *Proc Staff Meet Mayo Clin* 1958; 33:458-59.

70 D. Brown, A. Winnie. Biography of Louis Gaston Labat. *Reg Anesth* 1992; 17:249-62.

71 W. Salter. Cited by L. Vandam, "The Origin and Development of the Journal *Anesthesiology*," in Polpitto, Vandam, 1982, pp. 228-29.

72 Between 1936 and 1968, for example, membership in the American Society of Anesthesiologists increased from 487 to 9549 (J. Bunker, *The Anesthesiologist and the Surgeon* [Boston: Little, Brown and Company, 1972], p. 63).

73 G. Weisz. *Divide and Conquer: A Comparative History of Medical Specialization* (Oxford: Oxford University Press, 2006), p. xix.

74 J. Fulton. The vision and daring of youth: The story of the introduction of surgical anesthesia. *Anesthesiology* 1947; 8:464-70. (An article with the same title but different wording was published in the *Yale Journal of Biology and Medicine*.)

75 Eckenhoff, 1978.

76 H. Ruth. Anesthesia travel clubs. *Anesthesiology* 1947; 8:402-03.

77 C. R. Stephen. "Anaesthetists'Travel Club, 1929-1952: An Historical Review." Privately printed, n. d., p. 28

78 A. Betcher. "Historical Development of The American Society of Anesthesiologists, Inc.," in Volpitto, Vandam, 1982, pp. 185-211.

79 Bacon, 2005, p. 76.

80 T. Seldon. "Francis Hoeffer McMechan, in Volpitto, Vandam, 1982, pp. 5-18.

81 Waters, 1946.

82 Betcher, 1982, p. 188.

83 D. Bacon. "The Creation of the American Society of Anesthesiologists: An Intriguing Decade," in Bacon, McGoldrick, and Lema, 2005, p. 19.

84 Ibid.

85 Ibid.

86 Betcher, 1982, p. 191.

87 Bacon, 2005, pp. 20-21.

88 Bacon, 2005, p. 21.

89 D. Bacon. White knight: ASRA, ASA, and the formation of the ABA. *Reg Anesth Pain Med* 2006; 31:66-70.

90 Betcher, 1982, p. 193.

91 Ibid., p. 193.

92 Bacon, 2005, p. 20.

93 Bacon, 2005, p. 36.

94 Ibid., pp. 36-37.

95 Ibid., pp. 37-38.

96 Ibid., p. 38.

97 Waters, 1951.

[98] J. Bunker. *The Anesthesiologist and the Surgeon: Partners in the Operating Room* (Boston: Little, Brown and Company, 1972), p. 17.

[99] O. Cope, J. Hedley-White, R. Kitz et al. "Henry Knowles Beecher: Pioneer in Anaesthesiology and Medical Ethics," cited in R. Kitz (ed.), *'This Is No Humbug': Reminiscences of the Department of Anesthesia at the Massachusetts General Hospital—A History* (no publishing details: ISBN 0-9715376-0-7)

[100] R. Stevens. *Medical Practice in Modern England: The Impact of Specialization and State Medicine* (New Haven: Yale University Press, 1960), p. 33.

[101] Hewitt, 1896.

[102] Ibid., p. 202.

[103] G. Rushman, N. Davies, R. Atkinson. *A Short History of Anaesthesia: The First 150 Years* (Oxford: Butterworth Heinemann, 1996), p. 193.

[104] Ibid., p. 196. 433

[105] bid., p. 198.

[106] D. S. Lewis. *The Royal College of Physicians and Surgeons of Canada 1920-1960* (Montreal: McGill University Press, 1962), p. 5.

[107] Ibid., p. 5.

[108] Ibid., p. 5.

[109] Ibid., p. 11.

[110] D. Shephard. *The Royal College of Physicians and Surgeons of Canada 1960-1980: The Pursuit of Unity* (Ottawa: The Royal College of Physicians and Surgeons of Canada, 1985), p. 11.

[111] E. S. Ryerson. The qualification of specialists in Canada. *Canad Med Ass J* 1933; 29:72-73.

[112] Lewis, p. 158.

[113] Ibid., p. 162

[114] D. Shephard. *Watching Closely Those Who Sleep: A History of the Canadian Anaesthetists' Society 1943-1993* (Toronto: Canadian Anaesthetists' Society, 1993).

[115] R. Gordon, D. Craig, D. Bevan. "The Society's Journal," in Shephard, 1993, pp. 160-69.

[116] Shephard, 1985, pp. 231-32. 434

[117] W. Bourne, B. Raginsky. The effects of avertin upon the normal and impaired liver. *Amer J Surg* 1931; 14:653-56.

[118] H. Griffith. Intratracheal gas-oxygen anesthesia. *Anesth Analg* 1929; 8:387-89.

[119] H. Griffith. Safety factors in spinal anesthesia. *Anesth Analg* 1952; 31:367-71.

[120] H. Griffith. Cyclopropane anesthesia. *Anesth Analg* 1935; 14:253-56.

[121] H. Griffith, E. Johnson. The use of curare in general anesthesia. *Anesthesiology* 1942; 3:418-20.

[122] W. E. Brown. Preliminary report; experiments with ethylene as a general anesthetic. *Canad Med Ass J* 1923; 13:210.

[123] A. Luckhardt, J. Carter. Ethylene as a gas anesthetic; preliminary communication. *JAMA* 1923; 80:1440-42.

[124] G. Lucas, V. Henderson. A new anaesthetic gas: Cyclopropane—a preliminary report. *Canad Med Ass J* 1929; 21:173-75.

[125] S. Gelfan, I. Bell. The anesthetic action of divinyl oxide on humans. *J Pharmacol Exp Ther* 1933; 47:1-3.

[126] W. Schwarz. "Attempts to Establish Anaesthesiology as a Specialty in German Medicine," in R. Atkinson, T. Boulton, 1989, pp. 170-75.

[127] E. von der Porten. Die Frage des Narkoticums. *Zentralbl Chir* 1922; 49:830-33.

[128] H. Killian. Ueber amerikanische Narkoseverhaltnisse. *Narkose Anaesth* 1928; 1:448-63.

[129] H. Schmidt. "Gruss und Hans Killian," in R. Frey, J. Bonica, F. Foldes et al. (eds.), *Erlebte Geschicte der Anaesthesie* (Mainz:1972), pp. 23-26.

[130] Schwarz, 1989.

[131] Bundesarztekammer. *Stenografischer Wortbericht des Arztetages* vom 15 bis 20 September 1953 in Lindau. (Koln: Arzte-Verlag, 1953), pp. 22-24.

[132] H. Schmidt. Die Gasnarkose vom Standpunkt des amerikanischen Narkosespezialisten. *Narkose Anaesth* 1928; 1:530-40.

Chapter 9

[1] K. Sykes, J. Bunker. *Anaesthesia and the Practice of Medicine: Historical Perspectives* (London: Royal Society of Medicine Press Ltd., 2007), p. 73

[2] Ibid., pp. 75-76.

[3] Ibid., pp. 85-86.

[4] V. Maddox. "The Historical Development of Phencyclidine," in E. Domino (ed.), *PCP (Phencyclidine): Historical and Current Perspectives* (Ann Arbor: NPP Books, 1981).

[5] M. Thuillier, R. Domenjoz. Zur pharmakologie der intravenosen kurznarkose mit 2-methoxyl-4-allylphenoxyessigsaeure-N, N-diathylamide (G29, 505). *Anaesthetist* 1957; 6:1263-70.

[6] J. E. Wynands, M. Burfoot. A clinical study of propanidid (FBA 1420). *Can Anaesth Soc J* 1963; 12:587-90.

[7] B. Orser. Lifting the fog around anesthesia. *Sci Amer* 2007; 256 (6):54-61.

[8] G. Crile. Psychogenic association, in relation to certain medical problems. *Boston Med Surg J* 1910; 163:893-984.

[9] J. Lundy. Balanced anesthesia. *Minn Med* 1926; 9:399-404.

[10] S. Courvoisier, J. Fournel, R. Ducrot et al. Pharmacodynamic properties of hydrochloride of 3-chloro-(dimethylamino-3'-propyl-10 phenothiazine. *Arch Int Pharmacodyn* 1953; 92; 305-61.

[11] E. Lear, I. Pallin, A. Chiron et al. Comparative studies of tranquillizers used in anesthesia. *JAMA* 1958; 166:1438-44.

[12] H. Laborit. *Pratique de l'Hibernation en Chirurgie et en Medecine* (Paris, 1954).

[13] J. Dundee. "Historical Vignettes and Classification of Intravenous Anesthetics," in J. Aldrete, T. Stanley (eds.), *Trends in Intravenous Anesthesia* (Chicago: Year Book Medical Publishers, 1980), p. 4.

[14] P. Huguenard. "A Historical View: Neuroleptanalgesia," in O. H. G. Wilder-Smith, E. Tassonyi, *Intravenous Anesthesia and Antinociception: A New Philosophy of Anesthetic Control* (Geneva: Editions Medecine et Hygiene, SA, 1995), pp. 19-21.

[15] G. Organe, R. Broad. Pentothal with nitrous oxide and oxygen. *Lancet* 1938; 2:1170-72.

[16] T. C. Gray, J. Halton. A milestone in anaesthesia (d-tubocurarine hydrochloride). *Proc Roy Soc Med* 1946; 34:400-06.

[17] W. Neff, E. Mayer, M. Perales. Nitrous oxide and oxygen anesthesia with curare relaxation. *Calif Med* 1947; 66:67-69.

[18] Lear et al., 1958.

[19] L. Sternbach. "The Benzodiazepine Story," in E. Jucker (ed.), *Drug Research*, 1978; 22 (Basel: Birkhauser).

[20] A. Brandt, S. Liu, B. Briggs. Trial of chlordiazepoxide as a preanesthetic medication. *Anesth Analg* 1962; 41:557-64.

[21] J. DuCailar, J. Rious, A. Bellanger, D. Grolleau. Utilisation du diazepam (Valium) en premedication. *Ann Anesth Fr* 1964; 5:706-10.

[22] L. Campan, L. Espagno. Note sur le diazepam en anesthesiology. *Ann Anesth Fr* 1964; 5:711-17.

[23] J. Stovner, R. Andresen. Diazepam in intravenous anesthesia. *Lancet* 1965; 2:1298-99.

[24] J. Reves, G. Corssen, C. Holcome. Comparison of two benzodiazepines for anesthesia induction: diazepam and midazolam. *Can Anaesth Soc J* 1978; 25:211-14.

[25] D. McCarthy, G. Chen. General anesthetic action of 2-(o-chlorophenyl)-2-methylamino cyclohexanone HCl (CI-581) in the Rhesus monkey. *Fed Proc* 1965; 24:268.

[26] E. Domino, P. Chodoff, G. Corssen. Pharmacologic effects of CI-581, a new dissociative anesthetic, in man. *Clin Pharm Ther* 1965; 6:279-91.

[27] H. Selye. Anesthetic effect of steroid hormones. *Proc Soc Exp Biol* 1941; 46:116.

[28] H. Selye. Studies concerning the correlation between anesthetic potency, hormonal activity and clinical structure among steroid compounds. *Anesth Analg* 1942; 21:41-52.

[29] S. P'An, J. Gardocki, D. Hutcheon et al. General anesthetic and other pharmacologic properties of a soluble steroid, 21-hydroxypregomedione sodium succinate. *J Pharmacol Exp Ther* 1955; 115:432-37.

[30] F. Murphy, N. Guadagni, F. DeBon. Use of steroid anesthesia in surgery. *JAMA* 1955; 156:1412-14.

[31] B. Davies, D. Pearce. "An Introduction to Althesin (CT 1341)," in *Proceedings of Conference at Royal College of Physicians*, London, 1972; 40.

[32] J. van Hemelrijck, I. Kissin. "History of Intravenous Anesthesia," in P. White (ed.), *Textbook of Intravenous Anesthesia* (Baltimore: Williams & Wilkins, 1977), pp. 1-9.

[33]

[34] J. E. Wynands, M. Burfoot. A clinical study of propanidid (FBA 1420). *Can Anaesth Soc J* 1963; 12:587-90.

35 E. Godefroi, P. Janssen, C. van Der Eycken et al. Dl-1-(1-arylalkyl) imidazole-5 carboxylate ester. *J Med Chem* 1965; 8:222-28.

36 A. Doenicke. Etomidate, a new intravenous hypnotic. *Acta Anaesthesiol Belg* 1974; 25:307-15.

37 R. Wagner, P. White, P. Kan et al. Inhibition of adrenal steroidogenesis by the anesthetic etomidate. *New Engl J Med* 1984; 310:1415-21.

38 B. Kay, G. Rolly. ICI 35868, a new intravenous induction agent. *Acta Anaesthesiol Belg* 1977; 28:303-16.

39 P. Sebel, J. Lowdon. Propofol: A new intravenous anesthetic. *Anesthesiology* 1989; 71:260-77.

40 L. Lasagna, H. Beecher. The analgesic effectiveness of nalorphine and nalorphine-morphine combinations in man. *J Pharmacol Exp Ther* 1954; 112:356-63.

41 T. Stanley, T. Egan, H van Aken. A tribute to Dr Paul A. J. Janssen: Entrepreneur extraordinaire, innovative scientist, and significant contributor to anesthesiology. *Anesth Analg* 2008; 106:451-62.

42 P. Janssen. A review of the chemical features associated with strong morphine-like activity. *Brit J Anaeth* 1962; 34:260-68.

43 P. Janssen. Potent, new analgesics, tailor-made for different purposes. *Acta Anaesth Scand* 1982; 26:262-68.

44 G. Corssen, J. Reves, T. Stanley. "History of Narcotics in Anesthesiology," in P. White (ed.), *Textbook of Intravenous Anesthesia* (Baltimore: Williams & Wilkins, 1997), p. 18.

45 P. Feldman, M. James, M. Brackeen et al. Design, synthesis, and pharmacological evaluation of ultrashort to long-acting opioid analgesics. *J Med Chem* 1991; 34:2202-08.

46 T. Egan, H. Lemmens, P. Fiset et al. The pharmacokinetics of the new short-acting opioid remifentanil (GI 87084B) in healthy adult male volunteers. *Anesthesiology* 1993; 79:881-92.

47 W. R. Martin, C. Eades, H. Fraser, A. Wikler. Use of hindlimb reflexes of the chronic spinal dog for comparing analgesics. *J Pharmacol Exp Ther* 1964; 144:8-11.

48 K. Tsou, C. Zhang. Studies on the site of analgesic action of morphine by intracerebral microinjection. *Scientia Sinica* 1964; 13:1099-1109.

49 Lasagna, Beecher, 1954.

50 W. Martin. Opioid antagonists. *Pharmacol Rev* 1967; 19:464-515.

51 H. Akil. "The Dawn of Endorphins," in M. Meldrum (ed.), *Opioids and Pain Relief: A Historical Perspective* (Seattle: IASP Press, 2003), pp. 99-110.

52 Tsou, Zhang, 1964.

53 D. Mayer, T. Wolfle, H. Akil et al. Analgesia from electrical stimulation in the brainstem of the rat. *Science* 174:1351-54.

54 Akil, 2003, p. 101.

55 H. Akil, D. Mayer, J. Liebeskind. Comparison in the rat between analgesia induced by stimulation of periaqueductal gray matter and morphine analgesia. *Compt Rend Hebd Seances Acad Sci D Sci Nat* 1972; 274:3603-05.

56 M. Meldrum, "The Search for the Opiate Receptor," in Meldrum, 2003, pp. 131-39.

[57] S. Snyder. Opiate receptors and internal opiates. *Sci Amer* 1977; 236 (3):44-56.

[58] A. Goldstein, L. Lowney, B. Pal. Stereospecific and nonspecific interactions of the morphine congener levorphanol in subcellular fractions of mouse brain. *ProcNnat Acad Sci USA* 1971; 68:1742-476.

[59] M. Cousins. "History of the Development of Pain Management with Spinal Opioid and Non-opioid Drugs," in Meldrum, 2003, p. 146.

[60] L. Terenius. Characteristics of the 'receptor' for narcotic analgesics in synaptic plasma membrane fraction from rat brain. *Acta Pharmacol Toxicol* 1973; 33:377-84.

[61] S. Snyder, C. Pert. Opiate receptor: Demonstration in nervous tissue. *Science* 1973; 179:1011-14.

[62] E. Simon, J. Hiller, I. Edelman. Stereospecific binding of the potent narcotic analgesic (3) etorphine to rat brain homogenate. *Proc Nat Acad Sci USA* 1973; 70:1947-1949.

[63] Akil, 2003, p. 105.

[64] J. Hughes, T. Smith, H. Kosterlitz. Identification of two related *pentapeptides* from the brain with potent opiate agonist activity. *Nature* 1975; 278:577-80.

[65] S. Snyder, 1977.

[66] S. Snyder, G. Pasternak. Historical review: Opioid receptors. *TRENDS Pharmacol Sci* 2003; 24:198-205.

[67] Hughes, Smith, Kosterlitz et al., 1975.

[68] W. Martin, G. Eades, J. Thompson et al. The effects of morphine- and nalorphine-like drugs in the dependent chronic spinal dog. *J Pharmacol Exp Ther* 1976; 197; 517-32.

[69] Much of this discussion has been facilitated by study of the chapter "A Brief History of Synapses and Synaptic Transmission" by Maxwell Cowan and Eric Kandel, in W. M. Cowan, T. Sudhoff, C. Stevens (eds.), and K. Davies, *Synapses* (Baltimore: Johns Hopkins University Press, 2001), pp. 1-87.

[70] A. Crum Brown, T. Fraser. On the connection between chemical constitution and physiological action. Part I. On the physiological action of the salts of the ammonium bases derived from strychnia, brucia, thebaia, codeia, morphia, and nicotia. *Trans Roy Soc Edin* 1868; 25:151-203.

[71] R. Barlow, H. Ing. Curare-like action of polymethylamine *bis*-quarternary ammonium salts. *Nature* 1948; 161:718.

[72] W. Paton, E. Zaimis. Curare-like action of polymethylamine *bis*-quarternary ammonium salts. Ibid., 718-19.

[73] R. Hunt, R. de M. Taveau. On the physiological action of certain cholin derivatives and new methods for detecting cholin. *Brit Med J* 1906; 2:1788-91.

[74] J. Le Heux. Cholin als hormone der Darmbewegung. III Mitteilung: Die Beteilung des Cholin an der Wirkung verschneidener Sauren auf den Darm. *Pflugers Arch Ges Physiol* 1921; 196:280-300.

[75] D. Glick. Some additional observations on the specificity of cholinesterase. *J Biol Chem* 1941; 137:357-62.

[76] D. Bovet, F. Bovet-Nitti, S. Guarino, V. Longo. Proprieta farmacodinamiche di alcuni derivati delola succinilcoline dotati di azioe curarca. *Rec 1ˢᵗ Sup Sanita, Roma* 1949; 12:106-37.

[77] G. Buttle, E. Zaimis. The action of decamethonium iodide in birds. *J Pharm Pharmac* 1949; 1:991-92.

[78] A. Phillips. Synthetic curare substitutes from aliphatic dicarboxylic acid aminoethyl esters. *J Amer Chem Soc* 1949; 71:3264.

[79] J. Castillo, A. Phillips, E. de Beer. The curariform action of decamethylen-1, 10-*bis*-trimethylammonium bromide. *J Pharm Exp Ther* 1949; 97:150-56.

[80] O. von Dardell, S. Thesleff. Kliniska erfarenheter med succinylkolinjodid, ett mytt medel som ger muskelavslappning. *Nord Med* 1951; 46:1308-11.

[81] O. Mayrhofer, M. Hassfurther. Kurzwirkende Muskelerschlaffungsmittel. *Wien Klin Wchsr* 1951; 47:885-89.

[82] R. Ottolenghi, C. Manni, P. Mazzoni. A new short-acting curarizing agent. *Anes Analg* 1952; 31:243-50.

[83] C. Scurr. A relaxant of very brief action. *Brit Med J* 1952; 2:831-32.

[84] F. Foldes, P. McNall, J. Borrego-Hinojosa. Succinylcholine: A new approach to muscular relaxation in anesthesiology. *New Engl J Med* 1952; 247:596-600.

[85] S. Love. Prolonged apnoea following Scoline. *Anaesthesia* 1952; 7:113-14.

[86] R. Gould. Succinylcholine chloride. *Brit Med J* 1952; 1:440.

[87] J. Harper. Prolonged respiratory paralysis after succinylcholine. Ibid., 886.

[88] C. L. Hewer. Prolonged respiratory paralysis after succinylcholine. Ibid., 1952; 1:971-72.

[89] H. Dorkins. Suxamethonium—the development of a modern drug from 1906 to the present day. *Med Hist* 1982; 26:145-68.

[90] D. Bovet, F. Depierre, Y. Lestrange. Propriets curarisantes des ethers phenoliques a functions ammonium quarternaires. *Compt Rend Acad Sci* 1947; 225:74-76.

[91] D. Bevan, J. Bevan, F. Donati. *Muscle Relaxants in Clinical Anesthesia* (Chicago: Year Book Medical Publishers, 1988), p. 133.

[92] V. Stoelting, J. Graf, Z. Viera. Bimethyl ether of *d*-tubocurarine as an adjunct to anesthesia. *Proc Soc Exp Biol Med* 1948; 69:565-66.

[93] P. Huguenard, A. Boue. Un nouvel ortho-curare francais de synthese, le 3697 RP. Rapport a la Societe d'Anesthesie de Paris, 1948, Séance de 17 Juin.

[94] R. Paez. *Wild Scenes in South America, or Life in the Llanos of Venezuela* (New York: Charles Scribner, 1868), pp. 206-08.

[95] A. Quevauviller, F. Laine. Sur la toxicite et la pouvoir curarisant du chlorure de malouetine. *Ann Pharmaceut Fran* 1960; 18:678-80.

[96] A. McKenzie. Prelude to pancuronium and vecuronium. *Anaesthesia* 2000; 55:551-56.

[97] M. Alauddin, B. Caddy, J. Lewis et al. Non-depolarizing neuromuscular blockade by 3 [alpha], 17 [alpha]-androstanes. *J Pharmacy Pharmacol* 1965; 17:55-58.

[98] W. Burkett, C. Hewitt, D. Savage. Pancuronium bromide and other steroidal neuromuscular blocking agents containing acetylcholine fragments. *J Med Chem* 1973; 16:116-24.

[99] J. Crul, L. Booij. First clinical experience with ORG NC 45. *Brit J Anaesth* 1990; 52:49-52S.

[100] A. Koopman. Sugammadex: A revolutionary approach to neuromuscular antagonism. *Anesthesiology* 2006; 104:631-33.

[101] R. Calverley. Fluorinated anesthetics. I. The early years 1932-1946. *Surv Anesthesiol* 1986; 30:170-73.

[102] H. Booth, E. M. Bixby. Fluorine derivatives of chloroform. *J Ind Eng Chem* 1932; 24:637-41.

[103] Calverley, 1986.

[104] B. Robbins. Preliminary studies of the anesthetic activity of fluorinated hydrocarbons. *J Pharmacol Exp Ther* 1946; 86:197-204.

[105] J. Krantz. Anesthesia XL: The anesthetic action of trfluormethyl vinyl ether. *J Pharmacol Exp Ther* 1953; 108:487-95.

[106] R. Calverley. "Anesthesia as a Specialty: Past, Present, and Future," in P. Barash, B. Cullen, R. Stoelting (eds.), *Clinical Anesthesia* (Philadelphia: J. B. Lippincott Company, 1989), p. 23.

[107] C. Suckling. Some chemical and physical features in the development of Fluothane. *Brit J Anaesth* 1957; 29:466-70.

[108] J. Raventos. The action of Fluothane, a new volatile anaesthetic. *Brit J Pharmacol* 1956; 11:394-410.

[109] M. Johnstone. The human cardiovascular response to Fluothane anaesthesia. *Brit J Anaesth* 1956; 28:392-410.

[110] H. Bryce-Smith, H. O'Brien. Fluothane: A nonexplosive volatile anaesthetic agent. *Brit Med J* 1956; 2; 969-72.

[111] J. Bunker, C. Blumenfeld. Liver necrosis after halothane anesthesia. *New Engl J Med* 1963; 268:531-34.

[112] J. Bunker, W. Forrest, F. Mosteller, L. Vandam (eds.). *The National Halothane Study* (Bethesda: National Institutes of Health, 1969).

[113] J. Bunker. *The Anesthesiologist and the Surgeon: Partners in the Operating Room* (Boston: Little Brown and Company, 1972), p. 104.

[114] F. Artusio, A. van Poznak. A clinical evaluation of methoxyflurane in man. *Anesthesiology* 1960; 21:512-17.

[115] J. Vitcha. A history of Forane. *Anesthesiology* 1971; 35:4-7.

[116] A. Dobkin, P. Byles, S. Ghanoomi, D. Valbuena. Clinical and laboratory evaluation of a new inhalation anesthetic: Forane. *Can Anaesth Soc J* 1971; 18:264-71.

[117] W. Stevens, E. Eger, T. Joas et al. Comparative toxicity of isoflurane, halothane, fluroxene and diethyl ether in human volunteers. *Can Anaesth Soc J* 1973; 20:357-68.

[118] B. Cason, E. Verrier, M. London et al. Effects of isoflurane and halothane on coronary vascular resistance and collateral myocardial blood flow: Their capacity to induce coronary steal. *Anesthesiology* 1987; 67:665-75.

[119] R. Wallin, B. Regan, M. Napoli, I Stern. Sevoflurane: a new inhalational anesthetic agent. *Anesth Analg* 1975; 54:758-65.

[120] R. Jones, J. Cashman, T. Mant. Clinical impressions and cardiorespiratory effects of a new fluorinated inhalation anesthetic, desflurane (I-653), in volunteers. *Brit J Anaesth* 1990; 64:11-15.

[121] R. M. Jones. Desflurane and sevoflurane: Inhalation agents for this decade? *Brit J Anaesth* 1990; 65:527-36.

Chapter 10

[1] J. Comroe, S. Botelho. The reliability of cyanosis in the recognition of arterial anoxemia. *Am J Med Sci* 1947; 214:1-5.

[2] J. Cooper, R. Newblower, C. Long, B. McPeek. Preventable anesthesia mishaps: A study of human factors. *Anesthesiology* 1978; 49:399-406.

[3] H. J. Bigelow. Insensibility during surgical operations produced by inhalation. *Boston Med Surg J* 1846; 35:309-17.

[4] P. Hutton. "Monitoring: Perspectives and Philosophy," in P. Hutton, C. Prys-Roberts (eds.), *Monitoring in Anaesthesia and Intensive Care* (London: W. B. Saunders Company, 1994), p. 1.

[5] Snow, 1858, pp. 123-27.

[6] M. Bliss. *Harvey Cushing: A Life in Surgery* (Oxford: Oxford University Press, 2005), p. 82.

[7] H. Beecher. The first anesthesia records (Codman, Cushing). *Surg Gynecol Obst* 1940; 71:689-93.

[8] J. Fulton. *Harvey Cushing: A Biography* (Springfield: Charles C. Thomas, 1946), p. 457.

[9] Bliss, 2005, pp. 129-52.

[10] S. Riva-Rocci. Un nuevo sfigmomanometro. *Gaz Med Torino* 1896; 47:981-96.

[11] H. Cushing. On the avoidance of shock in major amputations by cocainization of large nerve-trunks preliminary to their division. With observations on blood-pressure changes in surgical cases. *Ann Surg* 1902; 36:321-45.

[12] H. Cushing. On routine determinations of arterial tensions in operating-room and clinic. *Boston Med Surg J* 1903; 148:250-56.

[13] D. Shephard. Harvey Cushing and anaesthesia. *Can Anaes Soc J* 1965; 12:31-42.

[14] S. Hales. *Statical Essays: Containing Haemastatics; Or, an Account of Some Hydraulic and Hydrostatical Experiments made on the Blood and Blood-vessels of Animals* . . . . (London, 1733).

[15] J. Faivre. Etudes experimentales sur les lesions organiques du Coeur. *Gaz Med Paris* 1856; 726-30.

[16] P. Hutton, T. Clutton-Brock. "The Non-invasive Measurement of Blood Pressure," in. Hutton and Prys-Roberts, 1994, p. 106.

[17] N. Korotkoff. To the question of methods of determining the blood pressure. *Reports of the Imperial Military Academy* 1905; 11:365-67.

[18] H. Cushing. Some principles of cerebral surgery. *JAMA* 1909; 52:184-94.

[19] E. McKesson. Blood pressure under anesthesia from records of 6, 000 personal observations. *The American Year-book of Surgery* (New York: Surgery Publishing Company, 1916), pp. 87-94.

[20] C. Blitt. "A Philosophy of Monitoring," in Casey Blitt and R. Hines (eds.), *Monitoring in Anesthesia and Critical Care Medicine* (New York: Churchill Livingstone, 1995, 3rd edition), p. 1.

[21] W. Einthoven. Die galvanometrische registrirung des menschlichen capillary-elektrometers in der physiologie. *Arch Gen Physiol* 1903; 99:472-80.

[22] W. Rollason, J. Hough. *Electrocardiography for the Anaesthetist* (Oxford: Blackwell Scientific Publications, 1964).

[23] A. Guedel. Third stage ether anesthesia: A subclassification regarding the significance of the position and movement of the eyeball. *Am J Surg Q Suppl Anesth Analg* 1920; 53-57.

[24] N. Gillespie. The signs of anesthesia. *Anesth Analg* 1943; 22:275-82.

[25] F. Gibbs, E. Gibbs, W. Lennox. Effect on the electro-encephalogram of certain drugs which influence nervous activity. *Arch Int Med* 1937; 60:154-66.

[26] A. Faulconer, J. Pender, and R. Bickford. The classification and significance of electro-encephalographic patterns produced by nitrous oxide-ether anesthesia during surgical operation. *Proc Staff Meet Mayo Clin* 1950; 25:197-206.

[27] P. Southorn, M. Warner, A. Sessler, K. Rehder. The legacy of Albert Faulconer, Jr. *Anesth Analg* 2003; 95:1108-11.

[28] A. Faulconer, R. Bickford. *Electroencephalography in Anesthesiology* (Springfield: Charles C Thomas, 1960).

[29] Southorn et al, 2003.

[30] J. A. Lee. *A Synopsis of Anaesthesia* (Bristol: John Wright & Sons, 1947).

[31] D. Harken. Foreign bodies in, and in relation to, thoracic blood vessels and heart. I. Techniques for approaching and removing foreign bodies from chambers of the heart. *Surg Gynecol Obst* 1946; 83:117-25.

[32] L. Clark. Monitor and control of oxygen tension. *Trans Am Soc Artif Organs* 1956; 2:41-48.

[33] M. Johnstone. The human cardiovascular response to Fluothane anesthesia. *Brit J Anaesth* 1956; 28:392-410.

[34] J. Severinghaus, P. Astrup. History of blood gas analysis. IV. Leland Clark's oxygen electrode. *J Clin Monit* 1986; 2:125-39.

[35] H. Daneel. Uber den durch differndierende gase hervorgern fenen restroom. *Z Elektrochem* 1897/98; 4:227-42.

[36] J. Heyrovsky. Electrolysis with the dropping mercury electrode. *Chemicke Listy* 1922; 16:256-304.

[37] H. Beecher, R. Follansbee, A. J. Murphy et al. *J Biol Chem* 1942; 146:197-206.

[38] D. Bronk, F. Brink, C. Connelly et al. The time course of recovery of oxygen consumption in nerve. *Fed Proc* 1947; 6:83.

[39] Clark, 1956.

[40] Ibid.

[41] Severinghaus, Astrup, 1986.

[42] D. van Slyke, J. Neill. The determination of gases in blood and other solutions by various extraction and manometric measurements. *J Biol Chem* 1924; 61:523-73.

[43] C. G. Douglas, R. Havard. The changes in the carbon dioxide pressure and hydrogen ion concentrations of the arterial blood of man which are associated with hyperpnea due to carbon dioxide. *J Physiol* 1932; 74:471-89.

[44] J. Severinghaus, P. Astrup. History of blood gas analysis. II. pH and acid-base measurements. *J Clin Monit* 1985; 1:259-77.

[45] P. Astrup. A new approach to acid-base metabolism. *Clin Chem* 1961; 7:1-15.

[46] R. Gesell, D. McGinty. Regulation of respiration. VI. Continuous electrometric methods of recording changes in expired carbon dioxide and oxygen. *Am J Physiol* 1926; 79:72-90.

[47] R. Stow, R. Baer, B. Randall. Rapid measurement of the tension of carbon dioxide in blood. *Arch Phys Med Rehabil* 1957; 38:646-50.

[48] J. Severinghaus, A. Bradley. Electrodes for blood Po_2 and Pco_2 determination. J Appl Physiol 1958; 13:515-20.

[49] J. Severinghaus, P. Astrup. History of blood gas analysis. VI. Oximetry. *J Clin Monit* 1986; 2:270-88.

[50] G. Stokes. On the reduction and oxygenation of the colouring matter of the blood. *Dublin Philosophical Magazine* 1864; 28:391.

[51] F. Hoppe-Seyler. Uber die chemischen und optischen eigenschafter des blutfarbstoffs. *Arch Gen Pathol Anat Physiol* 1864; 29:233-51.

[52] K. Mathes. Untersuchungen uber die sauerstoffsatugungen des menschlichen arterienbluten. *Arch Exp Pathol Pharmacol* 1935; 176:685-96.

[53] G. Millikan, J. Pappenheimer, A. Rawson et al. Continuous measurement of oxygen saturation in man. *Am J Physiol* 1941; 133:390.

[54] R. D. McClure, V. Behrmann, F. Hartman. The control of anoxemia during surgical anesthesia with the aid of an oxyhemograph. *Ann Surg* 1948; 128:685-707.

[55] G. Millikan. Oximeter, instrument for measuring continuously oxygen saturation of arterial blood in man. *Rev Sci Instrum* 1942; 13:434-44.

[56] E. Goldie. Device for continuous indication of oxygen saturation of circulating blood in man. *J Sci Instrum* 1942; 19:23-25.

[57] J. R. Squire. Instrument for measuring quantity of blood and its degree of oxygenation in the web of the hand. *Clin Sci* 1940; 4:331-34.

[58] A. B. Hertzman. Photoelectric plethysmography of the finger and toes in man. *Proc Soc Biol Exp Med* 1937; 37:529-34.

[59] J. Severinghaus, Y. Honda. History of blood gas analysis. VII. Pulse oximetry. *J Clin Monit* 1987; 3:135-38.

[60] J. West, K. Fowler, H. Jones et al. Measurement of the ventilation-perfusion ratio inequality in the lung by the analysis of a single expirate. *Clin Sci* 1957; 16:529-45.

[61] D. Westenkow, D. Coleman. Raman scattering for respiratory gas monitoring in the operating-room: Advantages, specifications, and future advances. *Biomed Instr Tech* 1989; 23:485-88.

[62] B. Ibsen. The anaesthetist's viewpoint on the treatment of respiratory complications in poliomyelitis during the epidemic in Copenhagen, 1952. *Proc Roy Soc Med* 1954; 47:72-74.

[63] D. Swerdlow. Capnometry and capnography: The anesthesia disaster early warning system. *Sem Anesth* 1986; 5:194-205.

[64] *ibid.*

[65] J. Phillips, D. Keith, J. Hulka et al. Gynecologic laparoscopy in 1975. *J Reprod Med* 1976; 16:205-17.

[66] J. Penaz. "Photoelectric Measurement of Blood Pressure, Volume and Flow in the Finger," in A. Roald (ed.), *Digest of the 10th International Conference on Medicine and Biological Engineering* (International Federation of Medical and Biological Engineering, Dresden, 1973), 104.

[67] M. Ramsey. Non-invasive automatic determination of mean arterial pressure. *Med Biol Eng Comput* 1979; 17:11-14.

[68] E. H. Lambert, E. Wood. The use of resistance wire strain gauge manometer to measure intraarterial pressure. *Proc Soc Exp Biol Med* 1947; 64:186-90.

[69] L. H. Peterson, R. Dripps, G. Risman. A method for recording the arterial pressure pulse and blood pressure in man. *Am Heart J* 1949; 37:771-82.

[70] D. Massa, J. Lundy, A. Faulconer. A plastic needle. *Proc Staff Meet Mayo Clin* 1950; 50:413-15.

[71] S. Seldinger. Catheter replacement of the needle in percutaneous arteriography: A new technique. *Acta Radiol* 1953; 39:368-76.

[72] P.-O. Barr. Percutaneous puncture of the radial artery with a multipurpose Teflon catheter for indwelling use. *Acta Physiol Scand* 1961; 51:343-47.

[73] W. Ganz, R. Donoso, H. Marcus et al. A new technique for measurement of cardiac output by thermodilution in man. *Am J Cardiol* 1971; 27:392-96.

[74] M. Lategola, H. Rahn. A self-guiding catheter for cardiac and pulmonary catheterization and occlusion. *Proc Soc Biol Exp Med* 1953; 84:667-68.

[75] H. J. Swan, W. Ganz, J. Forrester. Catheterization of the heart in man with use of a flow-directed balloon-tipped catheter. *New Engl J Med* 1970; 283; 447-52.

[76] R. L. Hines, P. Barash. "Pulmonary Artery Catheterization," in Casey D. Blitt, R. Hines (eds.), *Monitoring in Anesthesia and Critical Care Medicine* (New York: Churchill Livingstone, 3rd edition, 1995), p. 213.

[77] I. C. W. English, R. Frew, J. Piggott et al. *Anaesthesia* 1969; 24:521-31.

[78] Cooper et al., 1978.

[79] J. Eichorn, J. Cooper, D. Cullen et al. Standards for patient monitoring during anesthesia at Harvard Medical School. *JAMA* 1986; 256:1017-20.

[80] American Society of Anesthesiologists. Standards for bacic intraoperative monitoring, 1986.

[81] J. Tinker, D. Dull, R. Caplan et al. Role of monitoring devices in prevention of mishaps: A closed-claims analysis. *Anesthesiology* 1989; 71:541-46.

[82] L. Kohn, J. Corrigan, M. Donaldson (eds.). *To Err Is Human: Building a Safer Health System* (Washington: US Institute of Medicine, Committee on Quality of Health Care in America, and National Academy Press, 2000).

[83] J. Davies, L. Strunin. Anaesthesia in 1984: How safe is it? *Can Med Ass J* 1984; 131:437-41.

[84] C. J. Cote, E. Goldstein, M. Cote et al. A single blind study of pulse oximetry in children. *Anesthesiology* 1988; 68:184-88.

[85] P. Duncan, M. Cohen. Pulse oximetry and capnography in anaesthetic practice: An epidemiological appraisal. *Can J Anaesth* 1991; 38:619-25.

[86] J. Moller, T. Pedersen, L. Rasmullen et al. Randomized evaluation of pulse oximetry in 20, 082 patients. I. Design, demography, pulse oximetry failure rate, and overall complication rate. *Anesthesiology* 1993; 78:436-44.

[87] Ibid. II. Perioperative events and postoperative complications, 454-53.

[88] J. Eichorn. Pulse oximetry as a standard of practice in anesthesia. *Anesthesiology* 1993; 78:423-26.

[89] F. Orkin, M. Cohen, P. Duncan. The quest for meaningful outcomes. *Anesthesiology* 1993; 78:417-22.

[90] Duncan, Cohen, 1991.

[91] J. Eichorn. Prevention of intraoperative anesthesia accidents and related severe injury through safety monitoring. *Anesthesiology* 1989; 71:572-77.

[92] R. L. Keenan. American Society of Anesthesiologists Refresher Course #114, New Orleans, October 1989.

[93] J. Tinker, D. Dull, R. Caplan et al. Role of monitoring devices in prevention of anesthetic mishaps: A close claims analysis. *Anesthesiology* 1989; 71:541-46.

[94] F. Block. We don't monitor enough. *J Clin Monit* 1986; 2:267-79.

[95] J. Moyers. Does monitoring have an effect on patient safety? *J Clin Monit* 1988; 4:107-11.

[96] E. C. Pierce. Monitoring instruments have significantly reduced anesthetic mishaps. *J Clin Monit* 1988; 4:111-14.

[97] F. Block. A proposed standard for monitoring equipment: What equipment should be included? *J Clin Monit* 1988; 4:1-4.

[98] Bigelow, 1846.

Chapter 11

[1] J. Clark. *An Account of Plans for the Internal Improvement and Extension of the Infirmary at Newcastle* (Newcastle: Edward Walker, 1801), p.13.

[2] F. Nightingale. *Notes on Hospitals* (London: Longman, Green, Longman, Roberts & Green, 1863), p. 89.

3   A. M. Harvey. Neurosurgical genius—Walter Edward Dandy. *J Hopk Med J* 1974;
    135; 358-68.

4   M. Kirschner. Zum Neubau der Chirurgischen UniversitatsklinikTuebingen. *Der
    Chirurg* 1930; 2:54-61.

5   J. Lundy. 'P.A.R.' spells better care for postanesthesia patients. *Mod Hosp* 1944;
    63(Nov.):63-64.

6   P. Lowenthal, A. Russell. Recovery Room: Life saving and economical. *Anesthesiology*
    1951; 12:470-76.

7   B. Ibsen. Intensive therapy: Background and development. *Int Anesthesiol Clin* 1999;
    37:1-14.

8   H. Gordon. "Perspectives in Neonatology—1980," in G. Avery (ed.), *Neonatology*
    (Philadelphia: J. B. Lippincott, 1981), p. 3.

9   P. Drinker, C. McKhann. The use of a new apparatus for the prolonged administration
    of artificial respiration. I. A fatal case of poliomyelitis. *JAMA* 1929; 92:1658-60.

10 H. Lassen. A preliminary report on the 1952 epidemic of poliomyelitis with special
    reference to the treatment of respiratory insufficiency. *Lancet* 1953; 1:37-41.

11 B. Ibsen. The anaesthetist's viewpoint on the treatment of respiratory complications
    in poliomyelitis in Copenhagen, 1952. *Proc Roy Soc Med* 1954; 47:72-75.

12 Lassen, 1953.

13 See W. Mushin, L. Rendell-Baker, P. Thompson *et al. Automatic Ventilation of the
    Lungs* (Oxford: Blackwell Scientific Publications, 1969[2nd ed.]) for detailed account
    of ventilators.

14 M. Hilberman. The evolution of intensive care units. *Crit Care Med* 1975; 3:159-65.

15 P. Safar, T. DeKornfeld, J. Pearson *et al.* The intensive care unit: A three-year
    experience at Baltimore City Hospitals. *Anaesthesia* 1961; 16:275-84.

16 P. Berthelsen, M. Cronqvist. The first intensive care unit in the world: Copenhagen
    1953. *Anesthesiology* 2003; 47:190-95.

17 M. Ambiavagar, R. McConn. Intensive therapy—a modern necessity. *Surg Clin N
    Amer* 1978; 58:1031-44.

18 P. Safar, A. Grenvik. Critical care medicine: organizing and staffing intensive care
    units. *Chest* 1971; 59:535-47.

19 J. Brown, G. Sullivan. Effect on ICU mortality of a full-time critical care specialist.
    Chest 1989; 96:127-29.

20 M. Murray, R. Pollack, M. Katz. Improving the outcome and efficiency of intensive
    care: The impact of an intensivist. *Crit Care Med* 1988; 16:11-17.

21 C. Hanson, C. Deutschman, E. Behringer *et al.* Do intensivists make a difference?
    Crit Care Med 1996; 24: A56.

22 S. Ghorra, S. Reinert, W. Cioffi *et al.* Analysis of the effect of the conversion from
    open to closed intensive care unit. *Ann Surg* 1999; 229:163-71.

23 W. Knaus, E. Draper, D. Wagner *et al.* An evaluation of outcome from intensive
    care in major medical centers. *Ann Int Med* 1986; 104:410-18.

24 Ibid.

25 P. Safar, A. Grenvik. Organization and physician education in critical care medicine. *Anesthesiology* 1977; 47:82-95.

26 B. Ibsen. From anaesthesia to anaesthesiology: Personal experiences in Copenhagen during the past 25 years. *Acta Anaesthesiol Scand* 1975; Suppl 61, p. 33.

27 J. Downes. The historical evolution, current status, and prospective development of pediatric critical care. *Crit Care Clinics* 1992; 8(1):1-22.

28 V. Apgar. A proposal for a new method of evaluation of the newborn infant. *Anesth Analg* 1953; 32:260-67.

29 P. Smythe, A. Bull. Treatment of tetanus neonatorum with intermittent positive pressure respiration. *Brit Med J* 1953; 32:260-67.

30 Downes, 1992.

31 G. Gregory, J. Kitterman, R. Phibbs *et al*. Treatment of the idiopathic respiratory distress syndrome with continuous positive airway pressure. *New Engl J Med* 1971; 284:1333-40.

32 Downes,1992.

33 Lassen, 1953.

34 H. Pontoppidan. "The Development of Respiratory Care and the Respiratory Intensive Care Unit (RICU)," in R. Kitz (ed.), *'This Is No Humbug': Reminiscences of the Department of Anesthesia at the Massachusetts General Hospital—A History* (Boston: Massachusetts General Hospital, n.d., ISBN 0-9715376-0-7), p. 159.

35 A. C. Smith, J. Spalding, W. R. Russell. Artificial respiration by intermittent positive pressure. *Lancet* 1954; 1:939-45.

36 A. C. Smith, E. Hill, J. Hopson. Treatment of severe tetanus with d-tubocurarine chloride and intermittent positive pressure respiration. *Lancet* 1956; 2:550-53.

37 W. Mushin, G. van Weerden. The assisted respiration unit. *Int Anesth Clin* 1999; 37:15-33.

38 H. Barber, R. Chambers, H. B. Fairley *et al*. A respiratory unit: The Toronto General Hospital unit for the treatment of severe respiratory insufficiency. *Canad Med Ass J* 1959; 81:97-101.

39 M. Holmdahl. The respiratory care unit. *Anesthesiology* 1962; 23:559-68.

40 H. Pontoppidan, R. Wilson, M. Rie *et al*. Respiratory intensive care. *Anesthesiology* 1977; 23:559-68.

41 C. Beck, W. Pritchard, H. Feil. Ventricular fibrillation of long duration abolished by electric shock. *JAMA* 1947; 135:985-86.

42 G. Biorck, cited by D. Julian. The history of coronary care units. *Brit Heart J* 1987; 57:497-502.

43 L. Goldman, E. Cook. The decline in ischemic heart disease mortality rates: An analysis of the comparative effects of medical interventions and changes in life style. *Ann Int Med* 1984; 101:825-36.

44 Julian, 1987.

[45] D. Julian. Treatment of cardiac arrest in acute myocardial ischemia and infarction. *Lancet* 1961; 2:840-44.

[46] H. W. Day. History of coronary care units. *Amer J Cardiol* 1972; 30:405-07.

[47] *ibid.*

[48] K. Brown, R. MacMillan, N. Forbeth *et al.* Coronary care unit: An intensive care unit for acute myocardial infarction. *Lancet* 1963; 2:349-52.

[49] K. Khush, E. Rapaport, D. Waters. The history of the coronary care unit. *Can J Cardiol* 2005; 21:1041-45.

[50] E. Braunwald. Evolution of the management of acute myocardial infarction: A 20th century saga. *Lancet* 1998; 352:1771-74.

[51] T. Killip, J. Kimball. Treatment of myocardial infarction in a coronary care unit: A two-year experience with 250 patients. *Amer J Cardiol* 1967; 20:457-64.

[52] Goldman, Cook, 1984.

Chapter 12

[1] J. Snow. *On Chloroform and Other Anaesthetics: Their Action and Administration* (London: John Churchill, 1858), pp. 329-344.

[2] Snow, 1858, p. 19.

[3] C. Koller. On the use of cocaine for producing anaesthesia on the eye. *Lancet* 1884; 2:990-92.

[4] R. Descartes. *L'Homme* (Paris: E. Angot, 1664).

[5] R. Melzack. "Toward a New Concept of Pain for the New Millennium," in S. Waldman (ed.), *Interventional Pain Management* (Philadelphia: W. B. Saunders Company, 2nd ed., 2001), p. 9.

[6] G. Crile. *An Experimental and Clinical Research into Certain Problems Relating to Surgical Operations* (Philadelphia: J. B. Lippincott, 1901).

[7] J. Gwathmey. *Anesthesia* (New York: D. Appleton and Company, 1914), p. 371.

[8] G. Labat. *Regional Anesthesia* 1922, p. 348.

[9] D. Bacon. Regional anesthesia and chronic pain management in the 1920s and 30s. *Reg Anesth* 1995; 20:185-92.

[10] J. Bonica. Evolution of pain concepts and pain clinics. *Clin Anesthesiol* 1985; 3:1-16.

[11] J. C. White, P. D. White. Angina pectoris: Treatment with paravertebral alcohol injections. *JAMA* 1928; 90:1099-1103.

[12] R. Leriche. Osteoporoses douloureuses posttraumatiques. *Presse Medicale* 1930; 38:617-21.

[13] A. Dogliotti. Traitement des syndromes douloureux de la peripherie par l'alcoholisation sub-arachnoidienne. *Presse Medicale* 1931; 39:1249-52.

[14] R. Minnitt. Self-administration of analgesia for the midwifery of general practice. *Proc Roy Soc Med* 1934; 27:1313-18.

[15] J. Lundy. *Clinical Anesthesia: A Manual of Clinical Anesthesiology* (Philadelphia: W. B. Saunders Company, 1942), p. 575.

16 Lundy, 1942, p. 576.

17 Ibid., p. 576.

18 R. C. Adams. *Intravenous Anesthesia* (New York: P. B. Hoeber, Inc., 1944), p. 329.

19 P. Woodbridge. Therapeutic nerve block with procaine and alcohol. *Am J Surg* 1930; 9:278-88.

20 H. Ruth. Diagnostic, prognostic and therapeutic block. *JAMA* 1934; 102:419.

21 E. Rovenstine, H. Wertheim. Therapeutic nerve block. *JAMA* 1941; 117:1599-1603.

22 J. Bonica. Evolution of pain concepts and pain clinics. *Clinics in Anesth* 1985; 3:1-16.

23 R. Marks, E. Sachar. Undertreatment of medical inpatients with narcotic analgesics. *Ann Int Med* 1973; 78:173-81.

24 Bonica, 1985.

25 F. Alexander. "The Genesis of the Pain Clinic," in *Pain Abstracts*, vol. 1, Second World Congress on Pain, Seattle. International Association for the Study of Pain, 1970, p. 250.

26 Bonica, 1985.

27 M. Swerdlow. The early development of pain relief clinics in the United Kingdom. *Anaesthesia* 1992; 47:977-80.

28 J. Penman. Pain as an old friend. *Lancet* 1954; 1:633-36.

29 H. Flor, T. Fydrich, D. Turk. Efficacy of multidisciplinary pain treatment centers: A meta-analytic review. *Pain* 1992; 49:221-30.

30 L. B. Ready, R. Oden, H. Chadwick et al. Development of an anesthesiology-based postoperative pain management service. *Anesthesiology* 1988; 68:100-06.

31 J. Bonica. *The Management of Pain* (Philadelphia: Lea & Febiger, 1953).

32 R. Melzack, 2001, p. 1.

33 Melzack, Wall, 1965.

34 W. K. Livingston. *Pain Mechanisms: Physiologic Interpretation of Causalgia and Its Related States* (New York: Macmillan, 1943).

35 W. Noordenbos. *Pain* (Amsterdam: Elsevier, 1959).

36 N. Lofgren. *Studies on Local Anesthetics. Xylocaine: A New Synthetic Drug* (Stockholm: Hoeggstroms, 1948).

37 B. Covino. One hndred years plus two of regional anesthesia. 1986; 11:105-17.

38 Covino, 1986.

39 F. Reynolds. Ropivacaine. *Anaesthesia* 1991; 46:339-40.

40 P. Sechzer. Patient-controlled analgesia (PCA): A retrospective. *Anesthesiology* 1990; 72:735-36.

41 P. Sechzer. Objective measurement of pain. *Anesthesiology* 1968; 29:209-10.

42 Minnitt, 1934.

43 T. Jeffcoate, K. Baker, R. Martin. Inefficient uterine action. *Surg Gynec Obstet* 1952; 95:257-73.

44 B. Roe. Are postoperative narcotics necessary? *Arch Surg* 1963; 87:912-15.

45 P. Sechzer. Objective measures of pain and pain relief following cardiovascular surgery. *Rev Argent Angiology* 1967; 1:9-12.

[46] J. Scott. Obstetric analgesia. *Am J Obs Gynecol* 1970; 106:959-78.

[47] W. Forrest, P. Smethurst, M. Kienitz. Self-administration of intravenous analgesics. *Anesthesiology* 1970; 33:363-65.

[48] M. Keeri-Szanto. Apparatus for demand analgesia. *Can Anaesth Soc J* 1971; 18:581-83.

[49] P. Sechzer. Studies in pain with the analgesic-demand system. *Anesth Analg* 1971; 50:1-10.

[50] J. Evans, J. MacCarthy, M. Rosen et al. Apparatus for patient-controlled administration of intravenous narcotics during labour. *Lancet* 1976; 1:17-18.

[51] J. Ballantyne, D. Carr, T. Chalmers et al. Postoperative patient-controlled analgesia: Meta-analyses of initial randomized control trials. *J Clin Anesth* 1993; 5:182-93.

[52] A. Matsuki. Nothing new under the sun—a Japanese pioneer in the clinical use of intrathecal morphine. *Anesthesiology* 1983; 58:289-90.

[53] S. Snyder, G. Pasternak. Historical review: Opioid receptors. *TRENDS Pharmacol Sci* 2003; 24:198-205.

[54] S. Snyder. Opiate receptors and internal opiates. *Sci Amer* 1977; 236 (3):44-56.

[55] Snyder, Pasternak, 2003.

[56] H. Akil. "The Dawn of the Endorphins," in M. Meldrum, *Opioids and Pain Relief: A Historical Perspective* (Seattle: IASP Press, 2003), pp. 99-110.

[57] M. Meldrum. "The Opiate Receptor: Scientific Treasure Trove," in Meldrum, 2003, pp. 131-40.

[58] M. Cousins. "History of the Development of Pain Management with Spinal Opioid and Non-Opioid Drugs," in Meldrum, 2003, pp. 141-55.

[59] F. Pages. Anestesia metamerica. *Revista de la Sanidad Militar, Madrid,* 1921, s. 3, 11:351-65, 385-96.

[60] J. Bonica. *The Management of Pain* (Philadelphia: Lea & Febiger, 1953).

[61] P. Bromage. *Spinal Epidural Analgesia* (Edinburgh: E. & S. Livingstone, 1954).

[62] K. Tuman, R. McCarthy, R. March et al. Effects of epidural anesthesia and analgesia on coagulation and outcome after major vascular surgery. *Anesth Analg* 1991; 73:696-704.

[63] J. Ballantyne, D. Carr, S. DeFerranti et al. The comparative effects of postoperative analgesic therapies on pulmonary outcome: meta-analyses of randomized, controlled trials. *Anesth Analg* 1998; 86:598-612.

[64] S. Snyder, C. Pert. Opiate receptor: Demonstration in nervous tissue. *Science* 1973; 179:1011-14.

[65] J. Hughes, H. Kosterlitz et al. Identification of two related pentapeptides from the brain with potent opiate agonist activity. *Nature* 1975; 258:577-79.

[66] H. Akil, D. Mayer, J. Liebeskind. Antagonism of stimulation produced analgesia by naloxone, a narcotic antagonist. *Science* 1976; 191:961-62.

[67] A. Duggan, J. Hall, P. Headley. Morphine, enkephalin and the substantia gelatinosa. *Nature* 1976; 264:456-58.

[68] T. Yaksh, T. Rudy. Analgesia mediated by a direct spinal action of narcotics. *Science* 1976; 192:1357-58.

[69] M. Cousins, L. Mather, C. Glynn et al. Selective spinal analgesia. *Lancet* 1979; 1:1141-42.

[70] J. Wang, L. Nauss, J. Thomas. Pain relief by intrathecally applied morphine in man. *Anesthesiology* 1979:1:527-28.

[71] M. Behar, D. Olshwang, F. Magora et al. Epidural morphine in treatment of pain. *Lancet* 1979; 1:527-28.

[72] D. Moore. The role of the anesthesiologist in managing postoperative pain. *Reg Anesth* 1990; 15:223-31.

[73] J. D. Haddox, J. Bonica. "Evolution of the Specialty of Pain Medicine and the Multidisciplinary Approach to Pain," in M. Cousins, P. Bridenbaugh (eds.), *Neural Blockade in Clinical Anesthesia and Management of Pain* (Philadelphia: Lippincott-Raven Publishers, 1999), p. 1113.

Chapter 13

[1] M. Eisenberg. "The Quest to Reverse Sudden Death: A History of Cardio-pulmonary Resuscitation," in N. Paradis, H. Halperin, R. Nowak (eds.), *Cardiac Arrest: The Science and Practice of Resuscitation Medicine* (Baltimore: Williams & Wilkins, 1996), pp. 1-27.

[2] B. Meursing, D. Wulterkens, R. van Kesteren. The ABC of resuscitation and the Dutch (re)treat. *Resuscitation* 2005; 64:279-86.

[3] G. Ewy. Cardiac arrest—guideline changes urgently needed. *Lancet* 2007; 369:882-94.

[4] A. Lyons, R. Petrucelli. *Medicine: An Illustrated History* (New York: Abrams, 1978), pp. 78-79, citing W. Jayne, *The Healing Gods of Ancient Civilizations* (New Haven: Yale University Press, 1925), p. 65.

[5] II Kings 4:34-35.

[6] Exodus I:15-17.

[7] A. Hermwreck. The History of Cardiopulmonary Resuscitation. *Am J Surg* 1988; 156:430-36.

[8] A. Vesalius. *De Humani Corporis Fabrica*, Lib. Septem, cap. xix, "De vivorum sectione nonulle" (Basle: Oprina, 1543).

[9] W. Harvey. *The Works of William Harvey, M. D.* [transl. R. Willis] (London: The Sydenham Society, 1847), p. 28.

[10] J. T. Hughes. Miraculous deliverance of Anne Green: An Oxford case of resuscitation in the seventeenth century. *Brit Med J* 1982; 285:1792-93.

[11] A. Johnson. *An Account of Some Societies in Amsterdam and Hamburg for the Recovery of Drowned Persons* (London, 1773).

[12] R. Lee. Cardiopulmonary resuscitation in the eighteenth century: An historical perspective on present practice. *J Hist Med All Sci* 1972; 27:418-33.

[13] E. Thompson. The role of physicians in the humane societies of the eighteenth century. *Bull Hist Med* 1963; 37:43-51.

[14] W. Tossach. A man dead in appearance recovered by distending the lungs with air. *Med Essays Observations* 1744; 5:605-08.

[15] H. Liss. A history of resuscitation. *Ann Emerg Med* 1986; 15:65-72.

[16] S. Hales. *Statical Essays* (London: W. Innys, R. Manby, T. Woodward, 1733), pp. 323-24.

[17] S. Hales. *A Description of Ventilators* (London, 1743)., pp. 252-56.

[18] J. Fothergill. Observations on a case published in the last volume of *Medical Essays, etc.* of recovering a man dead in appearance, by distending the lungs with air. *Phil Trans* 1745; 43:275.

[19] B. Pugh. *A Treatise of Midwifery* (London: J. Buckland, 1754).

[20] J. Hunter. Proposals for the recovery of persons apparently drowned. *Phil Trans* 1776; 66:412-25.

[21] Ibid.

[22] C. Kite. *An Essay on the Recovery of the Apparently Dead* (London: C. Dilly, 1788).

[23] W. Cullen. *A Letter to Lord Cathcart, President of the Board of Police in Scotland Concerning the Recovery of Persons Drowned and Seemingly Dead* (Edinburgh, 1774).

[24] J. Herholdt, C. Rrafn. *An Attempt at an Historical Survey of Life-saving Measures for Drowning Persons and Information of the Best Means by Which They Can Again be Brought Back to Life* Copenhagen: H. Tikiob, M. Seest, 1796). (See also Reprint, 1960.)

[25] D. Schecter. Early experience with resuscitation by means of electricity. *Surgery* 1971; 69:36-72.

[26] G. Bianchi. Response a la letter du Docteur Bassini. *Jour de Med* 1756; 4:46.

[27] *Registers of the Royal Humane Society of London*, 1774-1784 (London: Nichols & Sons). Cited by Schecter, 1971.

[28] Hunter, 1776.

[29] Kite, 1788, opp. p. 192.

[30] J. Curry. *Observations on Apparent Death from Drowning, Hanging, Suffocation by Noxious Vapours, Fainting Fits, etc.* (London: E. Cox & Sons, 1815 [2nd edition]).

[31] R. Reece. *Medical Guide for the Use of the Clergy, Heads of Families, and Junior Practitioners in Medicine and Surgery* (London: Longman, Hurst & Co., 1824 [14th edition])

[32] Cited by Schechter, 1971.

[33] W. Channing. *The Medical Applications of Electricity* (Boston: T. Hall, 1865 [6th edition]).

[34] Schechter, 1971.

[35] J. MacWilliam. Fibrillar contraction of the heart. *J Physiol* 1887; 8:296-310.

[36] A. Hoffman. Fibrillation of the ventricles at the end of an attack of paroxysmal tachycardia in man. *Heart* 1912; 3:213-18.

[37] J. Prevost, F. Batelli. On some effects of electrical discharges on the hearts of mammals. *Compt Rend Acad Sci (Paris)* 1899; 129:1267.

[38] B. Brodie. "Effects of strangulation," Lecture, Royal College of Surgeons, London, in *The Works of Sir Benjamin Collins Brodie* (London: Longman, Green, Longman, Roberts & Green, 1865), vol. 1, p. 420.

39 L. d'Etiolles. Recherches sur l'asphyxie. *J de Physiol Exper* 1827; 7:45-65.

40 M. Hall. Asphyxia, its rationale and its remedy. *Lancet* 1856; 1:393-94.

41 H. Silvester. A new method of resuscitating stillborn children and of restoring persons apparently drowned or dead. 1858; 2:559-76.

42 B. Howard. The direct method of artificial respiration. *Lancet* 1877; 2:193-96.

43 E. Schafer. Description of a simple and efficient method of performing artificial respiration in the human subject. *Med Chir Trans* 1904; 87; 609-23.

44 H. Nielsen. Method of resuscitation. *Ugeskr Laeger* 1932; 50:1201.

45 F. Eve. Activation of the inert diaphragm by a gravity method. *Lancet* 1932; 2:995-97.

46 A. Gordon, M. Sadove, F. Ramon et al. Critical survey of manual artificial respiration. *JAMA* 1951; 147:1444-53.

47 J. Balassa. Jelvenyes gogvizdag fekelyes gogporckorilob kovetkezteben: tetszhalal megmentes gogmetszes altal (oedema glottidis symptomaticum ex perichondritde laryngeali ulceros-asphyxia—laryngotomia cum exitu fausto). *Orvosi Hetilap* 1858; 2:653-58. (See also S. Husveti, H. Ellis, Janos Balassa: pioneer of cardiac resuscitation, *Anaesthesia* 1969; 24:113-15.)

48 F. Maass. Die Methode der Wieder belebung bei Herztd nach Chloroformeinathung. *Ber Klin Wchsr* 1892; 29:265-68.

49 R. Boehm. Ueber Wiederbelebung nach Vergiftungen und Asphyxie. *Arch Exp Pathol Pharmacoker* 1878; 8:68-101.

50 G. Crile, D. Dolley. An experimental research into the resuscitation of dogs killed by anaesthetics and asphyxia. *J Exp Med* 1906; 8:713-20.

51 T. Hake. Studies on ether and chloroform from Prof. Schiff's physiological laboratory. 1874; 12:241-50.

52 W. Keen. Case of total laryngectomy and abdominal hysterectomy in both of which massage of the heart for chloroform collapse was employed with notes of 25 other cases of cardiac massage. *Ther Gaz* 1904; 28:212-30.

53 J. Elam. "Rediscovery of Expired Air Methods for Emergency Ventilation," in P. Safar, J. Elam (eds.), *Advances in Cardiopulmonary Resuscitation* (New York: Springer-Verlag, 1977), p. 263.

54 B. Ibsen. The anaesthetists's viewpoint on the treatment of respiratory complications in poliomyelitis in Copenhagen, 1952. *Proc Roy Soc Med* 195 4; 47:72-75.

55 J. Elam, E. Brown, J. Elder. Artificial respiration by mouth-to-mask method. A study of the respiratory gas exchange of paralyzed patients ventilated by operator's expired air. *New Engl J Med* 1954; 250:749-54.

56 P. Safar. "An Autobiographical Memoir," in B. R. Fink, K. McGoldrick (eds.), *Careers in Anesthesiology* (Park Ridge: Wood Library-Museum of Anesthesiology, 2000), p. 128.

57 Ibid., p. 129.

58 P. Safar. Mouth-to-mouth airway. *Anesthesiology* 1957; 18:904-06.

59 P. Safar, S. Tisherman, W. Behringer et al. Suspended animation for delayed resuscitation from prolonged cardiac arrest, unresuscitable by standard cardiopulmonary resuscitation. *Crit Care Med* 2000 ? ? ?

60 P. Safar, J. Elam. Manual versus mouth-to-mouth methods of artificial respiration. *Anesthesiology* 1958; 19:111-12.

61 P. Safar, L. Aguto-Escarraga, J. Elam. Upper airway obstruction in the unconscious patient. *J Appl Physiol* 1959; 14:760-64.

62 P. Safar, L. Escarraga, J. Elam. A comparison of the mouth-to-mouth and mouth-to-airway methods of artificial respiration with the chest-pressure arm-lift methods. *New Engl J Med* 1961; 258:671-77.

63 S. Morikawa, P. Safar, J. DeCarlo. Influence of head-jaw position upon upper airway patency. *Anesthesiology* 1961; 22:265-70.

64 A. Gordon, C. Frye, L. Gittelson et al. Mouth-to-mouth versus manual artificial respiration for children and adults. *JAMA* 1958; 167:320-28.

65 American Medical Association, Council on Medical Physics. Symposium on Mouth-to-Mouth Resuscitation (Expired Air Inflation). *JAMA* 1958; 167:317-19.

66 N. Roth. First stammering of the heart: Ludwig's kymograph. *Med Instrument* 1978; 13:348.

67 J. McWilliam. Cardiac failure and sudden death. *Brit Med J* 1889; 14:1843-49.

68 J. Prevost, F. Batelli. On some effects of electrical discharges on the heart of mammals. *Compt rend Acad Sci* 1899; 129:1267-68.

69 A. G. Levy. Sudden death under light chloroform anaesthesia. *J Physiol* 1911; 42: iii-iv.

70 D. Hooker, W. Kouwenhoven, O. Langworthy. The effect of alternating electrical currents on the heart. *Am J Physiol* 1933; 103:444-54.

71 W. Kouwenhoven, D. Hooker. Resuscitation by countershock. *Electr Engin* 1933; 52:475-77.

72 C. Beck, W. Pritchard, H. Feil. Ventricular fibrillation of long duration abolished by electric shock. *JAMA* 1947; 135:985-86.

73 D. Leighninger. "Contributions of Claude Beck," in P. Safar (ed.), *Advances in Cardiopulmonary Resuscitation* (New York: Springer-Verlag, 1975), pp. 259-62.

74 J. Meyer. Claude Beck and cardiac resuscitation. *Ann Thor Surg* 1988; 35:103-05.

75 W. Kouwenhoven, J. Kay. A simple electrical apparatus for the clinical treatment of ventricular fibrillation. *Surgery* 1951; 30:781-86.

76 W. Kouwenhoven. The development of the defibrillator. *Ann Int Med* 1969; 71:449-51.

77 P. Zoll, A. Linenthal, W. Gibson et al. Termination of ventricular fibrillation in man by externally applied countershock. *New Engl J Med* 1965; 254:727-32.

78 B. Lown, J. Neumann, R. Amaringham et al. Comparison of alternating-current with direct-current countershock across the closed chest. *Amer J Cardiol* 1962; 10:223-33.

79 W. Kouwenhoven, J. Jude, G. Knickerbocker. Closed-chest massage. *JAMA* 1960; 173:1064-67.

80 P. Safar, T. Brown, W. Holtey. Ventilation and circulation with closed chest cardiac massage in man. *JAMA* 1961; 176:574-76.

81 Kouwenhoven, 1969.

82 Kouwenhoven, Jude, Knickerbocker, 1960.

[83] P. Safar. "From Vienna to Pittsburgh for Anesthesiology and Acute Medicine," in B. R. Fink, K. McGoldrick (eds.), *Careers in Anesthesiology* (Park Ridge: Wood Library-Museum of Anesthesiology, 2000), vol. 5, p. 142.

[84] Safar, Brown, Holtey, 1961.

[85] P. Baskett, T. Baskett. *Resuscitation Greats* (Bristol: Clinical Press, Ltd., 2007).

[86] Z.-J. Zheng, J. Croft, W. Giles et al. Sudden cardiac death in the United States, 1989 to 1998. *Circulation* 2001; 104:2158-63.

[87] W. Roberts. Sudden cardiac death. *Circulation* 1998; 98:2334-51.

[88] M. Eisenberg, B. Howard, R. Cummins et al. Cardiac arrest and resuscitation." A tale of 29 cities. *Ann Emerg Med* 1990; 19:179-86.

[89] M. Eisenberg, T. Mengert. Cardiac resuscitation. *New Engl J Med* 2001; 344:1304-13.

[90] P. Safar. On the history of the Emergency Medical Services. *Bull Anesth Hist* 2001; 19 (3):4-9.

[91] E. Nagel. History of emergency medicine: A memoir. *Bull Anesth Hist* 2001; 19 (3):9-10.

[92] T. Bunch, R. White, B. Gersh et al. Long-term outcomes of out-of-hospital cardiac arrest after successful early defibrillation. *New Engl J Med* 2003; 348:2626-33.

[93] R. White, D. Snyder, R. D. White et al. Call-to-shock time versus a new ECG analysis for the prediction of resuscitation outcome (Abstract). *Resuscitation* 2006; 69:49.

[94] SOS-KANTO Study Group. Cardiopulmonary resuscitation by bystanders with chest compression only (SOS-KANTO): An observational study. *Lancet* 2007; 369:920-26.

[95] Ewy, 2007.

[96] A. Sanders, G. Ewy. Cardiopulmonary resuscitation in the real world: When will the guidelines get the message? *JAMA* 2005; 293:363-65.

[97] G. Ewy. Cardiocerebral resuscitation: The new cardiopulmonary resuscitation. *Circulation* 2005; 111:2134-42.

[98] The Hypothermia After Cardiac Arrest Study Group. Mild therapeutic hypothermia to improve the neurologic outcome after cardiac arrest. *New Engl J Med* 2002; 346:549-56.

[99] R. Robertson. Sudden death from cardiac arrest—improving the odds. *New Engl J Med* 2000; 343:1259-60.

[100] Safar, 2001.

Chapter 14

[1] E. A. Hessel. "Evolution of Cardiac Anesthesia and Surgery," in J. Kaplan, D. Reich, C. Lake, S. Konstadt (eds.), *Kaplan's Cardiac Anesthesia* (New York: Elsevier Saunders, 5th edition, 2003), pp. 3-32.

[2] M. Harmel, A. Lamont. Anesthesia in the surgical treatment of congenital pulmonic stenosis. 1946; 7:447-98.

[3] M. Bliss. *Harvey Cushing: A Life in Surgery* (Oxford: Oxford University Press, 2005 Press, 2005), p. 215.

[4]   A. Conn. Origins of paediatric anaesthesia in Canada. *Paediatr Anaesth* 1992; 2:179-89.

[5]   K. Sykes, J. Bunker. *Anaesthesia and the Practice of Medicine: Historical Perspectives* (London: Royal Society of Medicine Press, Ltd., 2007), p. 39.

[6]   In Canada, a committee that considered specialization was even named the Fragmentation Committee. See D. Shephard. *The Royal College of Physicians and Surgeons of Canada 1960-1980: The Pursuit of Unity* (Ottawa: The Royal College of Physicians and Surgeons, 1985), p. 340.

[7]   H. Cushing. The special field of neurological surgery. *Johns Hopkins Hospital Bulletin* 1905; 16:77-87.

[8]   S. Slogoff, A. Keats. Does perioperative myocardial ischemia lead to postoperative myocardial ischemia? *Anesthesiology* 1985; 62:107-14.

[9]   A. Merry, M. Ramage, R. Whitlock. First-time coronary artery bypass grafting: The anaesthetist as risk factor. *Brit J Anaesth* 1992; 68:6-12.

[10] J. Y. Simpson. *Anaesthesia, Hospitalism, Hermaphroditism* (Philadelphia: Lindsay and Blakiston, 1849), p. 83.

[11] D. Caton. *What a Blessing She Had Chloroform: The Medical and Social Response to the Pain of Childbirth From 1800 to the Present* (New Haven: Yale University Press, 1999), p. ix.

[12] Simpson, 1849, p. 90.

[13] D. Caton. Obstetric anesthesia: The First ten years. *Anesthesiology* 1970; 33:102-09.

[14] D. Caton. Obstetric anesthesia and concepts of placental transport: A historical review of the nineteenth century. *Anesthesiology* 1977; 46:132-37.

[15] D. Caton. "In the Present State of Our Knowledge": Early use of opioids in obstetrics. *Anesthesiology* 1995; 82:779-84.

[16] Caton, 1999.

[17] Caton, 1999, p. 53.

[18] D. Chestnut. *Obstetric Anesthesia: Principles and Practice* (Philadelphia: C. V. Mosby, 3rd edition, 2004), p. 369.

[19] D. Moir. *Obstetric Anaesthesia and Analgesia* (London: Bailliere Tindall, 1976), pp. 5-6.

[20] O. Kreis. Ueber Medullnarkose bei Gebarenden. *Zentralbl fur Gynakol* 1900; 24:724-29.

[21] G. Pitkin. Controllable spinal anesthesia. *Amer J Surg* 1928; 5:537-53.

[22] J. Adriani, D. Roman-Vega. Saddle block anesthesia. *Amer J Surg* 1946; 71:12-16.

[23] J. Cleland. Paravertebral anesthesia in obstetrics. *Surg Gynecol Obst* 1933; 57:51-62.

[24] R. Hingson, W. Edwards. Continuous caudal analgesia: an analysis of the first ten thousand confinements thus managed with the report of the authors' first thousand cases. *JAMA* 1943; 123:538-46.

[25] S. Hughes, G. Levinson, M. Rosen (eds.). *Shnider and Levinson's Anesthesia for Obstetrics* (Philadelphia: Lippincott Williams & Wilkins, 4th edition, 2002), p. 212.

[26] J. A. Lee. *A Synopsis of Anaesthesia* (Bristol: J. Wright, 1947), pp. 223-27.

[27] V. Apgar. A proposal for a new method of evaluation of the newborn infant. *Anesth Analg* 1953; 32:260-67.

28 R. Maltby (ed.). "Virginia Apgar (1909-1974)," in *Notable Names in Anaesthesia* (London: Royal Society of Medicine Press, Ltd., 2002), p. 5.

29 Caton, 1999, p. 8.

30 C. W. Long. An account of the first use of sulphuric ether by inhalation as an anesthetic in surgical operations. *South Med J* 1849; 5:705-13.

31 J. Snow. *On Chloroform and Other Anaesthetics* (London: John Churchill, 1858), pp. 123-27.

32 A. G. Levy. Sudden death under light chloroform anaesthesia. *J Physiol* 1911; 42:iii-iv.

33 L. Hewer. *Anaesthesia in Children* (London: H. K. Lewis, 1923).

34 R. Goldbloom. Halifax and the precipitate birth of pediatric surgery. *Pediatrics* 1986; 77:764.

35 A. Conn. Origins of paediatric anaesthesia in Canada. *Paediatr Anaesth* 1992; 2:179-89.

36 R. Smith, M. Rockoff. "History of Pediatric Anesthesia," in E. Motoyama, P. Davis (eds.), *Smith's Anesthesia for Infants and Children* (St Louis: Mosby Elsevier, 7th edition, 2006), p. 1175.

37 P. Ayre. Endotracheal anesthesia for babies with special reference to harelip and cleft palate operations. *Anesth Analg* 1937; 16:330-33.

38 Conn, 1992.

39 Obituary: M. Digby Leigh. *Canad Anaesth Soc J* 1976; 23:100.

40 M. D. Leigh, K. Belton. *Pediatric Anesthesia* (New York: Macmillan, 1948).

41 Smith, Rockoff, 2006, p. 1176.

42 R. Smith. *Anesthesia for Infants and Children* (St Louis: Mosby, 1959).

43 C. Smith. *The Physiology of the Newborn Infant* (Springfield: Charles C Thomas, 1945).

44 H. Taussig. *Congenital Malformations of the Heart* (New York: The Commonwealth Fund, 1947).

45 W. Nelson. *Nelson's Textbook of Pediatrics* (Philadelphia: W. B. Saunders, 1950).

46 J. Eckenhoff. Some anatomic considerations of the infant larynx influencing tracheal intubation. *Anesthesiology* 1951; 12:401-10.

47 M. D. Leigh, D. McCoy, K. Belton et al. Bradycardia following intravenous administration of succinylcholine to infants and children. *Anesthesiology* 1957; 18:698-702.

48 E. Macon, H. Bruner. The scientific aspect of endotracheal tubes. *Anesthesiology* 1950; 11:313-20.

49 A. Stead. The response of the newborn to muscle relaxants. *Anesthesiology* 1955; 27:124-30.

50 G. J. Rees. Anaesthesia in the newborn. *Brit Med J* 1952; 2:1419-22.

51 G. J. Rees. An early history of paediatric anaesthesia. *Paediatric Anaesthesia* 1991; 1:3-11.

52 G. Gregory, E. Eger, E. Munson. The relationship between age and halothane requirement in man. *Anesthesiology* 1969; 30:488-91.

[53] E. Salanitre, H. Rackow. The pulmonary exchange of nitrous oxide and halothane in infants and children. *Anesthesiology* 1969; 30:388-94.

[54] Snow, 1858, p. 49.

[55] H. Nicodemus, C. Nassiri-Rahimi, L. Bachman et al. *Anesthesiology* 1969; 31:344-48.

[56] Gregory et al, 1969.

[57] E. Motoyama. Pulmonary mechanics during early postnatal years. *Pediatr Res* 1977; 11:220-23.

[58] N. Goudsouzian, J. Donlon, J. Savarese, J. Ryan. Re-evaluation of dosage and duration of action of d-tubocurarine in the pediatric age group. *Anesthesiology* 1975; 43:416-25.

[59] H. Churchill-Davidson, R. Wise. Neuromuscular transmission in the newborn infant. *Anesthesiology* 1963; 24:271-78.

[60] R. McIntyre, A. Laws, P. Ramachandran. Positive expiratory pressure plateau: improved gas`exchange during mechanical ventilation. *Can Anaesth Soc J* 1969; 16:477-86.

[61] J. Downes. The historical evolution, current status and prospective development of pediatric critical care. *Crit Care Clin* 1992; 8:1-22.

[62] Snow, 1858, p. 49.

[63] H. Weintraub, L. Kekoler. "Demographics of Aging," in C. McCleskey (ed.), *Geriatric Anesthesia* (Baltimore: Williams & Wilkins, 1997), p. 4.

[64] R. Suzman, K. Kinsella, G. Myers. "Demography of Older Populations in Developed Countries," in J. Evans, T. Williams (eds.), *Oxford Textbook of Geriatric Medicine* (London: Oxford University Press, 1992), p. 3.

[65] Weintraub, Kekoler, 1997, p. 4.

[66] D. Callahan. Aging and the ends of medicine. *Ann N Y Acad Sci* 1987; 530:125-32.

[67] W. Owens. Overview of anesthesia for the geriatric patient. *Int Anesthesthiol Clin* 1988; 26:96-97.

[68] R. Miller (ed.). *Anesthesia* (New York: Churchill Livingstone, 4th edition, 1986), p. 1802.

[69] C. R. Stephen. "The Risk of Anesthesia and Surgery in the Geriatric Patient," in S. Kretchel (ed.), *Anesthesia and the Geriatric Patient* (New York: Grune & Stratton 1984), p. 231.

[70] F. Fowkes, J. Lunn, S. Farrow et al. Epidemiology in anaesthesia III: Mortality risk in patients with coexisting disease. *Brit J Anaesth* 1982; 54:819-25.

[71] R. Roy. "Anesthetic Implications of the Rectangular Survival Curve," in McCleskey, 1997, p. 23.

[72] H. T. Davenport. Anaesthetics and elderly patients. *Brit Med J* 1991; 303:870-71.

[73] S. Shafer. "Pharmacokinetics and Pharmacodynamics of the Elderly," in McLeskey, 1997, pp. 123-42.

[74] K. Woodhouse. "The Pharmacology of Aging," in R. Tallis, H. Fillitt, J. Brocklehurst (eds.), *Brocklehurst's Geriatric Medicine and Gerontology* (Edinburgh: Churchill Livingstone, 5th edition, 1998), p. 171.

[75] Weintraub, Kekoler, 1997, p. 4.

[76] M. Warner, M. Hosking, C. Lobdell et al. Surgical procedures among those >/90 years of age: A population-based study in Olmsted County, Minnesota, 1975-1985. *Ann Surg* 1988; 207:380-386.

[77] R. Jones, D. Brown. "Risk Assessment and Outcome," in McCleskey, 1997, p. 213.

[78] Roy, 1997.

[79] Davenport, 1991.

[80] S. Slogoff, A. Keats. Does perioperative myocardial ischemia lead to postoperative myocardial infarction? *Anesthesiology* 1985; 62:107-14.

[81] M. Merry, M. Ramage, R. Whitlock et al. First-time coronary artery bypass grafting: The anesthetists as a risk factor. *Brit J Anaesth* 1992; 68:6-12.

[82] J. Michenfelder, G. Gronert, K. Rehder. Neuroanesthesia. *Anesthesiology* 1969; 30:65-100.

[83] E. Sachs. *Fifty Years of Neurosurgery: A Personal Story* (New York: Vantage Press, 1955), p. 68.

[84] J. Michenfelder. The past, present, and future of research in neuroanesthesia. *J Neurosurg Anesthesiol* 1993; 5:22-30.

[85] W. Cannon, 1901. Cited by E. Frost, "History of Neuroanesthesia," in M. Albin (ed.) *Textbook of Neuroanesthesia with Neurosurgical and Neuroscience Perspectives* (New York: McGraw-Hill, 1997), pp. 1-20.

[86] L. Weed, P. McKibben. Pressure changes in the cerebro-spinal fluid following intravenous injection of solutions of various concentration. *Amer J Physiol* 1919; 48:512-30.

[87] A. Guedel, D. Treweek. Ether apneas. *Anesth Analg* 1934; 13:263-64.

[88] J. Lundy. *Clinical Anesthesia* (Philadelphia: W. B. Saunders Company, 1942), p. 3.

[89] S. Kety, C. Schmidt. The effects of active and passive hyperventilation on cerebral blood flow, cerebral oxygen consumption, output, and blood pressure of normal young men. *J Clin Invest* 1945; 25:107-19.

[90] S. Kety, C. Schmidt. Determination of cerebral blood flow in man by the use of nitrous oxide in low concentrations. *Amer J Physiol* 1945; 143:53-66.

[91] M. Schapira. Evolution of anesthesia for neurosurgery. *New York State J Med* 1964; 64:1801-05.

[92] Michenfelder, 1993.

[93] Albin, 1997.

[94] A. Hunter. *Neurosurgical Anaesthesia* (Philadelphia: F. A. Davis Co., 1964).

[95] R. Gilbert, F. Brindle, A. Galindo. *Anesthesia For Neurosurgery* (Boston: Little, Brown, 1966).

[96] M. Albin. Celebrating silver: The genesis of a neuroanesthesiology society. *J Neurosurg Anesthesiol* 1997; 9:296-307.

[97] Ibid.

[98] Ibid.

[99] Ibid.

[100] Michenfelder, 1993.

[101] D. Harken. Foreign bodies in and in relation to the thoracic vessels and heart, I: Techniques for approaching and removing foreign bodies from the chambers of the heart. *Surg Gynecol Obst* 1946; 83:117-25.

[102] L. D. Vandam. Early American anesthetists: The origins of professionalism in anesthesia. *Anesthesiology* 1973; 38:264-74.

[103] E. Wilkins, H. Urschel. "General Thoracic Surgery: Its History and Development," in F. G. Pearson, J. Deslauriers, R. Ginsberg, C. Hiebert, M. McKneally, H. Urschel (eds.), *Thoracic Sugery* (New York: Churchill Livingstone, 1995), p. 1.

[104] F. Sauerbruch. Ueber die physiologischen und physikalischen Grundlagen bei intrathoakalen Eingriffen in meiner pneumaischen Operationskammer. *Arch Klin Chir* 1904; 77:977.

[105] N. Gillespie. *Endotracheal Anaesthesia* (Madison: University of Wisconsin Press, 1941), p. 20.

[106] V. Eisenmenger. *Wien Med Wchsr* 1893; 43:199, cited by B. Duncum, *The Development of Inhalation Anaesthesia With Special Reference to the Years 1846-1900* (Oxford: Oxford University Press and Wellcome Historical Medical Museum, 1947), p. 61.

[107] A. Guedel, R. Waters. A new intratracheal catheter. *Anesth Analg* 1928; 7:238-39.

[108] R. Waters. Clinical scope and utility of carbon dioxid filtration in inhalation anesthesia. *Anesth Analg* 1924; 20-22.

[109] J. Gale, R. Waters. Closed endobronchial anesthesia in thoracic surgery: Preliminary report. *Anesth Analg* 1932; 11:283-87.

[110] L. Rehn. Zur chirurgerie des herzens und des herzbeutels. *Zbl Chir* 1907; 36:305-60.

[111] Harken, 1946.

[112] W. Mushin, L. Rendell-Baker. *The Principles of Thoracic Anaesthesia: Past and Present* (Oxford: Blackwell Scientific Publications, 1953), pp. 56-57.

[113] L. Rendell-Baker, J. Pettis. The development of positive pressure ventilators. In R. Atkinson, T. Boulton (eds.), *The History of Anaesthesia* (London: Royal Society of Medicine Services, Ltd., 1989), pp. 402-25.

[114] Ibid., p. 190.

[115] Ibid., p. 191.

[116] H. Janeway. Intratracheal anaesthesia. *Ann Surg* 1913; 58:927-30.

[117] E. Cutler, S. Levine. Cardiotomy and valvulotomy for mitral stenosis. *Boston Med Surg J* 1923; 188:1023-27.

[118] H. Souttar. Surgical treatment of mitral stenosis. *Brit Med J* 1925; 2:603-06.

[119] E. Hessel. "Evolution of Cardiac Anesthesia and Surgery," in J. Kaplan, D. Reich, C. Lake, S. Konstadt (eds.), *Kaplan's Cardiac Anesthesia* (New York: Elsevier Saunders, 5th edition, 2003), p. 9.

[120] H. B. Shumacker. *The Evolution of Cardiac Surgery* (Bloomington: Indiana University Press, 1992).

[121] P. Drinker, C. McKhann. The use of a new apparatus for prolonged administration of artificial respiration. *JAMA* 1929; 92:1658-61.

[122] E. Andersen, C. Crafoord, P. Frencker. A new and practical method of producing rhythmic ventilation during positive pressure anaesthesia. *Acta Otolaryngolica* 1939; 28:95-102.

[123] B. Ibsen. The anaesthetist's viewpoint on the treatment of respiratory complications in poliomyelitis during the epidemic in Copenhagen, 1952. *Proc Roy Soc Med* 1954; 47:72-74.

[124] H. Beecher, D. Todd. A study of the deaths associated with anesthesia and surgery. *Ann Surg* 1954; 140:2-34.

[125] E. Lowenstein, P. Hallowell, F. Levine et al. Cardiovascular response to large doses of intravenous morphine in man. *New Engl J Med* 1969; 281:1389-93.

[126] E. Lowenstein. The birth of opioid anesthesia. *Anesthesiology* 2004; 100:1013-15.

[127] T. Stanley, L. Webster. Anesthetic requirements and cardiovascular effects of fentanyl-oxygen and fentanyl-diazepam-oxygen anesthesia in man. *Anesth Analg* 1978; 57:411-18.

[128] Wilkins, Urschel, 1995, p. 2.

[129] Ibid., p. 2.

[130] R. Gross, J. Hubbard. Surgical ligation of a patent ductus arteriosus. *JAMA* 1939; 112:729-36.

[131] Harmel, Lamont, 1946.

[132] J. Kaplan, S. King. The precordial electrocardiographic lead (V5) in patients who have coronary-artery disease. *Anesthesiology* 1976; 45:570-77.

[133] M. Matsumoto, Y. Oka, L. Strom et al. Application of transesophageal echocardiography to continuous intraoperative monitoring of left ventricular performance. *Am J Cardiol* 1980; 46:95-101.

[134] K. Keown, D. Grove, H. Ruth. Anesthesia for commissurotomy for mitral stenosis: Preliminary report. *JAMA* 1951; 146:446-50.

[135] J. O'Donnell, T. McDermott. Anesthetic problems of surgical correction of aortic insufficiency. *Anesthesiology* 1955; 163:343-54.

[136] K. Keown. *Anesthesia for Surgery of the Heart* (Springfield: Charles C Thomas, 1956).

[137] E. Gain. Anaesthetic experiences using extracorporeal circulation for open-heart surgery. *Can Anaes Soc J* 1957; 4:419-27.

[138] E. Wynands, C. Sheridan, K. Kakar. Coronary artery disease and anesthesia (experience in 120 patients for revascularization of the heart). *Can Anaesth Soc J* 1967; 14:382-98.

[139] J. Arens. Three decades of cardiac anesthesia. *Mount Sinai J Med* 1985; 52:516-20.

[140] C. Hogue, K. Tuman, G. Gravlee. Cardiovascular anesthesia: The Society of Cardiovascular Anesthesiologists, its journal and new opportunities. *Anesth Analg* 2004; 98:1200.

[141] E. Lowenstein, R. Miller. The International Anesthesia Research Society and the Society of Cardiovascular Anesthesiologists: A new partnership. *Anesth Analg* 1984; 78:1-3.

Conclusion

[1] F. Hewitt. The past, present, and future of anaesthesia. *Practitioner* 1896; 57:347-56.

[2] R. Ellis. *On Narcotism by the Inhalation of Vapours by John Snow MD* (London: Royal Society of Medicine Services, 1991), pp. xix-xxi.

[3] C. Bernard. *On the Effects of Toxic and Medicinal Substances* [1857]. Translated and reprinted in A. Faulconer, T. Keys (eds.), *The Foundations of Anesthesiology* (Springfield: Charles C Thomas, 1965), vol. 2, pp. 1142-50.

[4] G. Edwards. Frederic William Hewitt (1857-1916). *Ann Roy Coll Surg Engl* 1951; 8:233-45.

[5] S. Meltzer, J. Auer. Continuous respiration without respiratory movements. *J Exp Med* 1909; 11:622-25.

[6] H. Dale. Chemical transmission of the effects of nerve impulses. *Brit Med J* 1:835-41.

[7] N. Greene. *Anesthesia and the University* (Philadelphia: J. B. Lippincott Company, 1975), p. 27.

[8] L. D. Vandam. Early American anesthetists: The origins of professionalism in anesthesia. *Anesthesiology* 1973; 38:264-74. Vandam's definition is relevant to anesthesia in the latter part of the 19th century and the first half of the 20th, particularly as discussed by Greene (1975).

[9] S. Snow. *Operations Without Pain: The Practice and Science of Anesthesia in Victorian Britain* (Basingstoke: Palgrave Macmillan, 2006), p 154.

[10] K. Rehder, P. Southorn, A. Sessler. *Art to Science* (Rochester, MN: Department of Anesthesiology, Mayo Clinic, n. d.), p. 15.

[11] R. Wolfe. *Tarnished Idol: William T G Morton and the Introduction of Surgical Anesthesia A Chronicle of the Ether Controversy* (Norman Publishing: San Anselmo, 2000).

[12] J. Snow, 1852.

[13] Hewitt, 1896.

[14] S. O. Goldan. Anesthetization as a specialty: Its present and future. *Amer Med* 1901; 2:101-04.

[15] J. Gwathmey. A plea for the scientific administration of anesthetics. *JAMA* 1916; 47:1361-65.

[16] L. D. Vandam. Walter M. Boothby, M. D.—The wellsprings of anesthesiology. *New Engl J Med* 1967; 276:558-63.

[17] F. W. Clement. "Elmer I. McKesson," in P. Volpitto, L. D. Vandam (eds.), *The Genesis of Contemporary American Anesthesiology* (Springfield: Charles C Thomas, 1982), pp. 21-27.

[18] J. Stetson. "Dennis Emerson Jackson (1878-1980)," in R. Atkinson, T. Boulton (eds.), *The History of Anaesthesia* (London: Royal Society of Medicine, International Congress and Symposium Series No. 134, 1989), pp. 564-74.

[19] R. Maltby (ed.). "Boyle Machine: Henry Edmund Gaskin Boyle," in R. Maltby (ed.), *Notable Names in Anaesthesia* (London: Royal Society of Medicine Press, Ltd., 2002), pp. 25-27.

[20] Maltby, 2002, pp. 123-25.

[21] B. Bamforth, K. Siebecker. "Ralph M. Waters," in Volpitto, Vandam, 1982, pp. 51-68.

[22] W. Neff. "Arthur E. Guedel," in Volpitto, Vandam, 1982, pp. 29-32.

[23] J. Eckman. "John Silas Lundy," in Volpitto, Vandam, 1982, pp. 35-48.

[24] J. Bevan, M. Pacelli. *Quintessential Canadian Anaesthetist: Wesley Bourne* (Montreal: McGill-Queen's University Press, 1997).

[25] R. Maltby, D. Shephard (eds.). Harold R. Griffith—His Life and Legacy. *Can J Anesth* 1992; 32 (Suppl 1):1-145.

[26] K. Sykes, J. Bunker. *Anaesthesia and the Practice of Medicine: Historical Perspectives* (London: Royal Society of Medicine Press, Ltd., 2007), pp. 71-82.

[27] G. Rushman, N. Davies, R. Atkinson. *A Short History of Anaesthesia: The First 150 Years* (Oxford: Butterworth-Heinemann, 2007) p. 149.

[28] J. Bunker. *The Anesthesiologist and the Surgeon* (Boston: Little, Brown and Co., 1972), pp. 11-12.

[29] Greene, 1975, p. 44.

[30] T. H. Seldon. "Francis Hoeffer McMechan," in Volpitto, Vandam, 1982, pp. 5-18.

[31] Greene, 1975, pp. 44-46.

[32] R. Waters. Pioneering in anesthesiology. *Postgrad Med* 1948; 4:265-70.

[33] C. Leake, M. Y. Chen. The anesthetic properties of certain unsaturated ethers. *Proc Soc Exper Biol Med* 1930; 28:151-54.

[34] C. Suckling. Some chemical and physical features in the development of Fluothane. *Brit J Anaesth* 1957; 29:466-70.

[35] A. Koopman. Sugammadex: A revolutionary approach to neuromuscular antagonism. *Anesthesiology* 2006; 104:631-33.

[36] J. Bonica. *The Management of Pain* (Philadelphia: Lea and Febiger, 1953).

[37] B. Ibsen. The anaesthetist's viewpoint on the treatment of respiratory complications in poliomyelitis during the epidemic in Copenhagen, 1952. *Proc Roy Soc Med* 1954; 47:72-74.

[38] L. Acierno, L. T. Worrell. Peter Safar: Father of modern cardiopulmonary resuscitation. *Clin Cardiol* 2007; 30:52-54.

[39] D. Caton. *What a Blessing She Had Chloroform: The Medical and Social Response to the Pain of Childbirth from 1800 to the Present* (New Haven: Yale University Press, 1999), pp. 3-6, 15-19, 22-37, 63-65.

[40] Ibid., pp. 135-43, 149-51.

[41] J. Cooper, R. Newblower, C. Long et al. Preventable anesthesia mishaps. *Anesthesiology* 1978; 49:399-406.

[42] J. Eichorn, J. Cooper, D. Cullen et al. Standards for monitoring during anesthesia at Harvard Medical School. *JAMA* 1986; 256:1017-20.

[43] J. G. Reves, N. Greene. "Anesthesiology and the Academic Medical Center: Place and Promise at the Start of the New Millennium." *Int Anesthesiol Clin* 2000; 38, p. 46.

[44] Reves, Greene, 2000, p. 53.

[45] E. Campbell. Relationship between market competition and the activities and attitudes of medical school faculty. *JAMA* 1997; 278:222-26.

[46] Ibid., p. 53.

[47] L. D. Vandam. Early American anesthetists: The origins of professionalism in anesthesia. *Anesthesiology* 1973; 38:264-76.

[48] Greene, 1975, p. 26.

[49] ABIM Foundation, Medical Professionalism Project. Medical professionalism in the new millennium: A physician charter. *Ann Int Med* 2002; 136:243-46.

[50] ABIM Foundation, 2002.

[51] Cooper et al., 1978.

[52] Eichorn et al., 1986.

Index

Personal Names

www.ingramcontent.com/pod-product-compliance
Lightning Source LLC
Chambersburg PA
CBHW031813170526
45157CB00001B/44